DARSE QABALAT

Simplifying Syllabus. Amplifying Success.

A Comprehensive Textbook of Unani OBSTETRICS
Based on NCISM Final Year Syllabus

Dr. Misba Naim

notionpress.com

INDIA • SINGAPORE • MALAYSIA

ISBN

Hardcase 979-8-90362-5-116
Paperback 979-8-90362-5-109

Dedication

"For the voices that shaped me—and the learners I write for."

To the students of Unani medicine—
who sat puzzled before an exam paper...
This book is for you.
To my teachers and mentors—
whose wisdom lit every page I wrote.
Thank you for your guidance.
To my family and loved ones—
who offered unwavering support, faith and patience.
Your love gave me the strength to complete this mission.
And finally,
to the Unani system itself—
a science of healing that continues to enrich humanity.

Dr Misba Naim
Author | Educator | Guide

Contents

Preface

"Uniting scattered knowledge into one structured journey — aligned, accessible, exam-ready."

In the journey from student to educator, the pursuit of clarity becomes both a struggle and a calling. When I stood at the threshold of mastering Unani obstetrics, I faced the same dilemma that echoes among countless BUMS final prof students: Where do we begin, and how do we make sense of it all?

"Ilmul Qabalat" was born from that very need—a bridge between complexity and comprehension. This book is the first-ever textbook in Unani obstetrics designed to fully reflect the new curriculum proposed by NCISM. It is not just a personal milestone, but a collective resource for every student, educator and practitioner who seeks depth, clarity and exam-oriented preparation.

Every page reflects my experience of teaching and my memory of learning.

Breaking down intricate classical concepts into teachable units

- Structuring chapters that echo the rhythm of actual classroom hours
- Integrating questions, mnemonics, flowcharts and clinical relevance
- Creating a resource that speaks to final prof BUMS exams, government medical exams, PG entrance exam and upcoming NEXT exams.

If this book empowers even one student to feel confident on exam day... or helps one educator deliver a more engaging lecture then its purpose is fulfilled.

With reverence to Unani medicine, and love for the community that shaped me—this is my humble offering.

✦ Dr Misba Naim ✦

Author | Educator | Guide

July 2025

Acknowledgements

"With gratitude to the hands that lifted me, and to the legacy I carry forward."

All praise and gratitude belong to **ALMIGHTY**— the source of knowledge, mercy, and inspiration. It is by **HIS** will that this book came into existence, and through **HIS** guidance that I was able to persevere in its creation.

To my beloved parents and family, whose prayers built my foundation, whose sacrifice gave me strength, and whose unwavering love continues to shape the educator and student within me — this book is a reflection of your blessings.

To my loving husband and children, who walked this journey with me—patiently, lovingly, and with faith— your presence gave me strength when I was weary and purpose when I felt lost.

I extend heartfelt appreciation to my teachers and mentors, both in Aligarh Muslim University and National Institute of Unani Medicine, Bengaluru, whose wisdom and patience illuminated my academic path. You shaped my understanding of *Ilmul Qabalat* and instilled in me the reverence for our timeless Unani heritage.

To my students, past and present — your curiosity, your questions and your hunger to learn, pushed me to make this book a reality. You reminded me that every complicated topic deserves clarity, every question deserves compassion and every classroom deserves structure.

To my friends, colleagues and the Unani academic community, thank you for championing educational innovation, for keeping tradition alive through teaching, and for welcoming the idea of reform and reorganization in our shared curriculum.

To NCISM for shaping the future of Unani medical education through a unified syllabus — this textbook is my contribution toward that vision.

To my friends, for their silent strength, warm encouragement and space to dream aloud — thank you for being part of the roots from which this work grew.

And finally, to every student who struggled to make sense of this subject and to every teacher who longed for a consolidated book— *DARSE QABALAT* is written for you.

Dr Misba Naim

Author | Educator | Guide

01

Fundamentals of Reproduction

(Tauleed ke bunyadi Usul)

1.1 *Tabveez* (Ovulation)
1.2 *Amal-i-baaraawri* (Fertilization)
1.3 *Amal-i-tanseeb* (Implantation)
1.4 *Irteqa -i-janin* (Development of fetus)
1.5 *Janini daruan-i-khun* (Foetal Circulation)

Learning Objective (At the end of the session, the students should be able to)

Explain the mechanism of *Tabvez* (Ovulation), *Amal e Barawri* (Fertilization), *Amal e Tanseeb* (Implantation) and changes in deciduas.

Summarize the basic embryology of the fetus, enlist factors influencing the fetal growth and development & define teratogenicity.

Discuss *Janeeni doran-e-Khoon* (Foetal Circulation) & changes at birth.

1. Fundamentals of Reproduction

(*Tauleed ke bunyadi Usul*)

Definition

Reproduction is the biological process by which organisms produce offspring, ensuring the continuation of their species. In humans, sexual reproduction involves the union of male and female gametes (sperm and ovum) to form a zygote, which develops into a new individual.

Key Components

Gametes: Specialized reproductive cells (sperm in males, ova in females) produced through gametogenesis (spermatogenesis and oogenesis).

Gonads: Primary reproductive organs (testes in males, ovaries in females) responsible for gamete production and sex hormone secretion.

Sex Hormones: Estrogen, progesterone (females) and testosterone (males) regulate reproductive processes, secondary sexual characteristics and gametogenesis.

Reproductive Tract: Facilitates gamete transport, fertilization and embryonic development (e.g., fallopian tubes, uterus in females; epididymis, vas deferens in males).

Hypothalamic-Pituitary-Gonadal (HPG) Axis: Regulates reproduction via gonadotropin-releasing hormone (GnRH), follicle-stimulating hormone (FSH) and luteinizing hormone (LH).

Process Overview

1. Gametogenesis: Sperm and ova are produced in the gonads through meiosis, resulting in haploid cells (23 chromosomes).
2. Fertilization: Fusion of sperm and ovum to form a diploid zygote (46 chromosomes).
3. Embryonic Development: Zygote undergoes cleavage, implantation and differentiation to form an embryo, fetus and eventually a newborn.
4. Hormonal Regulation: Estrogen and progesterone prepare the female reproductive tract for pregnancy, while testosterone supports spermatogenesis and male reproductive function.

Clinical Relevance

Disorders of reproduction include infertility, polycystic ovarian syndrome (PCOS) and hypogonadism.

Assisted reproductive technologies (ART), such as in vitro fertilization (IVF), address reproductive challenges.

1.1 Ovulation (*Tabveez*)

Ovulation is the release of a mature ovum from the ovarian follicle into the peritoneal cavity, typically occurring midway of the menstrual cycle (around day 14 in a 28-day cycle).

Anatomy and Physiology

Ovarian Follicle: The functional unit of the ovary, consisting of an oocyte surrounded by granulosa and theca cells.

Menstrual Cycle Phases

Follicular Phase: FSH stimulates follicular growth; granulosa cells produce estrogen, promoting endometrial proliferation.

Ovulatory Phase: A surge in LH triggers ovulation.

Luteal Phase: Post-ovulation, the ruptured follicle forms the corpus luteum, secreting progesterone.

Mechanism of Ovulation

1. Follicular Development

Primordial follicles mature into primary, secondary and tertiary (Graafian) follicles under FSH stimulation. The dominant follicle produces high levels of estrogen, creating a positive feedback loop with the pituitary gland.

2. LH Surge

Rising estrogen levels trigger a surge in LH (and to a lesser extent, FSH) from the anterior pituitary, typically 24–36 hours before ovulation.

LH induces enzymatic breakdown of the follicular wall (via proteases and prostaglandins).

3. Ovum Release

The follicular wall ruptures, releasing the mature ovum and its surrounding cumulus oophorus into the peritoneal cavity.

The fimbriae of the fallopian tube capture the ovum, facilitating its entry into the tubal lumen.

4. Corpus Luteum Formation

The ruptured follicle transforms into the corpus luteum, which secretes progesterone and some estrogen to prepare the endometrium for implantation.

Molecular Events

LH upregulates cyclooxygenase-2 (COX-2), increasing prostaglandin synthesis, which weakens the follicular wall.

Matrix metalloproteinases (MMPs) degrade the extracellular matrix, aiding follicle rupture.

Cumulus expansion occurs due to hyaluronic acid production, facilitating ovum release.

Clinical Relevance

Ovulatory Disorders: Anovulation (e.g., in PCOS) is a common cause of infertility.

Ovulation Induction: Medications like clomiphene citrate or gonadotropins stimulate ovulation in assisted reproduction.

Signs of Ovulation: Mittelschmerz (ovulation pain), basal body temperature rise and cervical mucus changes are clinical indicators.

1.2 Fertilization (*Amal-i-baaraawri*)

Fertilization is the fusion of a sperm and ovum to form a zygote, typically occurring in the ampulla of the fallopian tube within 24–48 hours post-ovulation.

Anatomy and Physiology

Sperm Transport: After ejaculation, sperm travel through the cervix, uterus and into the fallopian tube, aided by cervical mucus and uterine contractions.

Ovum Transport: The ovum is transported by ciliary action and peristalsis in the fallopian tube toward the ampulla.

Mechanism of Fertilization

1. Sperm Capacitation

Sperm undergo capacitation in the female reproductive tract, involving membrane changes and hyperactivation, enabling them to penetrate the ovum's layers.(6-8 hours in fallopian tube)

Capacitation involves removal of seminal plasma proteins and cholesterol from the sperm membrane.

2. Penetration of Ovum Layers

Cumulus Oophorus: Sperm release hyaluronidase to disperse cumulus cells.

Zona Pellucida: Sperm bind to ZP3 receptors on the zona pellucida, triggering the acrosome reaction, where acrosomal enzymes (e.g., acrosin) digest the zona pellucida.

Perivitelline Space: Sperm enters the space between the zona pellucida and ovum membrane.

3. Sperm-Ovum Fusion

Sperm binds to the ovum's plasma membrane via integrins and fertilin.

The sperm's nucleus enters the ovum, and the ovum completes meiosis II, releasing the second polar body.

4. Cortical Reaction

Cortical granules in the ovum release enzymes that harden the zona pellucida (zona reaction), preventing polyspermy.

5. Zygote Formation

Sperm and ovum pronuclei fuse, forming a diploid zygote with 46 chromosomes.

The zygote begins cleavage (mitotic divisions) as it travels toward the uterus.

Clinical Relevance

Infertility Causes: Impaired sperm motility, abnormal zona pellucida or tubal blockages can prevent fertilization.

Intracytoplasmic Sperm Injection (ICSI): A technique in IVF where a single sperm is injected into the ovum to overcome fertilization barriers.

Ectopic Pregnancy: Fertilization in the fallopian tube with subsequent implantation outside the uterus is a medical emergency.

1.3 Implantation (*Amal-i-tanseeb*)

Definition

Implantation is the process by which the blastocyst embeds into the endometrium of the uterus, establishing a connection for embryonic development, typically occurring 6–10 days post-fertilization.

Anatomy and Physiology

Blastocyst: A fluid-filled embryo consisting of an inner cell mass (future fetus), trophoblast (future placenta) and blastocoel.

Endometrium: The uterine lining, prepared by estrogen and progesterone, enters the receptive "window of implantation" (days 20–24 of the menstrual cycle).

Mechanism of Implantation

1. Blastocyst Hatching

The blastocyst escapes the zona pellucida via enzymatic degradation (e.g., by trypsin-like enzymes) and mechanical expansion.

2. Apposition

The blastocyst contacts the endometrial epithelium, typically at the upper posterior uterine wall.

Adhesion molecules (e.g., integrins, selectins) facilitate loose attachment.

3. Adhesion

Stronger binding occurs via integrin receptors (e.g., $\alpha v \beta 3$) on the trophoblast and endometrial cells.

Cytokines (e.g., LIF, IL-1) and growth factors (e.g., HB-EGF) mediate endometrial receptivity.

4. Invasion

Trophoblast cells differentiate into cytotrophoblast (proliferative) and syncytiotrophoblast (invasive). Syncytiotrophoblast invades the endometrial stroma, penetrating maternal blood vessels to establish uteroplacental circulation. Matrix metalloproteinases (MMPs) degrade the extracellular matrix, facilitating invasion.

5. Decidualization

Endometrial stromal cells transform into decidual cells under progesterone influence, creating a supportive environment for the embryo.

Decidua secretes prolactin, IGFBP-1, and other factors to regulate trophoblast invasion.

Clinical Relevance

Implantation Failure: Inadequate endometrial receptivity or blastocyst quality can lead to early pregnancy loss.

Ectopic Implantation: Implantation outside the uterus (e.g., fallopian tube) requires urgent intervention.

Assisted Reproduction: Endometrial preparation with hormonal therapy improves implantation rates in IVF.

Placental Disorders: Abnormal invasion (e.g., placenta accreta) can result from dysregulated implantation processes.

Summary

Reproduction involves coordinated gamete production, fertilization and embryonic development, regulated by the HPG axis. Ovulation is a hormonally driven process essential for fertility, with clinical implications in anovulatory disorders. Fertilization requires precise sperm-ovum interactions, with ART addressing barriers to this process. Implantation establishes pregnancy, with molecular and immune interactions critical for success and abnormalities leading to pregnancy complications.

Further Reading

Williams Obstetrics (for clinical correlations).

Molecular Biology of the Female Reproductive System (for molecular mechanisms).

ART protocols and guidelines (e.g., ASRM, ESHRE) for assisted reproduction techniques.

1.4 Fetal Development (*Irteqa -i-janin*)

Definition

Fetal development is the process by which a zygote, formed by fertilization, progresses through embryonic and fetal stages to become a viable fetus capable of extrauterine life. Human gestation spans approximately 40 weeks (280 days) from the last menstrual period (LMP), divided into the embryonic period (weeks 1–8 post-fertilization) and the fetal period (weeks 9–birth).

Overview

Embryonic Period: Rapid cellular division, differentiation and organogenesis establish the basic body structure.

Fetal Period: Growth, maturation and functional development of organs prepare the fetus for birth.

Key Processes: Cell proliferation, differentiation, migration and apoptosis, regulated by genetic, hormonal and environmental factors.

Stages of Fetal Development

1. Pre-Embryonic Period (Weeks 1–2 Post-Fertilization)

This period encompasses fertilization, cleavage and implantation, setting the stage for embryonic development.

Fertilization

Sperm and ovum fuse in the fallopian tube to form a zygote (46 chromosomes).

The zygote undergoes cleavage (mitotic divisions) to form a morula (16–32 cells) by day 3–4.

Morula to Blastocyst

By day 5–6, the morula develops into a blastocyst, consisting of:

Inner cell mass: Forms the embryo proper.

Trophoblast: Forms part of the placenta.

Blastocoel: Fluid-filled cavity.

The blastocyst hatches from the zona pellucida by day 6.

Implantation

The blastocyst implants into the endometrium (days 6–10), with trophoblast invasion establishing uteroplacental circulation.

Human chorionic gonadotropin (hCG) is secreted to maintain the corpus luteum.

Molecular Events

Expression of genes like Oct4 and Nanog maintains pluripotency in the inner cell mass.

Trophoblast secretes proteases (e.g., MMP-9) for endometrial invasion.

Clinical Relevance

Implantation failure or ectopic implantation can lead to early pregnancy loss or ectopic pregnancy.

hCG levels are used to confirm pregnancy and monitor early development.

2. Embryonic Period (Weeks 3–8 Post-Fertilization)

This period is characterized by rapid organogenesis, establishing the basic body structure and major organ systems. It is highly sensitive to teratogens.

Week 3: Gastrulation and Germ Layer Formation

The bilaminar disc (epiblast and hypoblast) transforms into a trilaminar disc via gastrulation.

Three germ layers form:

Ectoderm: Gives rise to the nervous system, skin and sensory organs.

Mesoderm: Forms muscles, bones, heart, blood vessels and kidneys.

Endoderm: Develops into the gastrointestinal tract, lungs and liver.

The primitive streak, node and notochord form, guiding axial development. Neurulation begins: The neural plate folds into the neural tube (future brain and spinal cord).

Week 4: Organogenesis Begins

Cardiovascular System: Heart tube forms and begins beating by day 22–24; primitive blood vessels develop.

Nervous System: Neural tube closes (failure results in neural tube defects, e.g., spina bifida).

Somites: Paired mesodermal structures form, giving rise to vertebrae, ribs and skeletal muscles.

Pharyngeal Arches: Form structures of the face, neck and pharynx.

Limb buds and optic vesicles appear.

Weeks 5–8: Major Organ Systems Formation

Head and Face: Facial features (eyes, nose, mouth) develop; brain differentiates into forebrain, midbrain and hindbrain.

Cardiovascular: Heart septation forms four chambers; major vessels (aorta, pulmonary artery) develop.

Respiratory: Lung buds form from the foregut; diaphragmatic development begins.

Gastrointestinal: Gut tube forms; liver, pancreas and gallbladder bud from the foregut.

Urogenital: Kidneys (pronephros, mesonephros, metanephros) develop sequentially; gonadal ridges form.

Musculoskeletal: Limb buds elongate; cartilage models of bones form.

By week 8, the embryo is recognizable as human, measuring ~2.5–3 cm.

Clinical Relevance

Teratogens: Exposure to drugs (e.g., thalidomide), infections (e.g., rubella), or alcohol during this period can cause congenital anomalies (e.g., limb defects, heart malformations).

Neural Tube Defects: Folic acid deficiency increases risks; supplementation is necessary.

Ultrasound: Early ultrasound (6–8 weeks) confirms embryonic viability and detects anomalies.

3. Fetal Period (Weeks 9–Birth)

Overview: This period focuses on growth, organ maturation and functional development. The fetus grows from ~3 cm (week 9) to ~50 cm (term) and from ~8 g to ~3.2–3.5 kg.

Second Trimester (Weeks 9–24)

Growth: Rapid increase in size; crown-rump length (CRL) reaches ~23 cm by week 24.

Nervous System: Brain growth accelerates; cerebral cortex develops gyri and sulci; myelination begins.

Cardiovascular: Heart rate stabilizes (120–160 bpm); fetal circulation (via ductus venosus, foramen ovale) supports oxygenation.

Respiratory: Alveolar precursors form; surfactant production begins (~week 20), critical for lung maturity.

Gastrointestinal: Gut elongates; meconium accumulates.

Urogenital: Kidneys produce urine (contributes to amniotic fluid); external genitalia differentiate.

Musculoskeletal: Bones ossify; fetal movements (quickening) are felt by the mother (~18–20 weeks).

Skin: Lanugo (fine hair) and vernix caseosa (protective coating) form.

Sensory: Eyes migrate to frontal position; hearing develops (~week 18).

Third Trimester (Weeks 25–Birth)

Growth and Maturation: Weight triples; fat deposition enhances thermoregulation.

Nervous System: Rapid brain growth; reflexes (suckling, grasping) develop.

Respiratory: Surfactant production increases; lungs prepare for air breathing.

Cardiovascular: Ductus arteriosus and foramen ovale remain open until birth.

Immune System: Passive immunity via maternal IgG transfer across the placenta.

Endocrine: Fetal adrenal glands produce cortisol, aiding lung maturation.

Fetal Positioning: Cephalic presentation is typical by term.

Molecular Events

Insulin-like growth factors (IGFs) promote growth.

Surfactant proteins (SP-A, SP-B) enhance lung maturity.

Erythropoietin regulates fetal hematopoiesis.

Clinical Relevance

Preterm Birth: Delivery before 37 weeks; immature lungs (respiratory distress syndrome) are a major concern.

Intrauterine Growth Restriction (IUGR): Impaired growth due to placental insufficiency or maternal factors (e.g., hypertension).

Fetal Monitoring: Ultrasound, doppler and cardiotocography assess fetal well-being.

Congenital Anomalies: Detected via anomaly scans (~18–20 weeks); examples include congenital heart defects, cleft palate.

1.5 Fetal Circulation (*Janini daruan-i-khun*)

Definition

Fetal circulation is the specialized circulatory system in the fetus, designed to deliver oxygenated blood and nutrients from the placenta while bypassing the non-functional lungs and liver. It differs from adult circulation due to the presence of fetal shunts and the placenta as the primary organ for gas exchange, nutrient supply and waste elimination.

Overview

Fetal circulation relies on the placenta for oxygenation, as the fetal lungs are fluid-filled and non-functional. Three key shunts - ductus venosus, foramen ovale and ductus arteriosus - divert blood away from the lungs and liver, optimizing oxygen delivery. The system transitions to adult circulation at birth following umbilical cord clamping and lung expansion.

Anatomy of Fetal Circulation

1. Placenta: Acts as the primary organ for gas exchange, nutrient transfer and waste removal. Oxygenated blood enters the fetus via the umbilical vein, while deoxygenated blood returns to the placenta via two umbilical arteries.

2. Umbilical Vessels

Umbilical Vein: Carries oxygenated blood (80–90% oxygen saturation) from the placenta to the fetus.

Umbilical Arteries: Return deoxygenated blood from the fetus to the placenta.

3. Fetal Shunts

Ductus Venosus: Connects the umbilical vein to the inferior vena cava (IVC), bypassing the liver.

Foramen Ovale: An opening in the interatrial septum, shunting blood from the right atrium to the left atrium, bypassing the lungs.

Ductus Arteriosus: Connects the pulmonary artery to the descending aorta, diverting blood away from the lungs.

4. Fetal Heart: Four-chambered but functionally different due to high pulmonary vascular resistance and low systemic resistance in the placenta.

5. Liver and Portal Circulation: The liver receives some blood from the umbilical vein, but most is shunted via the ductus venosus to prioritize systemic circulation.

Blood Flow Characteristics

Fetal blood volume is approximately 80–100 mL/kg.

Fetal hemoglobin (HbF) has a higher oxygen affinity than adult hemoglobin, facilitating oxygen uptake from maternal blood.

Oxygen saturation in the umbilical vein (~80–90%) is higher than in umbilical arteries (~50–60%).

Pathway of Fetal Blood Flow

Step-by-Step Blood Flow

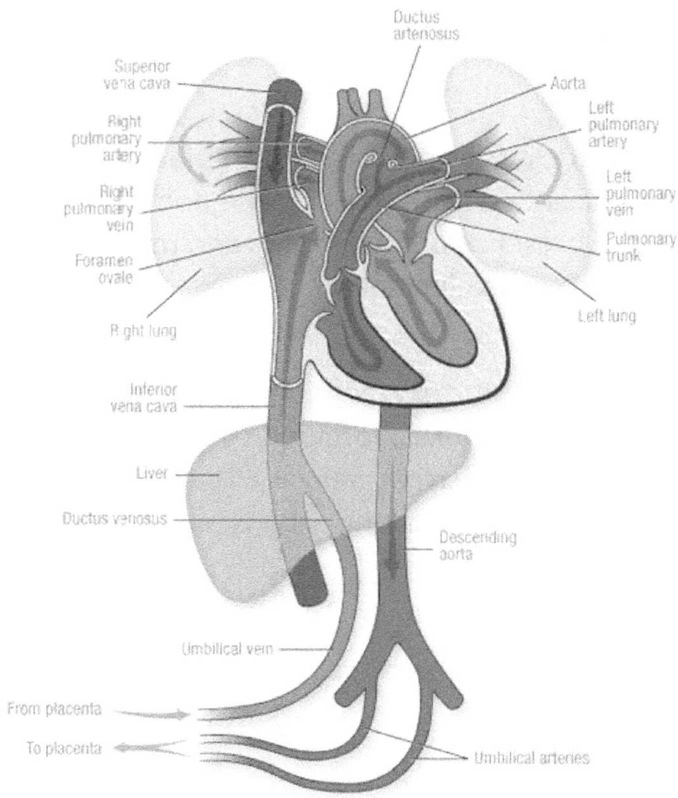

1. Oxygenated Blood from Placenta

Oxygenated blood from the placenta enters the fetus via the umbilical vein, traveling through the umbilical cord to the fetal liver.

2. Ductus Venosus

Approximately 50–60% of umbilical vein blood bypasses the liver through the ductus venosus, entering the inferior vena cava (IVC) . The remaining blood perfuses the liver via the portal sinus and hepatic veins, contributing to hepatic development.

3. Right Atrium

Blood from the IVC (oxygenated) and superior vena cava (SVC, deoxygenated from the upper body) enters the right atrium. The foramen ovale shunts ~30–40% of this blood directly to the left atrium, prioritizing oxygenated blood to the brain and coronary circulation.

4. Left Heart and Systemic Circulation

Blood in the left atrium flows into the left ventricle, which pumps it into the ascending aorta

This supplies oxygenated blood to the brain, heart (via coronary arteries) and upper body.

5. Right Heart and Pulmonary Bypass

Blood remaining in the right atrium flows into the right ventricle, which pumps it into the pulmonary artery. Due to high pulmonary vascular resistance, ~90% of pulmonary artery blood is shunted through the ductus arteriosus to the descending aorta, bypassing the lungs. A small amount (~10%) perfuses the lungs to support their development.

6. Descending Aorta and Umbilical Arteries

Blood in the descending aorta supplies the lower body and flows into the umbilical arteries, which return deoxygenated blood to the placenta for reoxygenation.

Oxygen Distribution

The brain and heart receive the most oxygenated blood (via the left ventricle).

The lower body and placenta receive less oxygenated blood (mixed blood from the ductus arteriosus).

The lungs receive minimal blood flow, sufficient only for growth and development.

Molecular and Physiological Regulation

Prostaglandins (e.g., PGE2) maintain patency of the ductus arteriosus and ductus venosus.

High pulmonary vascular resistance is due to low oxygen tension and compressed pulmonary vessels in fluid-filled lungs.

Low placental resistance facilitates blood flow to the placenta.

Transition to Neonatal Circulation

Changes at Birth

1. Umbilical Cord Clamping: Stops placental blood flow, increasing systemic vascular resistance.

2. Lung Expansion: The first breath lowers pulmonary vascular resistance, increasing pulmonary blood flow.

3. Shunt Closure

   a. Foramen Ovale: Increased left atrial pressure (from pulmonary venous return) and decreased right atrial pressure close the foramen ovale, forming the fossa ovalis.
   b. Ductus Arteriosus: Oxygenation and decreased prostaglandin levels cause constriction, forming the ligamentum arteriosum (functional closure within hours, anatomical closure in weeks).
   c. Ductus Venosus: Cessation of umbilical vein flow leads to closure, forming the ligamentum venosum (within days to weeks).

4. Umbilical Vessels: Umbilical arteries form the medial umbilical ligaments; the umbilical vein becomes the ligamentum teres hepatis.

Molecular Events

Increased oxygen tension inhibits prostaglandin synthesis, promoting ductus arteriosus closure.

Nitric oxide and prostacyclin in the lungs reduce pulmonary vascular resistance.

Endothelin-1 and other vasoconstrictors aid in shunt closure.

Clinical Relevance

1. Congenital Anomalies

a. Patent Ductus Arteriosus (PDA): Failure of ductus arteriosus closure post-birth, leading to left-to-right shunting and potential heart failure. Treated with indomethacin (prostaglandin inhibitor) or surgical ligation.

b. Persistent Foramen Ovale: Incomplete closure may cause atrial septal defects (ASDs).

c. Transposition of Great Arteries: Abnormal vessel connections disrupt fetal and neonatal circulation, requiring surgical correction.

2. Fetal Hypoxia

a. Placental insufficiency (e.g., in preeclampsia or IUGR) reduces oxygen delivery, detectable via abnormal Doppler studies (e.g., umbilical artery Doppler).

b. Fetal distress may necessitate urgent cesarean delivery.

3. Premature Infants

Preterm neonates may have delayed shunt closure due to immature prostaglandin metabolism, increasing PDA risk.

Respiratory distress syndrome (RDS) is common due to inadequate pulmonary blood flow and surfactant deficiency.

4. Fetal Monitoring

Doppler Ultrasound: Assesses umbilical artery, ductus venosus, and middle cerebral artery flow to evaluate fetal well-being.

Cardiotocography (CTG): Monitors fetal heart rate, reflecting oxygenation status.

5. Pharmacological Considerations

Prostaglandin analogs (e.g., alprostadil) maintain ductus arteriosus patency in congenital heart defects (e.g., tetralogy of Fallot).

NSAIDs (e.g., indomethacin) are used to close PDA in preterm infants.

Diagnostic and Monitoring Tools

Ultrasound (USG): Visualizes fetal heart, shunts and umbilical vessels; Doppler assesses blood flow velocity and direction.

Echocardiography (ECG): Detects congenital heart defects prenatally (e.g., ventricular septal defects).

Amniotic Fluid Volume (AFI): Reflects fetal renal perfusion and umbilical artery function.

Fetal Blood Sampling: Rarely used to assess oxygenation and acid-base status.

Summary

Fetal circulation is adapted to prioritize oxygen delivery to vital organs (brain, heart) while bypassing the lungs and liver via shunts (ductus venosus, foramen ovale, ductus arteriosus).

The placenta serves as the primary organ for gas exchange, with umbilical vessels facilitating blood flow.

Transition to neonatal circulation involves shunt closure and lung perfusion, driven by oxygenation and hemodynamic changes.

Obstetricians must recognize anomalies (e.g., PDA, ASD) and monitor fetal circulation (via Doppler, CTG) to manage complications like hypoxia or preterm birth.

Understanding fetal circulation is necessary for diagnosing congenital heart defects, managing preterm infants and optimizing perinatal outcomes.

Further Reading

Williams Obstetrics (for clinical correlations and management).

Langman's Medical Embryology (for developmental anatomy).

ACOG and ISUOG Guidelines (for fetal monitoring and ultrasound protocols).

Long Answer Questions (LAQs)

1. Describe the process of ovulation (Tabreez) in detail and explain its importance in reproduction.
2. Explain fertilization (Amal-e-Barāwari) with stages and site of fertilization.
3. Define implantation (Amal-e-Tanseeb) and describe its mechanism and significance.
4. Describe the development of fetus (Irteqa-e-Janīn) from fertilization to birth.
5. Explain fetal circulation (Jarīān-e-Daurān-e-Khūn-e-Janīn) with special reference to shunts.

Short Answer Questions (SAQs)

1. Define ovulation.
2. Mention the site of fertilization.
3. Define implantation.
4. Name the three fetal circulatory shunts.
5. Write two functions of fetal circulation.

Multiple Choice Questions (1 Mark Each)

1. Ovulation occurs from:

A. Uterus B. Cervix C. Ovary D. Vagina

Ans: C. Ovary

2. Fertilization usually occurs in:

A. Uterus B. Cervix C. Ampulla of fallopian tube D. Vagina

Ans: C. Ampulla of fallopian tube

3. Implantation normally occurs in:

A. Cervix B. Fundus of uterus C. Vagina D. Ovary

Ans: B. Fundus of uterus

4. Which hormone triggers ovulation?

A. FSH B. LH C. Estrogen D. Progesterone

Ans: B.LH

5. Ductus venosus connects:

A. Umbilical vein to IVC B. Umbilical artery to aorta

C. Pulmonary artery to aorta D. Right atrium to left atrium

Ans: A. Umbilical vein to IVC

6. Foramen ovale is present between:

A. Two ventricles B. Two atria

C. Aorta and pulmonary artery D. Umbilical vessels

Ans: B. Two atria

7. Ductus arteriosus connects:

A. Aorta and IVC B. Pulmonary artery and aorta

C. Umbilical vein and liver D. Umbilical artery and placenta

Ans: B. Pulmonary artery and aorta

8. Implantation occurs approximately on day:

A. 3 B. 7 C. 14 D. 21

Ans: B.7

9. Fetal blood is oxygenated mainly in the:

A. Liver B. Lungs C. Placenta D. Heart

Ans: C. Placenta

10. Development of fetus is called:

A. Ovulation B. Fertilization C. *Irteqa-e-Janin* D. Parturition

Ans: C. Irteqa-e-Janin

02

The placenta, Fetal Membranes, Amniotic fluid & Umbilical Cord

(Mashima, Aghshiya -i-Janin, Rutubat-i-Aminusiyya wa Hablussurrah)

2.1 *Tabi'I wa Ghayr Tabi'I Mashima* (Normal & Abnormal Placenta)
2.2 *Aghshiay -i-janin* (Foetal Membranes)
2.3 *Taba'I wa Gahyr Tabaiai Rutubat-i-Aminusiyya* (Amniotic Fluid & its Abnormalities)
2.4 *Taba'I wa Ghayr Taba'I Hablussurah* (Umbilical cord & its Abnormalities)

Learning Objective (At the end of the session, the students should be able to)

Explain the development, structure, circulation & functions of the normal placenta & define the types of Abnormal Placenta.

Explain the *Aghshiyae Janeen* (Foetal Membranes) and its function.

Summarize the characteristics of *Tabai wa Ghair Tabai Ratoobat-e-Aminoosi* (Amniotic Fluid & its Abnormalities) & enlist its function.

Explain the development, structure, and characteristics of the *Tabie wa Ghair Tabayi Hablussurah* (Umbilical Cord & its Abnormalities).

2.1 Normal & Abnormal Placenta

(Tabi'l wa Ghayr Tabi'l Mashima)

The placenta is a temporary, highly specialized organ that forms during pregnancy to mediate the exchange of oxygen, nutrients and waste products between the maternal and fetal circulations. It also functions as an endocrine organ, producing hormones needed for maintaining pregnancy and provides immunological protection to prevent fetal rejection.

Development

Origin: The placenta is a composite organ derived from both fetal and maternal tissues.

Fetal Contribution: Trophoblast cells from the blastocyst.

Maternal Contribution: Decidua basalis from the endometrium.

Timeline

Implantation (Day 6–7 post-fertilization): The blastocyst embeds in the endometrium and trophoblast cells begin to invade.

Week 2–3: Primary chorionic villi form as trophoblast proliferates, followed by secondary (with mesoderm) and tertiary villi (with fetal capillaries).

Week 12–14: The placenta becomes functionally mature, with the chorion frondosum (villous portion) forming the fetal placenta and the chorion laeve regressing.

Trophoblast Differentiation

Cytotrophoblast: Inner layer, mitotically active, regenerates syncytiotrophoblast.

Syncytiotrophoblast: Multinucleated outer layer, responsible for nutrient exchange, hormone production and maternal-fetal interface.

Decidualization: The maternal endometrium transforms into decidua, with the decidua basalis forming the maternal component of the placenta.

Structure

Shape and Size: Discoid in humans, typically 15–20 cm in diameter, 2–3 cm thick at the centre and weighs approximately 500–600 grams at term (about $1/6^{th}$ of fetal weight).

Surfaces

Fetal surface: Smooth, shiny and covered by the amnion. Umbilical cord inserts centrally or eccentrically, with umbilical vessels radiating beneath the amnion.

Maternal surface: Rough, lobulated, divided into 15–20 cotyledons (lobes) separated by decidual septa. Directly apposes the decidua basalis.

Anatomical Components

Chorionic Villi: Functional units of the placenta, consisting of fetal capillaries lined by endothelium. Surrounded by cytotrophoblast and syncytiotrophoblast layers. Bathed in maternal blood within intervillous spaces.

Intervillous Spaces: Lacunae where maternal blood pools for exchange with fetal blood.

Basal Plate: Maternal side, formed by decidua basalis, cytotrophoblast and fibrinoid material.

Chorionic Plate: Fetal side, formed by chorion and amnion, anchoring the umbilical vessels.

Layers of Placental Barrier (Hemochorial Placenta):

Syncytiotrophoblast.

Cytotrophoblast (diminishes as pregnancy progresses).

Villous connective tissue.

Fetal capillary endothelium.

By late pregnancy, the barrier thins to ~3–4 μm, enhancing exchange efficiency.

Blood Supply

Maternal Circulation

Source: Uterine arteries supply blood via ~80–100 spiral arteries.

Flow: Maternal blood enters intervillous spaces through spiral arteries, bathes villi and exits via endometrial veins.

Regulation: Spiral arteries remodel during pregnancy (trophoblast invasion reduces vascular resistance), ensuring low-pressure, high-flow perfusion (~600–700 mL/min at term).

Fetal Circulation

Source: Two umbilical arteries carry deoxygenated blood from the fetus to the chorionic villi (placenta); one umbilical vein returns oxygenated blood to the fetus.

Flow: ~300–400 mL/min at term, driven by the fetal heart.

Hemochorial Nature: Maternal and fetal blood do not mix; exchange occurs across the villous barrier via diffusion, active transport and pinocytosis.

Functions

1. Nutrient and Gas Exchange

Oxygen: Diffuses from maternal to fetal blood (gradient-driven).

Nutrients: Glucose, amino acids and lipids cross via facilitated diffusion or active transport.

Waste Removal: CO_2, urea and other metabolic wastes move from fetal to maternal blood.

Mechanism: The thin placental barrier and large surface area optimize exchange.

2. Endocrine Functions

Human Chorionic Gonadotropin (hCG): Maintains corpus luteum, detectable in early pregnancy for diagnosis.

Human Placental Lactogen (hPL): Promotes fetal growth, maternal lipolysis and glucose sparing.

Progesterone: Prevents uterine contractions and supports pregnancy maintenance.

Estrogens: Stimulate uterine growth and prepare breasts for lactation.

Other hormones: Placental growth hormone, corticotropin-releasing hormone (CRH).

3. Immunological Functions

Acts as a selective barrier, preventing direct mixing of maternal and fetal blood.

Expresses non-classical MHC molecules (e.g., HLA-G) to modulate maternal immune response and prevent fetal rejection.

Contains immune cells (e.g., Hofbauer cells) that protect against pathogens.

4. Metabolic Functions

Synthesizes glycogen, cholesterol and fatty acids for fetal use.

Metabolizes drugs and toxins to protect the fetus.

Clinical Significance

Placental Examination

Post-delivery inspection is critical to confirm completeness (retained fragments can cause postpartum hemorrhage or infection). Assess for size, weight, infarcts, calcifications or abnormal insertions.

Pathological Conditions

1. Placenta Previa

Placenta implants over or near the cervical os, causing painless vaginal bleeding.

Types: Complete, partial, marginal or low-lying.

Management: Cesarean section for complete previa; monitoring for low-lying.

2. Placental Abruption

Premature separation from the uterus, leading to hemorrhage, pain and fetal distress.

Risk factors: Hypertension, trauma, smoking.

Complications: Fetal hypoxia, maternal shock.

3. Placenta Accreta Spectrum

Abnormal invasion of trophoblast into myometrium (accreta), deeper layers (increta) or beyond (percreta).

Risk factors: Prior cesarean, placenta previa.

Management: Hysterectomy may be needed.

4. Placental Insufficiency

Impaired function due to infarcts, small size or vascular issues.

Leads to intrauterine growth restriction (IUGR) or fetal hypoxia.

5. Infections

Chorioamnionitis (bacterial infection) can ascend from the vagina, causing preterm labor or neonatal sepsis. Viral infections (e.g., CMV, Zika) may cross the placenta, affecting fetal development.

6. Tumors

Choriocarcinoma: Rare malignant tumor from trophoblast cells.

Hydatidiform Mole: Abnormal placental growth (complete or partial), associated with gestational trophoblastic disease.

Placental Variants

1. **Bilobed Placenta:** Two lobes of equal size, connected by membranes.

Multilobed Placenta may have three or more lobes of equal size.

Risk same as placenta succenruriata and risk of placenta previa and acreta are high.

2. **Succenturiate Placenta**: Accessory lobe(s) present, size of a cotyledon, may be present at varying distances from the margin. A leash of vessels connecting the main to the small lobe traverse through the membranes.

In case of absence of communicating vessels, it is called **Placenta Spuria**.

Risk of retained fragments: lead to PPH, subinvolution, uterine sepsis etc.

Management: Exploration of the uterus and removal of the lobe under general anesthesia is to be done.

3. **Placenta extrachorialis**: It may be of two types:

i) Circumvallate Placenta: This type of palcenta has a raised, rolled edge where the fetal membranes fold back, creating a 'pizza' look.

ii) Placenta Marginata: A thin fibrous ring is present at the margin of chorionic plate where fetal blood vessels appear to terminate.

There is increased chance of abortion, hydrorrhea gravidarum, antepartum hemorrhage, preterm delivery or retained placenta .

4. **Placenta Membranecea**: The placenta is unduly large and thin. Here, placenta develops not only from chorion frondosum but also from chorion leave. Large size may lead to placenta previa, imperfect separation in third stage leading to postpartum hemorrhage and chances of retained placenta.

Aging and Degeneration

At term, the placenta shows fibrinoid deposits, calcifications and infarcts (normal in small amounts). Excessive degeneration may impair function, necessitating early delivery.

Diagnostic Tools

Ultrasound: Assesses placental location, size and abnormalities (e.g., previa, abruption).

Doppler Studies: Evaluates umbilical and uterine artery blood flow for signs of insufficiency.

Histopathology: Post-delivery analysis for infarcts, infection or trophoblastic disease.

Biochemical Markers: hCG, alpha-fetoprotein and estriol levels in maternal serum reflect placental function.

Management

1. Antenatal Monitoring

Regular ultrasound to detect previa, growth restriction or abnormal flow.

Manage maternal conditions (e.g., hypertension, diabetes) to optimize placental function.

2. Intrapartum

Monitor for signs of abruption (e.g., uterine tenderness, fetal distress).

Prepare for cesarean section in cases of previa or accreta.

3. Postpartum

Inspect placenta for completeness and abnormalities.

Manage complications like retained placenta with manual removal or curettage under anesthesia.

Key Points

The placenta is a vital organ for fetal survival, integrating maternal and fetal systems.

Its hemochorial nature maximizes exchange efficiency but poses risks for hemorrhage or invasion.

Clinical vigilance for abnormalities (previa, abruption, accreta) is essential to prevent maternal and fetal morbidity.

Post-delivery placental examination is an essential obstetric skill to ensure maternal safety.

2.2 Foetal Membranes

(*Aghshiay -i-janin*)

Definition

The fetal membranes are extraembryonic structures that enclose the fetus and amniotic fluid, forming a protective sac. They consist of two primary layers: the amnion and the chorion, which together create a secure environment for fetal development.

Structure

1. Amnion

Composition: A thin, avascular, translucent membrane composed of:

A single layer of cuboidal epithelial cells facing the amniotic cavity.

Underlying connective tissue rich in collagen, providing tensile strength.

Location: Lines the inner surface of the amniotic cavity, directly surrounding the fetus and umbilical cord.

Properties: Elastic, smooth and resistant to rupture, yet thin enough to allow fluid exchange.

2. Chorion

Composition: A thick, bilayered membrane consisting of:

Trophoblastic layer (derived from the blastocyst's trophoblast).

Extraembryonic mesoderm (connective tissue layer).

Types

Chorion Frondosum: The villous portion that contributes to the fetal placenta, rich in chorionic villi.

Chorion Laeve: The smooth, non-villous portion that regresses as pregnancy progresses.

Location: Surrounds the amnion and interfaces with the maternal decidua.

Amniochorionic Membrane: By the second trimester, the amnion and chorion fuse, forming a single functional unit that encloses the amniotic cavity.

Development

Amnion: Arises from the inner cell mass of the blastocyst during implantation (around day 7–8 post-fertilization). Forms the amniotic cavity, which expands to surround the embryo. Initially separate, it fuses with the chorion by 12–16 weeks as the amniotic cavity enlarges.

Chorion: Develops from the trophoblast and extraembryonic mesoderm, forming the outer layer of the blastocyst. The chorion frondosum develops villi that interact with the decidua basalis to form the placenta, while the chorion leave regresses due to reduced vascularity.

Fusion: The amnion expands to contact the chorion, forming the amniochorionic membrane, which is essential for maintaining the integrity of the amniotic sac.

Functions

1. Protection

Act as a physical barrier, shielding the fetus from external trauma and ascending infections from the vaginal tract. The amnion's smooth surface minimizes friction against the fetus.

2. Containment

Enclose the amniotic fluid, maintaining a stable, fluid-filled environment for fetal development.

3. Immunological Role

The chorion expresses non-classical MHC molecules (e.g., HLA-G), suppressing maternal immune responses to prevent fetal rejection. Contains macrophages (Hofbauer cells) that combat pathogens.

4. Mechanical Role

Withstand intrauterine pressure during pregnancy. Facilitate labor by rupturing at term, releasing amniotic fluid ("water breaking").

5. Secretory Role

Contribute to amniotic fluid production (via amnion epithelial cells). Produce enzymes and cytokines that regulate intrauterine inflammation.

Clinical Significance

Premature Rupture of Membranes (PROM)

Definition: Rupture of membranes before the onset of labor, regardless of gestational age.

Preterm PROM (PPROM): Occurs before 37 weeks, increasing risks of preterm birth, chorioamnionitis and neonatal sepsis.

Diagnosis: Sterile speculum exam showing fluid pooling, positive nitrazine test (alkaline pH), or ferning pattern on microscopy.

Management: Depends on gestational age; may include antibiotics, corticosteroids for lung maturity, or delivery.

Chorioamnionitis

Bacterial infection of the membranes, often due to ascending pathogens (e.g., E. coli, Group B Streptococcus).

Clinical Features: Maternal fever, uterine tenderness, fetal tachycardia, foul-smelling amniotic fluid.

Complications: Preterm labor, neonatal sepsis, maternal endometritis.

Management: Antibiotics and prompt delivery.

Amnion Nodosum

Small, nodular deposits of squamous epithelial cells on the amnion, associated with oligohydramnios (e.g., due to fetal renal agenesis).

Differentiated from squamous metaplasia (benign) by histopathology.

Meconium-Stained Membranes

Indicates fetal passage of meconium, potentially signaling fetal distress.

May lead to meconium aspiration syndrome, if inhaled by the fetus.

Examination Post-Delivery

Inspect membranes for completeness, tears, staining (meconium, blood), or signs of infection (e.g., purulent discharge).

Retained membranes can cause postpartum hemorrhage or infection, requiring manual removal or curettage.

Pathological form

Membrane Abnormalities

Circumvallate Placenta: Folded membranes reduce placental surface area, linked to bleeding or preterm birth.

Amniotic Band Syndrome: Partial membrane rupture forms fibrous bands, potentially causing fetal amputations or craniofacial defects.

Infections

Viral infections (e.g., CMV, parvovirus) may cross membranes, affecting fetal development.

TORCH infections can lead to congenital anomalies or fetal loss.

Histopathology

Post-delivery analysis may reveal funisitis (umbilical cord inflammation), chorionitis or villitis, indicating infection or immune-mediated pathology.

2.3 Amniotic Fluid & its Abnormalities

(Taba'l wa Gahyr Tabaiai Rutubat-i-Aminusiyya)

Introduction

Amniotic fluid is the clear, slightly yellowish liquid that surrounds the fetus in the amniotic sac during pregnancy. It plays a critical role in fetal development, providing protection, nourishment and an environment conducive to growth. Abnormalities in amniotic fluid volume or composition can indicate underlying fetal or maternal pathology and require careful evaluation and management.

Physiology of Amniotic Fluid

Composition

Components: Amniotic fluid primarily consists of water (98–99%), with the remainder including electrolytes, proteins, carbohydrates, lipids, enzymes, hormones and fetal cells (e.g., squamous epithelial cells).

Fetal Contributions: Fetal urine, lung secretions and oral/nasal secretions contribute significantly to amniotic fluid after the first trimester.

Maternal Contributions: Transudation from maternal plasma across the placenta and fetal membranes also contributes.

Functions

1. Protection: Acts as a cushion, protecting the fetus from external trauma and maintaining a stable temperature.
2. Development: Allows free movement for musculoskeletal development and prevents limb contractures.
3. Respiratory: Facilitates lung development through fetal breathing movements.
4. Nutrition: Contains nutrients that the fetus may swallow.
5. Infection Barrier: Contains antimicrobial properties (e.g., lysozymes, immunoglobulins).

Volume Dynamics

First Trimester: Amniotic fluid is primarily a transudate of maternal plasma and fetal extracellular fluid across the fetal skin.

Second and Third Trimesters: Fetal urine becomes the primary source, balanced by fetal swallowing and intramembranous absorption (transfer of fluid across the amnion into the fetal circulation).

Volume Changes

50 mL at 12 weeks

400 mL at 20 weeks

Peaks at 800–1000 mL at 36–38 weeks

Declines to 500–600 mL at term

Regulation: Controlled by fetal urine production, swallowing, lung secretions and intramembranous absorption.

Assessment

Ultrasound: Amniotic fluid volume is measured using:

Amniotic Fluid Index (AFI): Sum of the deepest vertical pocket of fluid in each quadrant of the uterus (normal range: 5–25 cm).

Single Deepest Pocket (SDP): Depth of the largest fluid pocket (normal: 2–8 cm).

Abnormalities of Amniotic Fluid

Amniotic fluid abnormalities are primarily related to volume (too much or too little) or composition (e.g., meconium, blood). These conditions are associated with maternal, fetal or placental pathology and can impact pregnancy outcomes.

1. Oligohydramnios

Definition: It is the condition where the liquor amnii is deficient in amount to the extent of less than 200 ml at term. Sonographically, it is defined when amniotic fluid volume (AFI) < 5 cm or Single deepest pocket of amniotic fluid (SDP) < 2 cm. AFI between 5 and 8 is termed as borderline AFI or borderline oligohydramnios. (Dutta)

Etiology

Fetal Causes

Renal anomalies (e.g., bilateral renal agenesis, polycystic kidneys, urinary tract obstruction).

Fetal growth restriction (FGR) due to placental insufficiency.

Premature rupture of membranes (PROM).

Post-term pregnancy (>42 weeks).

Maternal Causes

Dehydration or hypovolemia.

Hypertensive disorders (e.g., preeclampsia).

Medications (e.g., ACE inhibitors, NSAIDs).

Placental Causes

Placental insufficiency.

Clinical Features

Reduced fundal height.

Fetal crowding or abnormal lie.

Ultrasound findings: Decreased fluid pockets, fetal compression.

Complications

Pulmonary Hypoplasia: Due to inadequate lung development.

Limb Deformities: From compression (e.g., clubfoot, contractures).

Cord Compression: Leading to fetal distress or hypoxia.

Meconium Aspiration Syndrome: Increased risk due to concentrated meconium.

Diagnosis

Ultrasound assessment of AFI or SDP.

Evaluate for underlying causes (e.g., fetal anomaly scan, Doppler studies).

Management

Mild Cases: Maternal hydration (oral or IV fluids), treat underlying cause (e.g., PROM management).

Severe Cases: Amnioinfusion (instilling saline into the amniotic cavity during labor), early delivery if fetal maturity permits.

Fetal Anomalies: Multidisciplinary approach, including neonatology and pediatric surgery consultation.

Monitoring: Serial ultrasounds, non-stress tests (NST) or biophysical profile (BPP).

2. Polyhydramnios

Definition: It is defined as a state where liquor amnii exceeds 2000 ml.

Clinical definition states- the excessive accumulation of liquor amnii causing discomfort to the patient and/or when an imaging help is needed to substantiate the clinical diagnosis of the lie and presentation of the fetus.

Sonographic diagnosis: when Amniotic fluid index (AFI) > 24 cm and deepest vertical pocket (SDP) > 8 cm. (Dutta)

Etiology

Fetal Causes

Gastrointestinal obstructions (e.g., esophageal or duodenal atresia).

Neuromuscular disorders impairing swallowing (e.g., anencephaly).

Congenital infections (e.g., parvovirus B19, cytomegalovirus).

Fetal anemia or hydrops fetalis.

Maternal Causes

Diabetes mellitus (poorly controlled).

Rh isoimmunization.

Idiopathic: Up to 50% of cases.

Other: Twin-to-twin transfusion syndrome (TTTS), chorioangiomas.

Clinical Features

Rapidly increasing fundal height.

Maternal discomfort (e.g., dyspnea, abdominal pain).

Preterm contractions or premature rupture of membranes.

Ultrasound findings: excessive fluid, floating fetus.

Complications

Preterm Labor: Due to uterine overdistension.

Cord Prolapse: During membrane rupture.

Placental Abruption: From sudden decompression.

Malpresentation: Due to excessive fetal mobility.

Postpartum Hemorrhage: Secondary to uterine atony.

Diagnosis

Ultrasound assessment of AFI or SDP.

Fetal anomaly scan, glucose tolerance test (for maternal diabetes), and infection screening.

Management

Mild Cases: Observation, control maternal diabetes if present.

Moderate to Severe Cases: Medications to reduce fetal urine output (e.g., indomethacin, with caution due to risk of premature ductal closure).

Amnioreduction (therapeutic removal of fluid via amniocentesis).

Treat underlying cause (e.g., laser therapy for TTTS).

Delivery Planning: Timing and mode depend on severity and gestational age.

3. Meconium-Stained Amniotic Fluid

Definition: Presence of fetal stool (meconium) in the amniotic fluid, giving it a greenish or brownish appearance.

Etiology

Fetal distress (e.g., hypoxia, cord compression).

Post-term pregnancy.

Normal in some term or post-term fetuses without distress.

Clinical Features

Visible during rupture of membranes or on ultrasound (particulate matter).

Complications

Meconium Aspiration Syndrome (MAS): Inhalation of meconium by the fetus, leading to respiratory distress, pneumonitis or persistent pulmonary hypertension.

Increased risk of neonatal sepsis or neurological injury if associated with hypoxia.

Diagnosis

Clinical observation during labor or delivery.

Ultrasound may detect particulate matter in severe cases.

Management

During Labor: Continuous fetal monitoring, avoid aggressive maneuvers (e.g., excessive fundal pressure).

Amnioinfusion: Dilutes meconium to reduce MAS risk.

Delivery: Pediatric team presence at delivery for airway management.

Postnatal: Neonatal resuscitation, suctioning below vocal cords if needed, and NICU care for MAS.

4. Chorioamnionitis

Definition: Infection of the amniotic fluid, membranes, or placenta, often due to ascending bacteria after prolonged rupture of membranes.

Etiology

Common pathogens: Escherichia coli, Group B Streptococcus, anaerobes.

Risk factors: PROM, prolonged labor, multiple vaginal examinations.

Clinical Features

Maternal fever, uterine tenderness, foul-smelling amniotic fluid.

Fetal tachycardia, leukocytosis.

Complications

Preterm labor, sepsis (maternal or neonatal), endometritis.

Diagnosis

Clinical criteria (Gibbs criteria): Maternal fever >38°C plus one or more of fetal tachycardia, maternal leukocytosis, uterine tenderness, or foul amniotic fluid.

Amniotic fluid analysis (culture, Gram stain) if feasible.

Management

Broad-spectrum antibiotics (e.g., ampicillin and gentamicin).

Expedited delivery (vaginal or cesarean, depending on clinical status).

Neonatal evaluation and treatment for sepsis.

5. Bloody Amniotic Fluid

Definition: Presence of blood in the amniotic fluid.

Etiology

Placental abruption.

Vasa previa or velamentous cord insertion.

Fetal or maternal bleeding (e.g., trauma, coagulopathy).

Clinical Features

Red or pink amniotic fluid during rupture of membranes.

Signs of fetal distress or maternal hemorrhage.

Complications

Fetal hypoxia, anemia, or demise.

Maternal shock or disseminated intravascular coagulation (DIC).

Diagnosis

Clinical observation, ultrasound, and fetal monitoring.

Kleihauer-Betke test to differentiate fetal vs. maternal blood.

Management

Emergency delivery for significant hemorrhage or fetal distress.

Blood transfusion for maternal or fetal anemia.

Address underlying cause (e.g., surgical intervention for vasa previa).

Diagnostic Techniques

1. Ultrasound

Primary tool for assessing amniotic fluid volume (AFI, SDP).

Detects fetal anomalies, placental issues, or Doppler abnormalities.

2. Amniocentesis

For infection (culture, PCR), genetic testing, or lung maturity assessment (e.g., lecithin/sphingomyelin ratio).

Risks: infection, membrane rupture, fetal injury.

3. Fetal Monitoring

Non-stress test (NST), contraction stress test (CST) or biophysical profile (BPP) to assess fetal well-being.

4. Laboratory Tests

Maternal: Glucose levels, infection markers (CRP, WBC).

Amniotic fluid: Analysis for infection, blood or meconium.

Management Principles

Individualized Care: Based on gestational age, severity and underlying cause.

Timing of Delivery

Preterm: Balance risks of prematurity vs. complications of abnormality.

Term: Expedite delivery, if fetal or maternal compromise.

Fetal Surveillance

Regular ultrasound, Doppler and fetal heart rate monitoring.

Biophysical profile for comprehensive assessment.

Maternal Support

Hydration, glucose control, infection treatment.

Psychological support for high-risk pregnancies.

Complications and Prognosis

Oligohydramnios: High risk of pulmonary hypoplasia, limb deformities and perinatal mortality, if severe and early-onset.

Polyhydramnios: Increased risk of preterm birth, abruption and postpartum hemorrhage; prognosis depends on underlying cause.

Meconium-Stained Fluid: Risk of MAS and neonatal morbidity; good outcomes with timely intervention.

Chorioamnionitis: Maternal and neonatal sepsis risk; prompt treatment improves prognosis.

Bloody Fluid: Potentially life-threatening; outcomes depend on cause and speed of intervention.

Preventive Measures

Maternal Health: Optimize control of diabetes, hypertension and infections.

Prenatal Care: Regular ultrasound monitoring for early detection of abnormalities.

Infection Control: Sterile technique during exams, timely management of PROM.

Patient Education: Awareness of symptoms (e.g., reduced fetal movements, vaginal leakage).

Conclusion

Amniotic fluid is essential for fetal development and its abnormalities can significantly impact pregnancy outcomes. Oligohydramnios, polyhydramnios, meconium-stained fluid, chorioamnionitis, and bloody amniotic fluid each requires prompt diagnosis and tailored management. Ultrasound, fetal monitoring and targeted interventions are necessary for optimizing maternal and fetal outcomes.

2.4 Umbilical cord and & its Abnormalities

(Taba'I wa Ghayr Taba'I Hablussurah)

Introduction

The umbilical cord is a flexible tube like structure, connecting the fetus to the placenta, facilitating the exchange of nutrients, oxygen and waste products. Abnormalities in its structure, length or function can lead to significant maternal and fetal complications.

Structure

Length: Average length at term is 50–60 cm (range: 30–100 cm).

Diameter: Approximately 1–2 cm, varying with Wharton's jelly content.

Insertion: Typically inserts centrally or eccentrically into the placenta; abnormal insertions are associated with complications.

Components: Vessels: Two umbilical arteries (carry deoxygenated blood from the fetus to the placenta) and one umbilical vein (carries oxygenated blood from the placenta to the fetus).

Wharton's Jelly: A gelatinous connective tissue matrix that surrounds the vessels, providing structural support and protection against compression.

Amniotic Covering: A single layer of amnion encases the cord, continuous with the fetal skin and amniotic membrane.

Functions

Nutrient and Oxygen Transport: The umbilical vein delivers oxygen-rich, nutrient-rich blood to the fetus, while the arteries return deoxygenated blood and waste to the placenta.

Protection: Wharton's jelly cushions the vessels, preventing compression during fetal movements or uterine contractions.

Fetal Circulation: The umbilical vein feeds into the fetal portal vein and ductus venosus, bypassing the liver to supply the heart and systemic circulation.

Blood Flow: Regulated by fetal cardiac output and placental resistance; assessed via Doppler ultrasound (e.g., umbilical artery Doppler for fetal well-being).

Development: Forms by 5–6 weeks of gestation from the yolk sac and allantois, fully functional by the end of the first trimester.

Assessment

Ultrasound: Evaluates cord structure, vessel number, insertion site, and blood flow (Doppler studies).

Gross Examination: Post-delivery inspection for length, coiling, knots, or abnormal insertions.

Coiling Index: Normal is 0.2–0.3 coils/cm; hypo- or hypercoiling may indicate pathology.

Abnormalities of the Umbilical Cord

Umbilical cord abnormalities can be classified based on structure, length, insertion, or complications during pregnancy or delivery. These conditions may lead to fetal distress, growth restriction or perinatal mortality if not managed appropriately.

1. Single Umbilical Artery (SUA)

Definition: Presence of only one umbilical artery instead of two, with one umbilical vein.

Prevalence: Occurs in 0.5–1% of singleton pregnancies; higher in twins or fetuses with anomalies.

Etiology: Agenesis or atrophy of one umbilical artery. Associated with congenital anomalies (20–30% of cases), especially cardiac, renal, or chromosomal abnormalities (e.g., trisomy 18).

Clinical Features: Often asymptomatic, detected on ultrasound or at delivery. May be associated with fetal growth restriction (FGR) or preterm birth.

Complications: Increased risk of congenital anomalies. Fetal hypoxia due to reduced placental perfusion. Perinatal mortality (higher in cases with associated anomalies).

Diagnosis: Ultrasound: Identifies two-vessel cord (one artery, one vein). Detailed fetal anomaly scan to rule out associated malformations. Karyotyping or genetic testing if anomalies are present.

Management: Serial ultrasound monitoring for fetal growth and well-being. Doppler studies to assess umbilical artery flow. Multidisciplinary approach if anomalies are detected. No specific intervention unless FGR or fetal distress is present.

2. Umbilical Cord Length Abnormalities

Short Cord (<35 cm)

Etiology: Unknown; may be associated with restricted fetal movement or oligohydramnios.

Complications

Placental abruption due to excessive tension.

Non-reassuring fetal heart rate patterns from cord stretching.

Inhibited fetal descent during labor.

Management: Monitor for fetal distress; cesarean delivery if complications arise.

Long Cord (>80 cm)

Etiology: Genetic predisposition or excessive fetal movement.

Complications

Cord prolapse or entanglement.

True knots or nuchal cords (cord around fetal neck).

Increased risk of thrombosis or compression.

Management: Ultrasound monitoring for cord position; careful labor management to avoid prolapse.

3. Abnormal Cord Insertion

Marginal Insertion (Battledore Placenta)

Definition: Cord inserts at the placental edge (margin)rather than centrally.

Prevalence: 5–7% of pregnancies.

Complications: Increased risk of fetal growth retardation or preterm birth due to reduced placental perfusion.

Management: Monitor fetal growth and Doppler flow; usually no specific intervention.

Velamentous Insertion

Definition: Cord inserts into the fetal membranes, with vessels traveling unprotected to the placenta.

Prevalence: 1% of singleton pregnancies; higher in twins.

Complications

Catastrophic fetal hemorrhage if membranes rupture.

Fetal death (50–60% mortality if undiagnosed).

Diagnosis: Transvaginal ultrasound with Doppler; high suspicion with low-lying placenta or velamentous insertion.

Management

Hospitalization at 30–32 weeks for close monitoring.

Corticosteroids for lung maturity.

Elective cesarean delivery at 34–36 weeks.

Emergency caesarean, if bleeding or membrane rupture occurs.

4. Umbilical Cord Coiling Abnormalities

Hypocoiling (<0.1 coils/cm)

Etiology: Unknown; may be associated with reduced Wharton's jelly.

Complications: Increased risk of fetal hypoxia, FGR, or stillbirth due to reduced protection against compression.

Management: Monitor fetal well-being with ultrasound and Doppler.

Hypercoiling (>0.3 coils/cm)

Etiology: Excessive fetal movement or genetic factors.

Complications: Risk of torsion, thrombosis, or fetal distress.

Management: Similar to hypocoiling; close fetal monitoring.

5. True Knots

Definition: A knot in the umbilical cord formed by fetal movement through a loop.

Prevalence: 0.3–2% of pregnancies.

Etiology: Long cord, excessive fetal movement, polyhydramnios, or small fetal size.

Complications: Cord occlusion leading to fetal hypoxia or demise. Risk increases if knot tightens during labor.

Diagnosis: Often incidental on ultrasound or at delivery. Doppler may show abnormal flow patterns.

Management: Antenatal: Monitor for fetal distress with NST or BPP. Intrapartum: Continuous fetal monitoring; cesarean delivery if knot causes distress.

6. Nuchal Cord

Definition: Umbilical cord wrapped around the fetal neck (single or multiple loops).

Prevalence: 15–30% at term; more common with long cords or polyhydramnios.

Complications: Usually benign, but tight nuchal cords may cause hypoxia or variable decelerations in labor. Rarely, neonatal morbidity or mortality if severe compression occurs.

Diagnosis

Ultrasound detection (loops around neck).

Fetal heart rate monitoring for decelerations.

Management

Most resolve spontaneously or are reducible at delivery.

Monitor during labor; cesarean delivery if persistent fetal distress.

7. Umbilical Cord Prolapse

Definition: Descent of the umbilical cord below the presenting part, with or without membrane rupture.

Prevalence: 0.1–0.6% of deliveries.

Etiology

Malpresentation (e.g., breech, transverse lie).

Polyhydramnios, preterm labor, or artificial rupture of membranes.

Long cord or low-lying placenta.

Complications

Cord compression causing fetal hypoxia or death.

Emergency situation with high perinatal mortality if not managed promptly.

Diagnosis

Palpation of cord in the vagina or visible after membrane rupture.

Fetal heart rate abnormalities (variable or prolonged decelerations).

Management

Immediate Actions

Elevate presenting part to relieve cord compression (e.g., knee-chest position).

Avoid cord manipulation to prevent vasospasm.

Administer oxygen and tocolytics if contractions persist.

Delivery: Emergency cesarean delivery (preferred); vaginal delivery only if imminent and cord compression is relieved.

Prevention: Avoid amniotomy in high-risk cases (e.g., malpresentation, unengaged head).

8. Umbilical Cord Cysts

Definition: Fluid-filled sacs in the umbilical cord, classified as true cysts (derived from embryonic remnants) or pseudocysts (fluid in Wharton's jelly).

Prevalence: Rare (1–3% of pregnancies).

Etiology

True cysts: Remnants of allantois or omphalomesenteric duct.

Pseudocysts: Degeneration of Wharton's jelly.

Complications

Usually benign, but large cysts may compress vessels, causing fetal distress.

Associated with chromosomal anomalies (e.g., trisomy 18) in some cases.

Diagnosis: Ultrasound detection of cystic structures; assess for associated anomalies.

Management

Monitor cyst size and fetal well-being.

Genetic testing if anomalies are present.

No intervention unless vascular compromise is evident.

9. Umbilical Cord Thrombosis

Definition: Formation of a thrombus in the umbilical vein or arteries.

Prevalence: Rare; exact incidence unknown.

Etiology

Cord compression, hypercoiling, or knots.

Maternal hypercoagulable states or fetal conditions (e.g., infection, hypoxia).

Complications

Fetal hypoxia, growth restriction, or demise.

High perinatal mortality if untreated.

Diagnosis

Ultrasound with Doppler showing absent or turbulent flow.

Often diagnosed postnatally on cord examination.

Management

Urgent delivery if detected antenatally with signs of fetal distress.

Evaluate for maternal thrombophilia if recurrent.

Diagnostic Techniques

1. Ultrasound

Primary tool for assessing cord structure, vessel number, insertion site, and Doppler flow.

Identifies knots, cysts, or abnormal insertions (e.g., velamentous, vasa previa).

2. Doppler Studies

Assesses umbilical artery and vein flow for signs of resistance or obstruction.

Useful in FGR, SUA, or suspected thrombosis.

3. Fetal Monitoring

Non-stress test (NST) or biophysical profile (BPP) for fetal well-being.

Intrapartum monitoring for decelerations suggestive of cord compression.

4. Post-Delivery Examination

Gross and histological analysis of the cord for anomalies or thrombosis.

5. Genetic Testing

Indicated for SUA, cord cysts, or associated fetal anomalies.

Management Principles

Antenatal Monitoring

Serial ultrasounds for growth, Doppler studies, and anomaly screening.

Biophysical profile or NST for high-risk cases.

Intrapartum Care

Continuous fetal heart rate monitoring to detect cord compression.

Avoid amniotomy in cases of malpresentation or suspected vasa previa.

Delivery Planning.

Elective cesarean for vasa previa, cord prolapse, or severe fetal distress.

Vaginal delivery feasible for minor abnormalities (e.g., nuchal cord) with no distress.

Maternal Counseling

Educate on signs of fetal distress (e.g., reduced movements).

Discuss risks and delivery plans for high-risk conditions.

Complications and Prognosis

Fetal Growth Restriction: Common with SUA, marginal insertion, or thrombosis.

Fetal Distress: Associated with cord prolapse, knots, or compression.

Perinatal Mortality: Highest with vasa previa, cord prolapse, or thrombosis if undiagnosed.

Congenital Anomalies: SUA and cord cysts may indicate underlying genetic or structural issues.

Prognosis: Varies by abnormality; early diagnosis and intervention (e.g., cesarean for vasa previa) improve outcomes significantly.

Preventive Measures

Prenatal Screening: Routine ultrasound to detect cord anomalies early.

Optimize maternal conditions (e.g., diabetes, thrombophilia).

Avoid premature amniotomy in high-risk cases.

Patient Education: Awareness of fetal movement monitoring and symptoms of complications.

Delivery Planning: Anticipate risks in cases of malpresentation or abnormal cord findings.

Conclusion

The umbilical cord is an important structure for fetal survival and development, and its abnormalities can pose significant risks to the fetus and mother. Conditions such as single umbilical artery, vasa previa, cord prolapse and thrombosis require prompt diagnosis and proper management to prevent adverse outcomes. Advances in ultrasound and Doppler technology have improved antenatal detection, enabling timely interventions.

Long Answer Questions (LAQs)

1. Describe the placenta (*Mashima*) with its formation, structure and functions.
2. Explain normal and abnormal placenta in detail.
3. Describe fetal membranes (*Aghshiya-e-Janīn*) and their functions.
4. Define amniotic fluid and describe its functions and abnormalities.
5. Describe the umbilical cord (*Habl-us-Surrah*) and its abnormalities.

Short Answer Questions (SAQs)

1. Define placenta.
2. Name the fetal membranes.
3. Define oligohydramnios.
4. How many vessels are present in umbilical cord?
5. Write two functions of amniotic fluid.

Multiple Choice Questions (1 Mark Each)

1. Placenta is formed from:

A. Maternal tissue only   B. Fetal tissue only

C. Both maternal and fetal tissue   D. Amniotic fluid

Ans: C. Both maternal and fetal tissue

2. Normal placenta is discoid in shape:

A. True B. False

Ans: A. True

3. Excess amniotic fluid is called:

A. Oligohydramnios B. Polyhydramnios

C. Hydramnios D. Anhydramnios

Ans: B. Polyhydramnios

4. Decreased amniotic fluid is called:

A. Polyhydramnios B. Oligohydramnios

C. Hydrops D. Ascites

Ans: B. Oligohydramnios

5. Umbilical cord normally contains:

A. 1 artery, 1 vein B. 2 arteries, 1 vein

C. 2 veins, 1 artery D. 1 artery only

Ans: B. 2 arteries, 1 vein

6. Amniotic fluid is mainly formed by:

A. Maternal blood B. Fetal urine

C. Placenta D. Cord blood

Ans: B. Fetal urine

7. Which membrane forms the amniotic sac?

A. Chorion B. Amnion

C. Decidua D. Peritoneum

Ans: B. Amnion

8. Placenta previa is:

A. Premature separation B. Low-lying placenta

C. Placental infarction D. Placental calcification

Ans: B. Low-lying placenta

9. Umbilical cord abnormality includes:

A. True knot B. Single umbilical artery

C. Cord prolapse D. All of the above

Ans: D. All of the above

10. Main function of placenta is:

A. Digestion B. Respiration and nutrition

C. Excretion only D. Protection only

Ans: B. Respiration and nutrition

03

Pregnancy

(*Haml*)

3.1 *Qabl az haml zehn saazi* (Preconceptional Counselling & care)
3.2 *Haml aur Wiladat se ma'qbl Tashkhisi zaray -i- aur mutalleqah qwaneen* (Preconception &Prenatal Diagnostic Techniques & PNDT Act)
3.3 *Ilm-al-Qabalat se mutaalliq qanooni aur akhlaqi masaayil* (Legal & Ethical Issues in Obstetric Practice)
3.4 *Haml ke taba'I taghayyurat* (Physiological Changes)
3.5 *Haml ki Alamat wa Nishaniyya wa Tashkhis-i-haml* (Signs & Symptoms & Diagnosis of pregnancy)
3.6 *Haml-i-Kadhib/Rijaa'* (Pseudocyesis / False Pregnancy)
3.7 *Hamla ki nigahdasht aur hamal ke daruan hone wale khafif amrad* (Antenatal care & Minor Ailments in pregnancy)
3.8 *Qaumi sehatee program braye qabalat* (National Health Programs in Obstetrics)

Learning Objective (At the end of the session, the students should be able to)

Describe the objectives & advantages of preconceptional counseling.
Explain PNDT act, preconceptional care and prenatal diagnosis.
Discuss the Legal and Ethical Issues in Obstetric Practices.
Explain the *Hamal ke Taba'I Taghayyurat* (Anatomical & Physiological changes during pregnancy).
Evaluate and assess the *Ḥamal Ki Alamat wa Nishaniyan* (Sings & Symptoms of Pregnancy) & *Ḥamal ki Tashkhees* (Diagnosis of Pregnancy).
Elicit & document Gestational Age, Expected Date of Delivery (EDD) & Obstetric Formula.
Define *Hamal-e- Kazib / Rijaa'* (Pseudocyesis /False Pregnancy).
Enumerate the objectives of *Ḥamla ki Nigahdasht* (antenatal care) & Illustrate the screening for high-risk factors, procedures of visits, antenatal advice & management of minor ailments in Pregnancy.
Enlist Various National Health Programs in Obstetrics.

3.1 Preconceptional Counseling & care

(*Qabl az haml zehn saazi*)

Introduction

Preconception counseling and care involve a proactive approach to optimizing maternal and fetal health before pregnancy. It aims to identify and mitigate risks, promote healthy behaviors and address medical, genetic and lifestyle factors that could impact pregnancy outcomes. This process is essential for reducing maternal and neonatal morbidity and mortality. It is a cornerstone of preventive obstetric care.

Purpose of Preconception Counseling

1. Risk Assessment: Identify medical, genetic, psychosocial and environmental factors that may affect pregnancy.
2. Health Optimization: Address chronic conditions, nutritional deficiencies and lifestyle risks to improve maternal and fetal outcomes.
3. Education: Provide women and their partners with information to make informed decisions about pregnancy planning.
4. Prevention: Reduce the incidence of congenital anomalies, preterm birth and maternal complications through early intervention.
5. Reproductive Planning: Discuss family planning, contraception and optimal timing of pregnancy.

Components of Preconception Counseling and Care

Preconception care is multidisciplinary, involving obstetricians, primary care providers, genetic counselors and other specialists as needed. It encompasses a thorough evaluation and tailored interventions.

1. Medical History Assessment

Chronic Conditions

Diabetes mellitus: Optimize glycemic control (target HbA1c <6.5%) to reduce risks of congenital anomalies and miscarriage.

Hypertension: Adjust medications to pregnancy-safe options (e.g., methyldopa, labetalol) and monitor blood pressure.

Thyroid disorders: Ensure euthyroid state (TSH 0.1–2.5 mIU/L in the first trimester) to support fetal neurodevelopment.

Seizure disorders: Optimize antiepileptic drugs (e.g., switch to lamotrigine or levetiracetam, avoid valproate due to teratogenicity).

Autoimmune diseases (e.g., lupus): Assess disease activity and adjust immunosuppressive therapy (e.g., hydroxychloroquine is safe).

Infectious Diseases

Screen for and treat infections (e.g., HIV, hepatitis B/C, syphilis, toxoplasmosis, cytomegalovirus).

Update vaccinations (e.g., rubella, varicella, influenza, Tdap) at least 1 month before conception.

Counsel on preventing sexually transmitted infections.

Mental Health

Screen for depression, anxiety or other psychiatric conditions.

Adjust psychotropic medications to pregnancy-safe options (e.g., SSRIs like sertraline) and coordinate with a psychiatrist.

Previous Pregnancy Complications

Review history of preterm birth, preeclampsia, gestational diabetes or fetal anomalies.

Plan interventions to reduce recurrence risk (e.g., low-dose aspirin for preeclampsia prevention).

2. Genetic and Family History

Screening

Obtain a detailed family history for genetic disorders (e.g., cystic fibrosis, sickle cell disease, thalassemia).

Offer carrier screening for common genetic conditions based on ethnicity (e.g., cystic fibrosis for Caucasians, sickle cell for African descent).

Discuss risks of consanguinity if applicable.

Counseling

Explain risks of inheritable conditions (e.g., autosomal recessive, dominant or X-linked disorders).

Offer preconception genetic counseling for couples with known risks or prior affected pregnancies.

Discuss options for preimplantation genetic diagnosis (PGD) or prenatal testing if indicated.

Age-Related Risks

Counsel women >35 years on increased risks of chromosomal abnormalities (e.g., Down syndrome) and pregnancy complications (e.g., gestational diabetes, preeclampsia).

3. Lifestyle and Behavioral Modifications

Nutrition

Assess body mass index (BMI)

Underweight (BMI <18.5): Recommend weight gain to reduce risks of preterm birth and low birth weight.

Overweight/Obese (BMI >25): Encourage weight loss to lower risks of gestational diabetes, hypertension and cesarean delivery.

Recommend a balanced diet rich in fruits, vegetables, lean proteins and whole grains.

Initiate folic acid supplementation (400–800 mcg daily for at least 1–3 months preconception) to reduce neural tube defects; higher doses (4 mg daily) for women with prior affected pregnancies or high-risk conditions (e.g., epilepsy, diabetes).

Screen for and correct nutritional deficiencies (e.g., iron, vitamin D, omega-3 fatty acids).

Substance Use

Tobacco: Counsel on smoking cessation; offer nicotine replacement therapy or behavioral support if needed. Smoking increases risks of miscarriage, FGR and preterm birth.

Alcohol: Advise complete abstinence, as no safe level exists in pregnancy; alcohol is linked to fetal alcohol spectrum disorders.

Recreational Drugs: Screen for and counsel against illicit drug use (e.g., marijuana, opioids, cocaine); refer to substance abuse programs if needed.

Exercise

Recommend 150 minutes/week of moderate aerobic exercise (e.g., brisk walking, swimming) unless contraindicated. Avoid high-risk activities (e.g., contact sports) during pregnancy planning.

Environmental Exposures

Advise avoidance of teratogens (e.g., radiation, certain chemicals, heavy metals like lead or mercury).

Counsel on safe handling of pets (e.g., avoid cat litter to prevent toxoplasmosis).

Discuss workplace hazards (e.g., prolonged standing, chemical exposures) and recommend modifications.

4. Reproductive Health and Family Planning

Contraception

Discuss current contraceptive use and plan for discontinuation when pregnancy is desired.

Ensure adequate time for fertility restoration (e.g., 1–3 months after stopping oral contraceptives).

Fertility Awareness

Educate on ovulation tracking (e.g., basal body temperature, ovulation predictor kits).

Address concerns about subfertility or infertility; refer to a reproductive endocrinologist if needed (e.g., history of irregular cycles, PCOS).

Interconception Interval

Recommend at least 18–24 months between pregnancies to reduce risks of preterm birth and low birth weight.

Sexual Health

Screen for and treat sexually transmitted infections.

Counsel on safe sexual practices to prevent infections during conception.

5. Psychosocial and Socioeconomic Factors

Screening

Assess for intimate partner violence, financial stressors or lack of social support.

Evaluate access to healthcare and insurance coverage.

Interventions

Refer to social workers, counselors or community resources as needed.

Address barriers to care (e.g., transportation, language).

Partner Involvement

Encourage partner participation in counseling to address shared risks (e.g., genetic screening, lifestyle changes). Discuss paternal health (e.g., smoking, obesity) as it may impact sperm quality and pregnancy outcomes.

6. Immunizations

Preconception Vaccines

Rubella and Varicella: Confirm immunity (IgG testing); vaccinate non-immune women and delay conception for 1 month post-vaccination.

Tdap: Administer to protect against pertussis (neonatal protection via maternal antibodies).

Influenza: Recommend annual flu vaccine, safe in any trimester and preconception.

Hepatitis B: Vaccinate high-risk women (e.g., healthcare workers, multiple sexual partners).

HPV: Offer to women ≤ 45 years if not previously vaccinated, though not urgent for pregnancy planning.

Counseling: Discuss importance of maintaining up-to-date vaccinations to prevent congenital infections.

7. Screening and Laboratory Tests

Routine Tests

Complete blood count (CBC) to detect anemia.

Blood type and Rh status; screen for Rh isoimmunization risk.

Thyroid function tests (TSH, free T4) if indicated.

Hemoglobin A1c for women with diabetes or at risk.

Lipid profile for women with cardiovascular risk factors.

Infectious Disease Screening

HIV, syphilis, hepatitis B/C, and rubella serology.

Urine or cervical screening for chlamydia and gonorrhea in high-risk women.

Toxoplasmosis or CMV testing if high-risk (e.g., exposure to raw meat, cat litter).

Genetic Screening

Carrier screening for conditions like cystic fibrosis, spinal muscular atrophy, or hemoglobinopathies based on ethnicity or family history.

Clinical Approach to Preconception Care

1. Initial Visit

Obtain a detailed history (medical, obstetric, family, social).

Perform a physical exam, including BMI, blood pressure, and pelvic exam if indicated.

Order baseline laboratory tests and screenings.

2. Counseling Session

Use a patient-centered approach to discuss findings and risks.

Provide written materials or resources for lifestyle changes.

Address questions about fertility, pregnancy planning, and risks.

3. Follow-Up

Schedule follow-up visits to monitor chronic conditions, confirm vaccination status, or assess lifestyle changes.

Reassess genetic risks or refer to specialists as needed.

4. Documentation

Record all findings, recommendations, and patient education in the medical record.

Provide a preconception care plan summarizing interventions and follow-up.

Special Cases

1. Women with Chronic Conditions

Diabetes: Achieve HbA1c <6.5% before conception; counsel on risks of congenital anomalies (e.g., neural tube defects, cardiac defects).

Hypertension: Transition to pregnancy-safe antihypertensives; monitor for preeclampsia risk.

Epilepsy: Optimize seizure control with low-risk antiepileptics; supplement with high-dose folic acid (4 mg daily).

2. Women with Prior Adverse Outcomes

History of preterm birth: Consider progesterone supplementation in future pregnancies.

Recurrent pregnancy loss: Screen for antiphospholipid syndrome, uterine anomalies, or chromosomal issues.

Prior congenital anomalies: Offer genetic counseling and high-dose folic acid.

3. Adolescents

Address unique psychosocial needs (e.g., education, family support).

Emphasize contraception until ready for pregnancy.

4. Advanced Maternal Age (>35 years)

Discuss increased risks of aneuploidy, miscarriage, and medical complications.

Offer early genetic screening or diagnostic testing options.

5. Women with Obesity

Counsel on weight loss (5–10% reduction can improve outcomes).

Screen for comorbidities (e.g., diabetes, sleep apnea).

Discuss risks of macrosomia, cesarean delivery, and congenital anomalies.

Management Strategies

Plan interventions based on risk factors, medical history and patient preferences.

Use shared decision-making to set realistic goals (e.g., weight loss, smoking cessation).

Involve specialists (e.g., endocrinologists, geneticists, dietitians) for complex cases.

Coordinate with primary care for chronic disease management.

Promote preconception care in community settings (e.g., family planning clinics, primary care).

Advocate for policies improving access to preconception services (e.g., insurance coverage for genetic screening).

Use electronic health records for risk assessment checklists.

Complications / Outcomes

Maternal

Reduced risk of gestational diabetes, preeclampsia and cesarean delivery through optimized health.

Improved management of chronic conditions, reducing exacerbations in pregnancy.

Fetal

Decreased incidence of neural tube defects (e.g., spina bifida) with folic acid supplementation.

Lower risk of congenital anomalies through control of maternal diabetes or avoidance of teratogens.

Reduced preterm birth and low birth weight with lifestyle interventions.

Neonatal

Decreased neonatal infections (e.g., congenital syphilis, hepatitis B) through maternal screening and treatment. Improved neurodevelopmental outcomes with optimized maternal thyroid function.

Prognosis

Evidence-Based Impact

Folic acid supplementation reduces neural tube defects by 50–70%.

Glycemic control in diabetic women lowers congenital anomaly rates from 10–20% to 2–3%.

Smoking cessation reduces preterm birth and FGR risk by up to 30%.

Preconception weight loss in obese women decreases gestational diabetes risk by 20–40%.

Long-Term Benefits

Healthier pregnancies lead to reduced maternal and neonatal healthcare costs.

Improved maternal health enhances future reproductive and overall health outcomes.

Conclusion

Preconception counseling and care are essential components of obstetric practice, offering a critical opportunity to optimize maternal and fetal health before pregnancy. By addressing medical, genetic, lifestyle and psychosocial factors, clinicians can reduce the risk of adverse pregnancy outcomes and promote healthy pregnancies.

3.2 Preconception & Prenatal Diagnostic Techniques & PNDT Act

(*Haml aur Wiladat se ma'qbl Tashkhisi zaray -i- aur mutalleqah qwaneen*)

Introduction

Preconception and prenatal diagnostic techniques are necessary tools in obstetrics for assessing maternal and fetal health, identifying genetic or structural abnormalities and guiding clinical management. These techniques enable early detection of risks, allowing for informed decision-making and interventions to optimize pregnancy outcomes. However, their use, particularly for fetal sex determination, has raised ethical and social concerns, leading to regulatory frameworks like the Pre-Conception and Pre-Natal Diagnostic Techniques (Prohibition of Sex Selection) Act, 1994 in India.

Preconception Diagnostic Techniques

Preconception diagnostics focus on assessing maternal and paternal health, genetic risks and reproductive potential before conception to optimize pregnancy outcomes.

Medical and Reproductive History

Purpose: Identify risk factors for adverse pregnancy outcomes.

Components

Maternal history: Chronic conditions (e.g., diabetes, hypertension), previous pregnancy complications (e.g., preterm birth, preeclampsia), infections and medication use.

Paternal history: Genetic disorders, substance use, or occupational exposures affecting sperm quality.

Family history: Genetic conditions (e.g., cystic fibrosis, thalassemia), consanguinity.

Clinical Application: Guides further testing (e.g., genetic screening) and lifestyle interventions.

Genetic Screening

Carrier Screening

Tests for autosomal recessive or X-linked disorders (e.g., cystic fibrosis, spinal muscular atrophy, sickle cell disease) based on ethnicity or family history.

Methods: Blood or saliva-based DNA testing (e.g., next-generation sequencing, PCR).

Indications: Couples with a family history of genetic disorders or high-risk ethnic groups (e.g., Ashkenazi Jews for Tay-Sachs, South Asians for thalassemia).

Expanded Carrier Screening: Screens for multiple genetic conditions simultaneously, regardless of ethnicity.

Preimplantation Genetic Testing (PGT)

Used in assisted reproductive technologies (e.g., IVF).

Types: PGT-M: For monogenic disorders (e.g., cystic fibrosis).

PGT-A: For aneuploidy (e.g., Down syndrome).

PGT-SR: For structural chromosomal rearrangements.

Procedure: Embryo biopsy at the blastocyst stage, followed by genetic analysis.

Counseling: Essential to explain risks, benefits and implications of testing.

Laboratory Tests

Maternal: Complete blood count (CBC) for anemia.

Blood type and Rh status to assess isoimmunization risk.

Thyroid function tests (TSH, free T4) for hypothyroidism or hyperthyroidism.

Hemoglobin A1c for diabetes screening.

Serology for infections (e.g., rubella, varicella, HIV, hepatitis B/C, syphilis).

Paternal: Semen analysis if subfertility is suspected.

Clinical Application: Identifies treatable conditions (e.g., iron deficiency, thyroid dysfunction) to optimize maternal health.

Infectious Disease Screening

Tests: HIV, hepatitis B/C, syphilis, toxoplasmosis, cytomegalovirus (CMV) and rubella serology.

Purpose: Prevent congenital infections (e.g., congenital rubella syndrome, neonatal HIV).

Interventions: Vaccination (e.g., rubella, varicella) at least 1 month before conception, treatment of active infections (e.g., syphilis with penicillin).

Imaging and Other Tests

Pelvic Ultrasound: Assesses uterine or ovarian abnormalities (e.g., fibroids, polycystic ovaries) in women with irregular cycles or infertility.

Hysterosalpingography: Evaluates tubal patency in cases of subfertility.

Clinical Application: Identifies structural barriers to conception or pregnancy maintenance.

Prenatal Diagnostic Techniques

Prenatal diagnostics aim to assess fetal health, detect congenital anomalies and monitor pregnancy progression. These techniques are divided into non-invasive and invasive methods.

1. Non-Invasive Prenatal Diagnostic Techniques

Ultrasound

First Trimester (11–14 weeks)

Nuchal translucency (NT) measurement: Screens for aneuploidy (e.g., Down syndrome).

Fetal anatomy scan: Assesses early structural anomalies.

Combined with maternal serum markers (e.g., PAPP-A, free β-hCG) for aneuploidy risk assessment.

Second Trimester (18–22 weeks)

Anomaly scan: Detects structural defects (e.g., neural tube defects, cardiac anomalies).

Assesses placental position, amniotic fluid volume and fetal growth.

Third Trimester

Monitors fetal growth, Doppler studies (umbilical and middle cerebral artery) for fetal well-being and assesses for late-onset anomalies.

Clinical Application: Routine screening for anomalies, growth restriction and placental issues; guides further testing or interventions.

Maternal Serum Screening

First Trimester Combined Screening

Measures PAPP-A and free β-hCG, combined with NT ultrasound.

Screens for trisomy 21 (Down syndrome), trisomy 18 and trisomy 13.

Sensitivity: ~85–90% for Down syndrome.

Second Trimester Quadruple Test

Measures α-fetoprotein (AFP), hCG, estriol and inhibin-A.

Screens for neural tube defects, aneuploidy and placental dysfunction.

Timing: 15–20 weeks.

Clinical Application: Risk stratification for aneuploidy; abnormal results prompt invasive testing.

Non-Invasive Prenatal Testing (NIPT)

Method: Analyzes cell-free fetal DNA (cffDNA) in maternal blood.

Indications: Screens for trisomy 21, 18, 13, and sex chromosome abnormalities; optional microdeletion screening.

Timing: After 10 weeks of gestation.

Advantages: High sensitivity (>99% for Down syndrome), low false-positive rate (~0.1%).

Limitations: Not diagnostic; requires confirmation with invasive testing (e.g., amniocentesis).

Clinical Application: Preferred for high-risk women (e.g., advanced maternal age, abnormal serum screening).

Fetal Heart Rate Monitoring

Non-stress test (NST): Assesses fetal heart rate reactivity in response to movements.

Biophysical profile (BPP): Combines ultrasound (fetal movement, tone, breathing, amniotic fluid) with NST.

Clinical Application: Monitors fetal well-being in high-risk pregnancies (e.g., FGR, diabetes).

2. Invasive Prenatal Diagnostic Techniques

Amniocentesis

Procedure: Ultrasound-guided aspiration of amniotic fluid (15–20 mL) at 15–20 weeks.

Indications

Karyotyping or microarray for chromosomal abnormalities.

Genetic testing for single-gene disorders.

Assess for congenital infections (e.g., CMV, toxoplasmosis).

Fetal lung maturity testing (lecithin/sphingomyelin ratio) in late pregnancy.

Risks: Miscarriage (0.1–0.3%), infection, membrane rupture, preterm labor.

Clinical Application: Diagnostic confirmation after abnormal screening results.

Chorionic Villus Sampling (CVS)

Procedure: Ultrasound-guided sampling of placental villi at 10–13 weeks (transcervical or transabdominal).

Indications: Same as amniocentesis but allows earlier diagnosis.

Risks: Miscarriage (0.5–1%), limb reduction defects (rare, if performed <10 weeks), infection.

Clinical Application: Preferred for early genetic diagnosis in high-risk cases.

Cordocentesis (Percutaneous Umbilical Blood Sampling, PUBS)

Procedure: Ultrasound-guided sampling of fetal blood from the umbilical cord, typically after 18 weeks.

Indication: Fetal anemia assessment (e.g., Rh isoimmunization, parvovirus B19).

Rapid karyotyping or genetic testing.

Fetal infection or metabolic disorder evaluation.

Risks: Fetal loss (1–2%), bleeding, cord hematoma, preterm labor.

Clinical Application: Used in specialized cases when other tests are inconclusive.

Fetal Biopsy or Aspiration

Rare procedures for specific anomalies (e.g., skin biopsy for genodermatoses, liver biopsy for metabolic disorders).

High risk of fetal loss; performed only in specialized centers.

3. Other Prenatal Diagnostic Techniques

Fetal MRI

Indications: Detailed evaluation of fetal brain, spine, or other anomalies when ultrasound is inconclusive.

Timing: Second or third trimester.

Advantages: High-resolution imaging without radiation risk.

Clinical Application: Used for complex anomalies (e.g., cortical malformations, congenital diaphragmatic hernia).

Fetoscopy

Procedure: Endoscopic visualization of the fetus via a small incision in the uterus.

Indications: Rare; used for laser therapy (e.g., twin-to-twin transfusion syndrome) or fetal surgery.

Risks: High risk of preterm labor, membrane rupture, or fetal loss.

Clinical Application: Limited to specialized fetal therapy centers.

Ethical and Social Considerations

Informed Consent: Patients must be counseled on the purpose, risks, benefits, and limitations of each test. Non-directive counseling ensures autonomy in decision-making.

Cultural Sensitivity: Address cultural or religious beliefs that may influence acceptance of testing or outcomes (e.g., termination of pregnancy).

Psychosocial Impact: Positive results for fetal anomalies can cause significant emotional distress; provide psychological support and referrals.

Sex Selection: Misuse of diagnostic techniques for fetal sex determination has led to skewed sex ratios in some regions, necessitating strict regulations like the PCPNDT Act.

Pre-Conception and Pre-Natal Diagnostic Techniques (PCPNDT) Act, 1994 (India)

Background

The PCPNDT Act was enacted in India to address the misuse of prenatal diagnostic techniques for sex determination, which contributed to female feticide and imbalanced sex ratios. Amended in 2003 to include preconception techniques (e.g., PGT for sex selection), the Act regulates the use of diagnostic technologies to prevent sex-selective abortions while ensuring access to legitimate medical testing.

Objectives

1. Prohibit sex selection before or after conception.
2. Regulate the use of preconception and prenatal diagnostic techniques for legitimate medical purposes (e.g., detecting genetic or congenital anomalies).
3. Prevent misuse of diagnostic technologies leading to female feticide.
4. Promote gender equality and improve sex ratios.

Provisions

1. Regulation of Diagnostic Facilities

All ultrasound clinics, genetic laboratories, and counseling centers must be registered with the Appropriate Authority (state or district level).

Facilities must maintain records of all procedures and submit them for inspection.

Only qualified personnel (e.g., registered medical practitioners, sonologists) can perform diagnostic tests.

2. Prohibited Activities

Sex determination of the fetus is strictly prohibited, except in cases of sex-linked genetic disorders (e.g., Duchenne muscular dystrophy).

Communication of fetal sex to the patient or family, directly or indirectly, is illegal.

Sex selection through preconception techniques (e.g., sperm sorting, PGT for non-medical reasons) is banned.

3. Indications for Diagnostic Techniques

Permitted only for

Chromosomal abnormalities (e.g., Down syndrome).

Genetic disorders (e.g., cystic fibrosis, hemophilia).

Congenital anomalies (e.g., neural tube defects).

Metabolic disorders or hemoglobinopathies.

Requires written consent and documentation of medical necessity.

4. Record-Keeping

Facilities must maintain detailed records (e.g., Form F for ultrasound) for at least 2 years.

Records must include indications, patient details, and procedure outcomes.

5. Public Awareness

Clinics must display signage stating that sex determination is illegal.

Educational campaigns to inform the public about the Act and its objectives.

6. Penalties

Violation (e.g., performing or aiding sex determination) is punishable with:

Imprisonment up to 3 years and/or fine up to ₹10,000 for the first offense.

Imprisonment up to 5 years and/or fine up to ₹50,000 for subsequent offenses.

Suspension or cancellation of medical registration for practitioners.

Patients or families seeking sex determination may also face penalties (imprisonment up to 3 years and/or fine up to ₹50,000).

Challenges

Illegal practices persist in some regions due to lax enforcement or societal demand. Limited awareness in rural areas and among underserved populations. Technological advancements (e.g., NIPT) pose new regulatory challenges.

Impact

Sex Ratio Improvement: The Act has contributed to stabilizing sex ratios in some Indian states, though disparities persist (e.g., national sex ratio at birth was 914 females per 1,000 males in 2011, improving to 929 by 2020).

Ethical Practice: Promotes ethical use of diagnostic technologies for medical purposes.

Challenges Remaining: Cultural preferences for male children and illegal practices require ongoing vigilance and education.

Clinical Approach to Preconception and Prenatal Diagnostics

1. Preconception

Conduct a thorough history and physical exam to identify risks.

Offer genetic and infectious disease screening based on individual risk factors.

Provide counseling on test results, implications and lifestyle modifications.

Ensure compliance with PCPNDT Act for any preconception testing (e.g., PGT).

2. Prenatal

Schedule routine ultrasounds (first trimester NT, second trimester anomaly scan, third trimester growth scan).

Offer maternal serum screening or NIPT for aneuploidy risk assessment.

Recommend invasive testing (amniocentesis, CVS) for high-risk cases, with informed consent.

Monitor fetal well-being with NST or BPP in high-risk pregnancies.

Adhere to PCPNDT Act regulations, avoiding any disclosure of fetal sex.

3. Counseling

Provide non-directive counseling to discuss risks, benefits and limitations of tests.

Address emotional and ethical concerns, especially for abnormal findings.

Refer to genetic counselors or fetal medicine specialists for complex cases.

Complications and Risks

Preconception: False-positive genetic screening results may cause anxiety; confirmatory testing is needed. Limited access to advanced testing (e.g., PGT) in low-resource settings.

Prenatal: Non-invasive tests (e.g., NIPT, serum screening) have false-positive/negative rates, requiring invasive confirmation.

Invasive tests carry risks of miscarriage, infection, or preterm labor.

Ethical dilemmas arise with abnormal findings, necessitating sensitive counseling.

Prognosis and Outcomes

Preconception

Early identification of genetic or medical risks improves pregnancy planning and outcomes.

Folic acid supplementation reduces neural tube defects by 50–70%.

Optimized chronic conditions (e.g., diabetes, thyroid) lower congenital anomaly rates.

Prenatal

Early detection of anomalies allows for timely interventions (e.g., fetal surgery, termination if chosen).

NIPT and ultrasound improve aneuploidy detection rates (>99% for Down syndrome).

Monitoring high-risk pregnancies reduces perinatal mortality.

PCPNDT Act

Contributes to ethical practice and gender equality.

Reduces sex-selective abortions, though cultural and enforcement challenges persist. Preventive Measures and Public Health Role

Education

Train healthcare providers on preconception and prenatal diagnostics and PCPNDT compliance.

Educate patients on the importance of early screening and legal restrictions on sex determination.

Conclusion

Preconception and prenatal diagnostic techniques are essential for optimizing maternal and fetal health, enabling early detection of risks, and guiding clinical management. Techniques range from non-invasive screenings (e.g., ultrasound, NIPT) to invasive diagnostics (e.g., amniocentesis, CVS), each with specific indications and risks. The PCPNDT Act in India regulates these technologies to prevent misuse for sex selection, promoting ethical practice and gender equality.

3.3 Legal & Ethical Isssues in Obstetric Practice

(Ilm-al-Qabalat se mutaalliq qanooni aur akhlaqi masaayil)

Introduction

Obstetric practice involves unique legal and ethical challenges due to the dual responsibility of caring for both the mother and the fetus. Obstetricians must navigate complex clinical decisions while adhering to legal frameworks, ethical principles and societal expectations. Legal issues often arise from malpractice claims, consent violations, or non-compliance with regulations, while ethical dilemmas stem from balancing maternal autonomy, fetal interests and resource constraints.

Ethical Principles in Obstetrics

Obstetric practice is guided by four core ethical principles:

1. Autonomy: Respecting the patient's right to make informed decisions about her care.
2. Beneficence: Acting in the best interest of the patient (mother and fetus).
3. Non-Maleficence: Avoiding harm to the mother and fetus.
4. Justice: Ensuring fair allocation of resources and equitable care.

These principles often conflict in obstetrics, requiring careful judgment to balance maternal and fetal interests, cultural sensitivities and legal obligations.

Legal Frameworks in Obstetric Practice

In India, obstetric practice is governed by a combination of national laws, medical regulations and international guidelines. Key legal frameworks include:

1. Pre-Conception and Pre-Natal Diagnostic Techniques (PCPNDT) Act, 1994

Purpose: Prohibits sex determination and sex-selective abortions to address female feticide and promote gender equality.

Provisions

Bans fetal sex determination except for medical indications (e.g., sex-linked disorders).

Requires registration of ultrasound and genetic testing facilities.

Mandates record-keeping (e.g., Form F for ultrasounds) and prohibits communication of fetal sex.

Penalties: Up to 3 years imprisonment and ₹10,000 fine for first offense; up to 5 years and ₹50,000 for subsequent offenses; medical license suspension.

Implications: Obstetricians must ensure compliance during ultrasound or genetic testing, maintain meticulous records, and avoid any actions that could be interpreted as aiding sex determination.

2. Medical Termination of Pregnancy (MTP) Act, 1971 (Amended 2021)

Purpose: Regulates abortion to ensure safe and legal access while preventing misuse.

Provisions

Allows termination up to 20 weeks by one registered medical practitioner (RMP) for conditions like risk to maternal life, fetal anomalies, or contraceptive failure.

Permits termination between 20–24 weeks for specific cases (e.g., rape, fetal anomalies, vulnerable women) with two RMPs' approval.

Beyond 24 weeks, requires approval from a medical board for severe fetal anomalies or maternal life-threatening conditions.

Protects patient confidentiality and requires informed consent.

Implications: Obstetricians must adhere to gestational limits, obtain proper consent, and document indications. Non-compliance risks legal penalties and ethical violations.

3. Consumer Protection Act (CPA), 2019

Purpose: Protects patients as consumers of medical services, allowing them to seek redress for deficient care.

Application in Obstetrics: Malpractice claims arise from negligence (e.g., failure to diagnose fetal distress, improper cesarean timing). Patients can file complaints with consumer courts for compensation.

Implications: Obstetricians must maintain high standards of care, document decisions thoroughly, and communicate risks clearly to avoid litigation.

4. Indian Medical Council (Professional Conduct, Etiquette, and Ethics) Regulations, 2002

Purpose: Governs ethical conduct of medical practitioners.

Provisions

Requires informed consent, confidentiality, and competence in practice.

Prohibits unethical practices (e.g., kickbacks, unnecessary procedures).

Implications: Non-compliance can lead to disciplinary action, including license suspension by the National Medical Commission (NMC).

5. Other Relevant Laws

Protection of Children from Sexual Offences (POCSO) Act, 2012: Applies to pregnant minors, requiring mandatory reporting of sexual abuse.

Mental Healthcare Act, 2017: Ensures mental health support for women with perinatal psychiatric conditions.

Domestic Violence Act, 2005: Addresses intimate partner violence, which may impact pregnant women.

Globally, obstetricians must also consider frameworks like the World Health Organization (WHO) guidelines and country-specific laws

Legal and Ethical Issues in Obstetric Practice

1. Informed Consent

Legal Requirement

Informed consent is mandatory for all obstetric procedures (e.g., cesarean section, amniocentesis, labor induction) under the Indian Medical Council Regulations and CPA.

Must include explanation of risks, benefits, alternatives, and consequences of refusal.

Consent must be voluntary, documented and obtained from a competent patient or legal guardian (e.g., for minors).

Ethical Considerations

Respecting autonomy requires clear communication, especially for high-risk procedures or fetal anomalies. Language barriers, low literacy, or cultural beliefs may complicate consent; use interpreters or visual aids as needed.

Challenges

Emergency situations (e.g., fetal distress) may limit time for full consent; implied consent may apply, but documentation is critical.

Coercion by family members (e.g., for cesarean or termination) violates autonomy.

Implications

Failure to obtain informed consent can lead to malpractice lawsuits or ethical complaints.

Example: A cesarean performed without consent due to family pressure could result in legal action under the CPA.

2. Fetal Sex Determination and the PCPNDT Act

Legal Issue

The PCPNDT Act prohibits fetal sex determination to prevent sex-selective abortions, which have contributed to skewed sex ratios (e.g., 914 females per 1,000 males in India, 2011). Obstetricians must avoid any direct or indirect disclosure of fetal sex during ultrasound or genetic testing.

Ethical Issue

Balancing patient curiosity about fetal sex with legal and ethical obligations.

Addressing societal gender biases that drive demand for sex determination.

Challenges

Patients or families may pressure clinicians for sex information, risking ethical violations.

Non-compliance (e.g., unregistered ultrasound machines, incomplete records) can lead to severe penalties.

Implications

Obstetricians must educate patients about the law, display PCPNDT compliance notices, and maintain meticulous records.

Example: An obstetrician inadvertently hinting at fetal sex during an ultrasound could face imprisonment and license suspension.

3. Medical Termination of Pregnancy (MTP)

Legal Issue

The MTP Act regulates abortion, specifying gestational limits, indications and provider qualifications.

Termination beyond 24 weeks requires medical board approval, adding complexity in cases of severe fetal anomalies.

Ethical Issue

Balancing maternal autonomy with fetal interests, especially in cases of late-term anomalies.

Religious or cultural objections to abortion may conflict with medical recommendations.

Challenges

Delayed diagnosis of fetal anomalies may push terminations beyond legal limits, requiring court intervention.

Access to safe abortion services is limited in rural areas, raising equity concerns.

Implications

Obstetricians must ensure compliance with MTP Act guidelines, provide non-directive counseling, and refer to medical boards when needed.

Example: Performing an unauthorized termination beyond 24 weeks could lead to criminal charges.

4. Maternal-Fetal Conflict

Legal Issue

No Indian law grants the fetus independent legal status; maternal autonomy takes precedence.

However, courts may intervene in extreme cases (e.g., refusal of life-saving cesarean for fetal distress).

Ethical Issue

Balancing maternal autonomy with beneficence toward the fetus.

Example: A woman refusing a cesarean for religious reasons despite fetal distress creates a dilemma between respecting her choice and preventing fetal harm.

Challenges

Coercing treatment violates autonomy but may be justified to save the fetus in emergencies.

Cultural or family pressures may influence maternal decisions, complicating ethical deliberations.

Implications

Obstetricians must engage in shared decision-making, document discussions, and seek legal/ethical consultation in complex cases.

Example: A court may order a cesarean if maternal refusal endangers a viable fetus, though this is rare.

5. Medical Negligence and Malpractice

Legal Issue

Negligence claims under the CPA arise from failure to meet the standard of care (e.g., delayed diagnosis of preeclampsia, improper fetal monitoring).

Elements of negligence: Duty of care, breach of duty, causation and damage.

Compensation can be sought for maternal or fetal harm (e.g., cerebral palsy due to hypoxic injury).

Ethical Issue

Maintaining competence and adhering to evidence-based guidelines (beneficence, non-maleficence).

Transparent communication after adverse events to maintain trust.

Challenges

High cesarean rates in private hospitals raise concerns about unnecessary procedures driven by financial incentives.

Defensive medicine (e.g., ordering excessive tests) may increase costs and patient anxiety.

Implications

Obstetricians must follow national guidelines (e.g., FOGSI, WHO), document care thoroughly, and disclose errors transparently.

Example: Failure to monitor fetal heart rate during labor leading to neonatal hypoxia could result in a multimillion-rupee lawsuit.

6. Confidentiality and Privacy

Legal Issue

The Indian Medical Council Regulations and CPA mandate patient confidentiality, except in cases required by law (e.g., POCSO Act for minors).

Breaches (e.g., disclosing pregnancy details to family without consent) can lead to legal action.

Ethical Issue

Respecting patient privacy while addressing family dynamics common in India (e.g., involvement of in-laws).

Protecting sensitive information (e.g., HIV status, fetal anomalies).

Challenges

Family members may demand information, especially in cases of fetal loss or termination.

Electronic health records increase the risk of data breaches.

Implications

Obtain explicit consent before sharing information, use secure systems, and counsel patients on privacy rights.

Example: Disclosing a patient's HIV status to her spouse without consent violates ethical and legal standards.

7. Reproductive Rights and Access to Care

Legal Issue

The MTP Act and Right to Health under Article 21 of the Indian Constitution ensure access to safe reproductive care.

Denial of care (e.g., refusing abortion for eligible cases) can be challenged in court.

Ethical Issue

Ensuring equitable access to care, especially for marginalized groups (e.g., rural women, low-income families).

Addressing conscientious objection (e.g., providers refusing to perform abortions due to personal beliefs).

Challenges

Limited access to ultrasound, genetic testing, or abortion services in rural India.

Stigma around pregnancy complications (e.g., miscarriage, anomalies) may deter women from seeking care.

Implications

Obstetricians must advocate for equitable access, refer patients to appropriate facilities, and respect reproductive choices.

Example: Denying a rape survivor an abortion within legal limits violates her rights and could lead to legal action.

8. Management of Fetal Anomalies

Legal Issue

The MTP Act allows termination for severe fetal anomalies, but late diagnoses (>24 weeks) require medical board approval.

Non-compliance with PCPNDT Act during anomaly screening risks penalties.

Ethical Issue

Counseling parents about fetal anomalies (e.g., anencephaly, trisomy 18) requires balancing hope with realistic outcomes.

Respecting parental decisions (e.g., continuation vs. termination) while providing non-directive support.

Challenges

Emotional distress and cultural stigma may complicate decision-making.

Limited access to advanced diagnostics (e.g., fetal MRI) in resource-poor settings.

Implications

Provide comprehensive, empathetic counseling, involve genetic counselors, and adhere to legal protocols for termination.

Example: Failing to offer termination for a lethal anomaly within legal limits could be seen as negligence.

9. Perinatal Mental Health

Legal Issue

The Mental Healthcare Act, 2017, mandates access to mental health services for pregnant women with conditions like postpartum depression.

Failure to screen or refer for mental health issues may constitute negligence.

Ethical Issue

Stigma around mental health in India may prevent women from seeking help.

Balancing maternal autonomy with the need for intervention in severe cases (e.g., suicidal ideation).

Challenges

Limited mental health resources in obstetric settings.

Family pressures may downplay maternal mental health concerns.

Implications

Screen for perinatal depression/anxiety, refer to psychiatrists, and ensure confidentiality.

Example: Ignoring signs of postpartum psychosis could lead to harm to the mother or infant, triggering legal action.

10. Resource Allocation and Justice

Legal Issue

The CPA and public health policies require equitable care, but resource disparities exist between public and private sectors.

Ethical Issue

Prioritizing care in resource-limited settings (e.g., NICU beds, ventilators).

Avoiding overtreatment in private settings driven by financial incentives.

Challenges

Rural hospitals may lack ultrasound or fetal monitoring, compromising care quality.

High costs of advanced diagnostics (e.g., NIPT) limit access for low-income patients.

Implications

Advocate for systemic improvements, prioritize evidence-based care, and ensure transparency in resource allocation.

Example: Performing unnecessary cesareans for profit violates justice and beneficence.

Complications and Consequences

Legal Consequences

Malpractice lawsuits under CPA can result in financial penalties and reputational damage.

PCPNDT violations lead to imprisonment, fines, and license suspension.

Non-compliance with MTP Act risks criminal charges.

Ethical Consequences

Breaches of autonomy or confidentiality erode patient trust.

Failure to address maternal-fetal conflicts may harm outcomes.

Inequitable care perpetuates health disparities.

Patient Outcomes

Legal/ethical lapses (e.g., missed diagnoses, unauthorized procedures) increase maternal and fetal morbidity/mortality.

Proper adherence improves trust, compliance and outcomes.

Preventive Measures

1. Education and Training

Incorporate medical law and ethics into obstetric curricula.

Conduct workshops on PCPNDT, MTP, and CPA compliance.

2. Patient Education

Inform patients about their rights, legal restrictions (e.g., sex determination), and care options.

Use multilingual materials to bridge communication gaps.

3. Systemic Improvements

Strengthen PCPNDT enforcement through regular audits and whistleblower protections.

Expand access to diagnostics and abortion services in rural areas.

4. Risk Management

Implement protocols for informed consent, documentation, and error disclosure.

Use electronic health records with secure privacy measures.

5. Advocacy

Promote gender equality and mental health awareness to reduce stigma.

Advocate for policies improving maternal healthcare access.

Conclusion

Legal and ethical issues in obstetric practice are complex, requiring obstetricians to balance clinical expertise with legal compliance and ethical integrity. The PCPNDT Act, MTP Act, and CPA provide critical frameworks in India to ensure safe and equitable care, while ethical principles guide decision-making in challenging scenarios like maternal-fetal conflicts or fetal anomalies. By prioritizing informed consent, confidentiality, and adherence to regulations, obstetricians can minimize legal risks, enhance patient trust, and improve maternal and fetal outcomes.

3.4 Physiological Changes

(*Haml ke taba'I taghayyurat*)

Introduction

Pregnancy induces profound physiological adaptations across multiple organ systems to support the developing fetus, prepare the mother for labor, and maintain maternal health. These changes are driven by hormonal, metabolic, and mechanical factors, beginning in the first trimester and continuing postpartum. Understanding these adaptations is essential to distinguish normal physiology from pathology and manage pregnancy effectively.

Hormonal Changes

Hormonal shifts orchestrate many physiological changes in pregnancy, primarily driven by the placenta, corpus luteum and maternal endocrine glands.

Human Chorionic Gonadotropin (hCG): Produced by the syncytiotrophoblast; peaks at 8–10 weeks (100,000–200,000 IU/L). Maintains corpus luteum to produce progesterone until placental production takes over.

Progesterone: Increases 10-fold (25 ng/mL in first trimester to 150 ng/mL at term). Functions: Maintains pregnancy by inhibiting uterine contractions, promotes myometrial growth, suppresses immune rejection of the fetus.

Estrogen (Estradiol, Estriol): Increases 100-fold (estriol dominates, produced by placenta using fetal adrenal precursors). Functions: Stimulates uterine growth, enhances uteroplacental blood flow, promotes breast development, and softens connective tissues (e.g., cervix, ligaments).

Human Placental Lactogen (hPL): Peaks in third trimester (5–7 µg/mL). Functions: Induces insulin resistance to prioritize glucose for the fetus, promotes lipolysis for maternal energy.

Other Hormones

Prolactin: Increases to prepare for lactation.

Cortisol and Thyroid Hormones: Rise to support metabolism and fetal development.

Relaxin: Softens cervix and pelvic ligaments, inhibits myometrial contractions.

Cardiovascular System

The cardiovascular system undergoes significant changes to meet the increased metabolic demands of pregnancy and ensure adequate uteroplacental perfusion.

Cardiac Output: Increases by 30–50% (from 4.5 L/min to 6–7 L/min) by the second trimester. Driven by increased stroke volume (early pregnancy) and heart rate (10–20 bpm increase). Peaks at 28–32 weeks, then plateaus; decreases slightly at term due to aortocaval compression.

Blood Volume: Plasma volume increases by 40–50% (1–2 L) by 32 weeks; red cell mass increases by 20–30%. Results in physiological hemodilution and a relative anemia (hemoglobin ~11–12 g/dL).

Blood Pressure: Decreases in first and second trimesters (systolic by 5–10 mmHg, diastolic by 10–15 mmHg) due to reduced systemic vascular resistance (SVR). SVR decreases by 20–30% due to vasodilation (progesterone, nitric oxide). Returns to pre-pregnancy levels by third trimester.

Heart: Heart shifts upward and left due to diaphragmatic elevation. Functional murmurs (e.g., systolic flow murmurs) common due to increased flow.

Aortocaval Compression: In the supine position (third trimester), the gravid uterus compresses the inferior vena cava and aorta, reducing venous return and cardiac output (supine hypotensive syndrome).

Clinical Implications

Increased cardiac output supports fetal oxygen delivery but may unmask underlying heart disease. Monitor for signs of heart failure in high-risk patients (e.g., pre-existing cardiac conditions). Avoid supine position in late pregnancy to prevent hypotension.

Hematological System

Hematological adaptations ensure oxygen delivery and prepare for potential blood loss during delivery.

Blood Volume and Composition

Plasma volume increases disproportionately to red cell mass, causing physiological anemia. White blood cell count rises (6,000–16,000/µL) due to increased neutrophils, peaking in labor. Platelet count may slightly decrease (150,000–400,000/µL) due to hemodilution and consumption.

Coagulation

Hypercoagulable state to prevent postpartum hemorrhage: Increased levels of clotting factors (I, VII, VIII, IX, X). Decreased fibrinolysis (reduced protein S, increased plasminogen activator inhibitor). Risk of thromboembolism increases 4–6-fold.

Iron Metabolism

Iron requirements increase (1,000–1,200 mg total for pregnancy) to support red cell mass expansion and fetal needs. Transferrin and ferritin levels adjust to meet demand; supplementation often required.

Clinical Implications

Monitor for pathological anemia (hemoglobin <10 g/dL) or thrombophilia.

Prophylactic anticoagulation may be needed in high-risk cases (e.g., history of DVT).

Respiratory System

Respiratory changes enhance oxygen delivery to the fetus and compensate for increased maternal metabolic demands.

Lung Mechanics: Diaphragm elevates 4–5 cm due to uterine growth, reducing functional residual capacity (FRC) by 20–25%. Chest wall compliance increases due to relaxin, maintaining total lung capacity.

Ventilation: Minute ventilation increases by 30–50% (from 7.5 L/min to 10–11 L/min) due to increased tidal volume (not respiratory rate). Progesterone stimulates the respiratory center, lowering $PaCO_2$ (from 40 mmHg to 30–32 mmHg), causing a compensated respiratory alkalosis (pH ~7.44).

Oxygenation: Oxygen consumption increases by 20–30% to meet fetal and maternal demands.

Oxygen dissociation curve shifts rightward, facilitating oxygen transfer to the fetus.

Clinical Implications

Dyspnea is common (60–70% of women) due to increased ventilation and diaphragmatic elevation. Reduced FRC increases risk of hypoxia in respiratory compromise (e.g., pneumonia, asthma).

Renal System

The renal system adapts to handle increased blood volume, waste clearance, and electrolyte balance.

Renal Blood Flow and Glomerular Filtration Rate (GFR)

Renal plasma flow increases by 50–80%; GFR increases by 50% (from 120 mL/min to 180 mL/min) by the second trimester. Results in lower serum creatinine (0.4–0.6 mg/dL) and urea (8–10 mg/dL).

Tubular Function

Increased glucose, amino acid, and protein reabsorption; mild glycosuria is common due to exceeding tubular reabsorption capacity. Sodium retention (900–1,000 mEq) due to aldosterone and renin-angiotensin system activation, despite increased GFR.

Anatomical Changes

Kidneys enlarge slightly; ureters dilate (right > left) due to progesterone and uterine compression, increasing risk of hydronephrosis and urinary tract infections.

Clinical Implications

Lower creatinine thresholds for diagnosing renal impairment in pregnancy.

Monitor for UTIs and pyelonephritis due to ureteral stasis.

Gastrointestinal System

Gastrointestinal changes support nutritional demands and accommodate the growing uterus.

Motility: Progesterone reduces smooth muscle tone, slowing gastric emptying and intestinal transit. Gastroesophageal sphincter tone decreases, leading to gastroesophageal reflux disease (GERD) in 50–80% of pregnancies.

Liver: Hepatic blood flow remains stable, but alkaline phosphatase increases (placental production). Serum albumin decreases (30–40 g/L) due to hemodilution; total protein remains stable. Gallbladder motility decreases, increasing risk of gallstones.

Nutritional Demands: Caloric needs increase by 300 kcal/day in the second and third trimesters. Increased absorption of iron, calcium, and folate to support fetal growth.

Clinical Implications

GERD and constipation are common; manage with lifestyle changes and safe medications (e.g., antacids, fiber). Monitor for cholestasis of pregnancy (elevated bile acids) or acute fatty liver.

Endocrine System

Endocrine adaptations support fetal development and maternal metabolism.

Thyroid: Thyroid-binding globulin (TBG) increases due to estrogen, raising total T3 and T4 levels; free T4 and TSH remain normal (TSH: 0.1–2.5 mIU/L in first trimester). hCG has thyrotropic activity, mildly suppressing TSH in early pregnancy.

Adrenal Glands: Cortisol levels increase 2–3-fold due to increased ACTH and CRH (placental production). Aldosterone rises to promote sodium retention.

Pancreas: Insulin resistance develops (hPL, cortisol, progesterone), increasing insulin secretion to maintain euglycemia. Glucose metabolism prioritizes fetal needs, increasing risk of gestational diabetes.

Calcium Metabolism: Increased 1,25-dihydroxyvitamin D enhances calcium absorption. Total calcium decreases due to hemodilution, but ionized calcium remains stable.

Clinical Implications: Screen for gestational diabetes (oral glucose tolerance test at 24–28 weeks). Monitor thyroid function in women with pre-existing thyroid disease.

Musculoskeletal System

Musculoskeletal changes accommodate the growing fetus and prepare for delivery.

Pelvis and Ligaments: Relaxin and estrogen soften pelvic ligaments and symphysis pubis, increasing joint laxity. Widening of the pubic symphysis (4–8 mm) facilitates delivery.

Spine: Lumbar lordosis increases to compensate for anterior uterine weight, leading to low back pain in 50–70% of women.

Weight Gain: Average weight gain: 11–16 kg (25–35 lbs) for normal BMI. Components: Fetus (~3.5 kg), placenta (~1 kg), amniotic fluid (~1 kg), uterine growth (~1 kg), maternal tissues, and fluid.

Clinical Implications

Counsel on posture, exercise, and weight management to reduce back pain and complications. Monitor for symphysis pubis dysfunction or diastasis recti.

Immune System

Immune adaptations balance maternal tolerance of the fetus with infection protection.

Immunosuppression: Shift toward Th2 immunity (anti-inflammatory) to prevent fetal rejection. Progesterone and hPL suppress maternal T-cell activity.

Inflammatory Response: Increased leukocytes and acute-phase reactants (e.g., C-reactive protein). Enhanced innate immunity to protect against infections.

Clinical Implications

Increased susceptibility to certain infections (e.g., influenza, listeriosis).Monitor for signs of chorioamnionitis or sepsis, especially with prolonged rupture of membranes.

Reproductive System

Reproductive organs undergo significant changes to support pregnancy and delivery.

Uterus: Grows from 70 g (pre-pregnancy) to 1,100 g at term; capacity increases from 10 mL to 5 L. Myometrial hypertrophy and hyperplasia driven by estrogen and progesterone. Blood flow to the uterus increases to 500–800 mL/min (10–15% of cardiac output).

Cervix: Softens (Goodell's sign) due to increased vascularity and collagen remodeling. Mucus plug forms to protect against ascending infections.

Vagina and Vulva: Increased vascularity causes bluish discoloration (Chadwick's sign). Vaginal pH becomes more acidic, reducing infection risk but increasing yeast infections.

Breasts: Estrogen and prolactin stimulate ductal and alveolar growth. Colostrum production begins in the second trimester.

Clinical Implications

Monitor uterine growth (fundal height) and cervical changes (e.g., preterm shortening). Screen for vaginal infections (e.g., bacterial vaginosis) to prevent preterm labor.

Skin and Integumentary System

Hormonal and mechanical changes affect the skin and connective tissues.

Skin: Hyperpigmentation (e.g., linea nigra, melasma) due to increased melanocyte-stimulating hormone. Areola and genital darkening common. Butterfly pattern pigmentation on face is called as pregnancy mask or chloasma of pregnancy.

Connective Tissue: Striae gravidarum (stretch marks) in 50–90% of women due to skin stretching and collagen breakdown. Increased vascularity causes spider angiomas and palmar erythema.

Hair and Nails: Hair growth increases (anagen phase prolonged); postpartum telogen effluvium causes hair loss. Nails may become brittle or grow faster.

Clinical Implications

Counsel on cosmetic changes and reassure about reversibility. Monitor for pruritic conditions (e.g., pruritic urticarial papules and plaques of pregnancy).

Neurological System

Neurological adaptations are minimal but significant for maternal well-being.

Central Nervous System: Progesterone may cause mild sedation, mood changes, or fatigue. Increased risk of carpal tunnel syndrome due to fluid retention compressing the median nerve.

Sleep: Disrupted by physical discomfort, urinary frequency, and hormonal changes.

Clinical Implications: Screen for perinatal mood disorders (e.g., depression, anxiety). Manage carpal tunnel with wrist splints and reassure about resolution postpartum.

Involution

Most changes reverse within 6–12 weeks postpartum.

Cardiovascular: Cardiac output and blood volume normalize by 6 weeks.

Hematological: Hypercoagulability persists for 6–8 weeks, increasing thromboembolism risk.

Renal: GFR returns to baseline by 6 weeks.

Reproductive: Uterus involutes (returns to pre-pregnancy size by 6 weeks); ovulation resumes based on breastfeeding status. Persistent changes (e.g., striae, pelvic floor laxity) may require long-term management.

Clinical Implications

1. Monitoring: Use pregnancy-specific reference ranges for laboratory tests (e.g., lower hemoglobin, creatinine).Regular ultrasound and Doppler to assess uteroplacental function.
2. Diagnosis: Distinguish physiological changes (e.g., dyspnea, edema) from pathology (e.g., heart failure, preeclampsia). Screen for gestational diabetes, hypertension, and infections.
3. Management: Tailor interventions to physiological changes (e.g., adjust medication doses for increased GFR). Counsel on expected symptoms (e.g., back pain, GERD) and when to seek care.
4. High-Risk Pregnancies: Chronic conditions (e.g., hypertension, diabetes) may be exacerbated by pregnancy adaptations. Monitor closely with multidisciplinary care (e.g., cardiology, endocrinology).

Conclusion

Physiological changes in pregnancy are complex and multisystemic, driven by hormonal, metabolic, and mechanical factors to support fetal development and maternal health. These adaptations, including increased cardiac output, hemodilution, hyperventilation and insulin resistance, are essential for a successful pregnancy but increase susceptibility to certain complications.

3.5 Signs & Symptoms & Diagnosis of pregnancy

(*Haml ki Alamat wa Nishaniyya wa Tashkhis-i-haml*)

Introduction

The diagnosis of pregnancy relies on a combination of clinical signs, symptoms and diagnostic tests to confirm the presence of a viable pregnancy and assess its progression. Early and accurate diagnosis is critical for initiating prenatal care, identifying complications and providing appropriate counseling. The signs and symptoms of pregnancy vary by trimester and are influenced by hormonal, physiological and anatomical changes.

Signs and Symptoms of Pregnancy

Pregnancy manifests through a constellation of symptoms and physical signs, categorized as presumptive, probable, and positive based on their diagnostic reliability. These manifestations are driven by hormonal changes (e.g., human chorionic gonadotropin [hCG], progesterone, estrogen) and the physical presence of a growing fetus.

1. Presumptive Signs and Symptoms

These are subjective or non-specific findings reported by the woman or observed clinically, which may suggest pregnancy but are not diagnostic due to overlap with other conditions.

Amenorrhea

Cessation of menstruation in a woman of reproductive age is often the earliest symptom.

Occurs after conception due to hCG maintaining the corpus luteum and progesterone suppressing ovulation.

Most reliable in women with regular cycles; less specific in irregular cycles, lactation, or perimenopause.

Differential Diagnosis: Stress, thyroid disorders, polycystic ovary syndrome (PCOS), or hormonal contraceptives.

Nausea and Vomiting (Morning Sickness)

Nausea, with or without vomiting, often worse in the morning but can occur anytime.

Begins at 4–6 weeks, peaks at 8–12 weeks, and usually resolves by 16–20 weeks.

Prevalence: Affects 70–80% of pregnant women.

Cause: Likely due to elevated hCG, estrogen, and progesterone affecting the gastrointestinal tract and central nervous system.

Differential Diagnosis: Gastroenteritis, hyperemesis gravidarum, peptic ulcer disease, or thyroid dysfunction.

Breast Changes

Tenderness, tingling, fullness, or enlargement of breasts; darkening of areolae; prominence of Montgomery tubercles (sebaceous glands on areolae).

Begins at 4–6 weeks due to estrogen, progesterone, and prolactin.

Prevalence: Common in early pregnancy.

Differential Diagnosis: Premenstrual syndrome, fibrocystic breast changes, or hormonal medications.

Fatigue

Profound tiredness or lethargy.

Common in the first trimester, resolving in the second trimester, and recurring in the third.

Cause: Increased metabolic demands, progesterone effects, and blood volume expansion.

Differential Diagnosis: Anemia, hypothyroidism, depression or chronic fatigue syndrome.

Urinary Frequency

Increased need to urinate, especially at night (nocturia).

Begins at 6–8 weeks due to increased renal blood flow and uterine pressure on the bladder; recurs in the third trimester due to fetal head compression.

Differential Diagnosis: Urinary tract infection (UTI), diabetes mellitus, or overactive bladder.

Pica

Altered taste or smell preferences, often for unusual foods .

Common in the first trimester.

Cause: hormonal; exact mechanism unclear.

Differential Diagnosis: Nutritional deficiencies or eating disorders.

Skin Changes

Hyperpigmentation (e.g., linea nigra, melasma), spider angiomas, or palmar erythema.

More prominent in the second and third trimesters.

Cause: Increased melanocyte-stimulating hormone and estrogen.

Differential Diagnosis: Chronic liver disease or hormonal medications.

2. Probable Signs

These are objective findings detected by a clinician, which are more specific to pregnancy but can still occur in other conditions (e.g., tumors, pseudocyesis).

Uterine Changes

Hegar's Sign: Softening of the lower uterine segment, palpable at 6–8 weeks.

Goodell's Sign: Softening of the cervix due to increased vascularity, evident by 4–6 weeks.

Chadwick's Sign: Bluish discoloration of the vagina and cervix due to vascular congestion, seen by 6–8 weeks.

Uterine Enlargement: Progressive growth; uterus is palpable abdominally by 12–14 weeks.

Cervical Mucus Plug

Formation of a thick mucus plug in the cervical canal to protect against infection.

Develops in the first trimester.

Ballottment

Palpation of the fetus bouncing within the amniotic fluid during bimanual examination.

Detectable by 16–20 weeks.

Braxton Hicks Contractions

Irregular, painless uterine contractions.

Begin in the second trimester, more noticeable in the third trimester.

Differential Diagnosis: Preterm labor or uterine fibroids.

Positive Pregnancy Test

Detection of hCG in urine or serum.

Urine tests are positive by 10–14 days post-conception; serum tests are more sensitive (detectable by 7–10 days).

Limitations: False positives in trophoblastic disease (e.g., molar pregnancy) or ectopic pregnancy; false negatives if tested too early.

3. Positive Signs

These are definitive indicators of pregnancy, confirming the presence of a fetus.

Fetal Heart Sound

Detection of fetal heart sounds.

Doppler ultrasound: Detectable by 10–12 weeks (120–160 bpm). Or by fetoscope: Detectable by 18–20 weeks.

Confirmation: Direct evidence of a viable fetus.

Fetal Movements

Palpable movements by the examiner or visualized on ultrasound.

Felt by the mother (quickening) at 16–20 weeks (primigravida) or 14–18 weeks (multigravida); confirmed by ultrasound or palpation by 20–22 weeks.

Ultrasound Visualization

Visualization of a gestational sac, yolk sac, embryo,or fetus.

Transvaginal ultrasound: Gestational sac by 4–5 weeks, fetal pole and heartbeat by 5–6 weeks. Transabdominal ultrasound: Detectable by 6–7 weeks.

Confirmation: Gold standard for diagnosing intrauterine pregnancy.

Diagnosis of Pregnancy

The diagnosis of pregnancy integrates clinical evaluation, laboratory tests and imaging to confirm pregnancy, determine gestational age, and rule out complications.

1. Clinical Evaluation

History

Assess for amenorrhea, nausea, breast tenderness, fatigue and urinary frequency.

Review menstrual history (last menstrual period [LMP]) to estimate gestational age.

Inquire about risk factors (e.g., irregular cycles, recent contraception use, history of ectopic pregnancy).

Physical Examination

General: Check for signs of anemia, thyroid enlargement or weight changes.

Abdominal: Palpate for uterine enlargement (fundal height measurable from 12 weeks).

Pelvic: Assess for Hegar's, Goodell's and Chadwick's signs; confirm uterine size.

Speculum Exam: Evaluate for vaginal/cervical changes or signs of infection.

Limitations: Clinical findings alone are not definitive; require confirmation with tests.

2. Laboratory Tests

Urine Pregnancy Test

Method: Detects hCG (sensitivity ~25 mIU/mL) using home or clinical kits.

Timings: Positive by 10–14 days post-conception (around missed period).

Accuracy: >99% if performed correctly; false negatives if tested too early or diluted urine.

Clinical Use: Quick, cost-effective screening tool.

Serum hCG Test

Method: Quantitative measurement of β-hCG in blood (sensitivity ~5 mIU/mL).

Timing: Detectable by 7–10 days post-conception.

Interpretation: Normal intrauterine pregnancy: hCG doubles every 48–72 hours in early pregnancy (peaks at 8–10 weeks).

Abnormal patterns: Slow rise (ectopic pregnancy), rapid rise (molar pregnancy), or decline (miscarriage).

Clinical Use: Confirms pregnancy, monitors progression, and evaluates for ectopic or trophoblastic disease.

Progesterone Levels

Use: Adjunct test in suspected ectopic pregnancy or miscarriage.

Interpretation: Levels >25 ng/mL suggest viable intrauterine pregnancy; <5 ng/mL indicate non-viable pregnancy.

Other Tests: CBC for anemia, blood type/Rh status and infection screening (e.g., rubella, HIV) as part of prenatal workup.

3. Ultrasound

Transvaginal Ultrasound

Indications: Confirm intrauterine pregnancy, assess viability, rule out ectopic pregnancy.

Findings

Gestational sac: Visible at 4–5 weeks (hCG ~1,500–2,000 mIU/mL).

Yolk sac: Seen at 5–6 weeks.

Fetal pole and heartbeat: Detectable at 5–6 weeks (hCG ~5,000–6,000 mIU/mL).

Advantages: High sensitivity for early pregnancy and complications.

Transabdominal Ultrasound

Indications: Used later (6–7 weeks onward) or when transvaginal is not feasible.

Findings: Confirms fetal number, location, and viability.

Clinical Use

Establishes gestational age (crown-rump length most accurate at 6–12 weeks).

Detects multiple gestations, molar pregnancy, or ectopic pregnancy.

Guides management in cases of vaginal bleeding or pain.

4. Gestational Age Assessment

Last Menstrual Period (LMP)

Calculate estimated due date (EDD) using Naegele's rule: EDD = LMP + 1 year – 3 months + 7 days.

Accuracy depends on regular cycles and accurate recall.

Ultrasound

First trimester crown-rump length (CRL) is the most accurate (±5–7 days).

Second trimester biparietal diameter (BPD) or femur length used if CRL unavailable (±10–14 days).

Clinical Correlation: Combine LMP and ultrasound for precise dating; ultrasound preferred if discrepancy >7 days.

Differential Diagnosis

1. Ectopic Pregnancy

Symptoms: Vaginal bleeding, pelvic pain, amenorrhea.

Diagnosis: Low or slowly rising hCG, empty uterus on ultrasound, or adnexal mass.

2. Molar Pregnancy

Symptoms: Vaginal bleeding, hyperemesis, uterine size > dates.

Diagnosis: High hCG, "snowstorm" appearance on ultrasound.

3. Miscarriage

Symptoms: Bleeding, cramping, loss of pregnancy symptoms.

Diagnosis: Declining hCG, absent fetal heartbeat, or empty gestational sac.

4. Pseudocyesis

Symptoms: False belief of pregnancy with amenorrhea, nausea, and abdominal distension.

Diagnosis: Negative hCG and ultrasound; psychological evaluation.

Other: Ovarian cysts, uterine fibroids, or endocrine disorders (e.g., PCOS, hypothyroidism).

Clinical Approach

1. Initial Assessment: Obtain a detailed history: LMP, symptoms, risk factors (e.g., prior ectopic, infertility). Perform physical exam to detect probable signs (e.g., uterine enlargement, cervical changes).
2. Confirm Pregnancy: Use urine or serum hCG test for initial confirmation. Perform transvaginal ultrasound if hCG >1,500 mIU/mL and pregnancy location is unclear.
3. Assess Viability and Location: Monitor hCG trends in early pregnancy if viability is uncertain. Use ultrasound to confirm intrauterine pregnancy and rule out ectopic or molar pregnancy.
4. Estimate Gestational Age: Combine LMP and ultrasound findings; prioritize CRL in the first trimester.
5. Screen for Complications: Evaluate vaginal bleeding, pain, or abnormal hCG patterns. Refer to specialists for high-risk cases.
6. Counseling: Educate patients on pregnancy symptoms, expected progression, and when to seek care. Address emotional concerns, especially in cases of uncertain viability.

Complications

False-Positive hCG

Causes: Trophoblastic disease, ectopic pregnancy, or hCG-secreting tumors.

Management: Correlate with ultrasound and clinical findings.

False-Negative Tests

Causes: Testing too early, dilute urine, or hook effect (very high hCG in molar pregnancy).

Management: Repeat test after 48–72 hours or use serum hCG.

Ectopic Pregnancy Risk

Prevalence: 1–2% of pregnancies.

High suspicion in women with pain, bleeding, or risk factors (e.g., prior ectopic, tubal surgery).

Legal and Ethical Considerations

PCPNDT Act (India)

Prohibits fetal sex determination during ultrasound or genetic testing to prevent sex-selective abortions.

Requires meticulous documentation (e.g., Form F) and compliance with regulations.

Penalties: Up to 3–5 years imprisonment and fines for violations.

Informed Consent

Obtain consent for diagnostic tests (e.g., ultrasound, amniocentesis), explaining risks and benefits.

Respect patient autonomy in decisions about testing or management.

Confidentiality

Protect patient privacy, especially in cases of unplanned pregnancy or complications.

Comply with laws (e.g., POCSO Act for pregnant minors).

Conclusion

The diagnosis of pregnancy involves integrating presumptive symptoms (e.g., amenorrhea, nausea), probable signs (e.g., uterine enlargement, positive hCG), and positive signs (e.g., fetal heartbeat, ultrasound visualization). Laboratory tests (hCG) and ultrasound are the cornerstones of diagnosis, enabling confirmation, gestational age assessment, and detection of complications like ectopic pregnancy or miscarriage. Early and accurate diagnosis facilitates timely prenatal care, improves maternal and fetal outcomes, and supports informed patient decision-making.

3.6 Pseudocyesis /False Pregnancy

(*Haml-i-Kadhib/Raja*)

Introduction

Pseudocyesis, also known as false pregnancy or phantom pregnancy, is a rare psychological condition in which a woman experiences signs and symptoms of pregnancy despite not being pregnant. This condition highlights the complex interplay between psychological, hormonal and physical factors, leading to a clinical presentation that mimics true pregnancy.

Definition

Pseudocyesis is defined as a clinical syndrome characterized by the false belief of being pregnant, accompanied by objective signs and symptoms mimicking pregnancy, in the absence of a viable intrauterine gestation.

Epidemiology

Prevalence: Rare, with an estimated incidence of 1–6 cases per 22,000 pregnancies in developed countries. Higher rates may occur in cultures where pregnancy carries significant social value.

Demographics

Primarily affects women of reproductive age (20–40 years), though cases have been reported in adolescents and postmenopausal women.

More common in regions with strong cultural emphasis on fertility or motherhood (e.g., parts of South Asia, Africa).

Risk Groups

Women with a history of infertility, miscarriage, or pregnancy loss.

Women under social or familial pressure to conceive.

Those with psychiatric disorders (e.g., depression, anxiety, schizophrenia).

Etiology and Pathophysiology

Pseudocyesis results from a complex interplay of psychological, neuroendocrine, and sociocultural factors:

1. Psychological Factors

Intense Desire or Fear: A strong desire to conceive (e.g., due to infertility or social pressure) or fear of pregnancy can trigger psychosomatic responses.

Psychiatric Conditions: Associated with depression, anxiety, personality disorders, or psychosis. In some cases, it may reflect unresolved trauma or grief from pregnancy loss.

Psychosomatic Mechanism: The brain's perception of pregnancy influences somatic symptoms via the hypothalamic-pituitary-ovarian axis.

2. Neuroendocrine Changes

Hormonal Dysregulation: Elevated prolactin levels, persistent corpus luteum activity, or increased sympathetic activity may mimic pregnancy-related hormonal changes.

Prolactin and Gonadotropins: Stress or psychological triggers can stimulate prolactin release, leading to amenorrhea and breast changes.

Sympathetic Activation: May cause abdominal distension or perceived fetal movements due to increased gastrointestinal motility.

3. Sociocultural Factors

Cultural emphasis on motherhood or fertility as a marker of identity (e.g., in patriarchal societies).

Social pressures, such as expectations from family or spouse, may exacerbate the condition.

Stigma around infertility or childlessness can contribute to psychological distress.

4. Historical Context

Historically reported in various books (e.g., Hippocrates documented cases in 300 BC).

Clinical Features

Pseudocyesis presents with signs and symptoms that closely resemble those of true pregnancy, categorized as presumptive and probable signs (positive signs of pregnancy, such as fetal heart tones, are absent).

1. Presumptive Symptoms

Amenorrhea: Cessation of menstruation, often the earliest symptom, due to stress-induced suppression of the hypothalamic-pituitary-ovarian axis or persistent corpus luteum activity.

Nausea and Vomiting: Mimics morning sickness, likely psychosomatic or due to heightened sympathetic activity.

Breast Changes: Tenderness, enlargement, or galactorrhea (milk secretion) due to elevated prolactin levels.

Fatigue: Subjective tiredness, possibly related to psychological stress or hormonal changes.

Food Cravings or Aversions: Altered taste preferences, similar to early pregnancy.

Urinary Frequency: Perceived need to urinate frequently, possibly due to pelvic congestion or psychological factors.

2. Probable Signs

Abdominal Distension

Progressive abdominal enlargement mimicking a pregnant uterus.

May result from gas accumulation, lordosis (exaggerated lumbar Curvature), or voluntary abdominal muscle contraction.

Can resemble a gravid abdomen, sometimes mimicking 6–9 months gestation.

Perceived Fetal Movements

Sensation of fetal movements (quickening), reported by the patient.

Likely due to intestinal peristalsis or muscle spasms misinterpreted as fetal activity.

Uterine Enlargement

Mild uterine enlargement may occur due to hormonal stimulation or pelvic congestion.

Uterus does not reach the size expected for gestational age in true pregnancy.

Cervical and Vaginal Changes

Softening of the cervix (Goodell's sign) or bluish discoloration (Chadwick's sign) may be present due to hormonal effects. Less pronounced than in true pregnancy.

Weight Gain

Weight gain due to fluid retention, overeating, or reduced physical activity.

Variable, often less than in true pregnancy.

3. Absence of Positive Signs

No fetal heart tones (by Doppler or fetoscope).

No visualization of a fetus on ultrasound.

No true uterine growth consistent with gestational age.

Diagnosis

Diagnosing pseudocyesis requires a careful, empathetic approach to confirm the absence of pregnancy while addressing psychological and social factors.

1. Clinical Evaluation

History

Assess for amenorrhea, pregnancy-like symptoms and psychological stressors (e.g., infertility, social pressure).

Explore psychiatric history (e.g., depression, anxiety, prior pregnancy loss).

Inquire about cultural or familial expectations regarding fertility.

Physical Examination

General: Evaluate for signs of pregnancy (e.g., breast changes, abdominal distension).

Abdominal: Palpate for uterine size (typically normal or minimally enlarged); no fetal parts or ballottement.

Pelvic: Assess for cervical softening or vaginal changes; uterus is non-gravid.

Psychiatric: Screen for signs of depression, anxiety or psychosis.

2. Laboratory Tests

Urine Pregnancy Test

Result: Negative in pseudocyesis (no hCG production).

Limitation: Rarely, low levels of hCG may be present due to persistent corpus luteum activity, requiring further evaluation.

Serum β-hCG

Result: Undetectable or very low (<5 mIU/mL), ruling out true pregnancy.

Use: Confirms absence of pregnancy and excludes ectopic pregnancy or trophoblastic disease.

Prolactin Levels

Result: May be elevated, contributing to amenorrhea and galactorrhea.

Use: Supports psychosomatic etiology but is non-specific.

Other Tests

Thyroid function tests to rule out hypothyroidism (can cause amenorrhea and fatigue).

Complete blood count (CBC) and metabolic panel to exclude systemic causes of symptoms.

3. Imaging

Ultrasound (Transvaginal or Transabdominal)

Findings: Empty uterus, no gestational sac, yolk sac, or fetus.

Use: Gold standard to confirm absence of pregnancy and rule out ectopic pregnancy or molar pregnancy.

Consideration: Perform with sensitivity, as patients may be emotionally invested in the belief of pregnancy.

Other Imaging (if indicated)

Abdominal X-ray or CT (rarely used) to exclude masses causing distension (e.g., ovarian cysts, fibroids).

Differential Diagnosis

True Pregnancy: Positive hCG, fetal heart tones and ultrasound confirmation.

Ectopic Pregnancy: Vaginal bleeding, pelvic pain, low/slowly rising hCG, adnexal mass on ultrasound.

Molar Pregnancy: High hCG, "snowstorm" ultrasound pattern, vaginal bleeding.

Ovarian Cysts or Tumors: May cause abdominal distension and hormonal changes; diagnosed by ultrasound or MRI.

Uterine Fibroids: Can mimic uterine enlargement; confirmed by imaging.

Endocrine Disorders: Hypothyroidism, hyperprolactinemia, or PCOS causing amenorrhea and symptoms.

Psychiatric Conditions: Delusional disorders or Munchausen syndrome; require psychiatric evaluation.

Management

Management of pseudocyesis requires a multidisciplinary approach, combining obstetric, psychiatric and social interventions with sensitivity to avoid stigmatizing the patient.

1. Confirming Non-Pregnancy

Gently present evidence of non-pregnancy (e.g., negative hCG, ultrasound findings).

Use empathetic, non-judgmental communication to avoid distress or denial.

Example: "The tests show that there is no pregnancy at this time, but we're here to understand what's causing your symptoms and support you."

Counseling

Acknowledge the patient's emotions and validate their experience.

Avoid confrontation, as denial may be a coping mechanism.

2. Psychiatric Evaluation and Treatment

Refer to a psychiatrist or psychologist for evaluation of underlying mental health conditions (e.g., depression, anxiety, somatic symptom disorder).

Assess for severe disorders (e.g., psychosis) requiring urgent intervention.

Cognitive Behavioral Therapy (CBT): Effective for addressing false beliefs and managing stress.

Supportive Psychotherapy: Helps patients process grief, infertility, or social pressures.

Medications (if indicated)

Antidepressants (e.g., SSRIs like sertraline) for depression or anxiety.

Antipsychotics (e.g., risperidone) for delusional disorders, used cautiously.

Dopamine agonists (e.g., bromocriptine) for persistent hyperprolactinemia causing galactorrhea.

3. Medical Management

Hormonal Correction

Address amenorrhea or galactorrhea if caused by hyperprolactinemia (e.g., cabergoline).

Rule out endocrine disorders (e.g., hypothyroidism) with appropriate treatment.

Symptom Relief

Manage nausea, bloating, or other symptoms symptomatically (e.g., antiemetics, dietary counseling).

Monitoring

Regular follow-up to assess resolution of symptoms and response to therapy.

4. Social Support

Address Social Pressures: Explore family or cultural expectations contributing to the condition (e.g., pressure to conceive). Involve family in counseling, if appropriate, to reduce stigma or blame.

Conclusion

Pseudocyesis is a rare but significant psychosomatic condition characterized by the false belief of pregnancy and associated physical symptoms. It arises from psychological, neuroendocrine, and sociocultural factors, requiring a compassionate, multidisciplinary approach to diagnosis and management. Obstetricians must confirm the absence of pregnancy using hCG tests and ultrasound, rule out organic causes, and address underlying psychological issues through psychiatric referral and counseling.

3.7 Antenatal care & Minor Ailments in pregnancy

(*Hamla ki nigahdasht aur haml ke dauran hone wale khafif amrad*)

Antenatal Care (ANC)

Introduction

Antenatal care refers to the systematic medical supervision, monitoring and support provided to pregnant women from conception to delivery to ensure optimal maternal and fetal health outcomes. ANC aims to prevent, detect and manage complications, promote healthy behaviors and prepare women for safe childbirth and the postpartum period.

Objectives of Antenatal Care

1. Promote Maternal Health: Monitor and maintain the physical and mental well-being of the pregnant woman.
2. Ensure Fetal Health: Assess fetal growth, development and well-being to prevent adverse outcomes.
3. Detect and Manage Complications: Identify high-risk pregnancies and manage conditions like anemia, hypertension, or infections early.
4. Prevent Maternal and Neonatal Mortality: Address preventable causes of mortality, such as hemorrhage, preeclampsia, or preterm birth.
5. Educate and Empower: Provide counseling on nutrition, birth preparedness, danger signs and family planning.
6. Facilitate Safe Delivery: Prepare for institutional delivery or skilled birth attendance and ensure access to emergency obstetric care.

Components of Antenatal Care

ANC involves a structured schedule of visits, clinical assessments, diagnostics, interventions and counseling. The WHO recommends a minimum of eight ANC contacts (updated from four visits in 2016) to reduce perinatal mortality and improve maternal outcomes.

1. ANC Visit Schedule

First Trimester (up to 12 weeks): Initial assessment and confirmation of pregnancy.

Second Trimester: Visit at 20, 26, and 30 weeks for monitoring and interventions.

Third Trimester: Visit at 34, 36, 38, and 40 weeks for delivery preparation and complication screening.

Frequency: More frequent visits for high-risk pregnancies (e.g., multiple gestation, diabetes, or hypertension).

2. Clinical Assessment

History Taking

Obstetric history: Previous pregnancies, miscarriages, preterm births, or cesarean sections.

Medical history: Chronic conditions (e.g., hypertension, diabetes), infections, or allergies.

Social history: Smoking, alcohol, domestic violence, or socioeconomic factors.

Physical Examination

Vital signs: Blood pressure, pulse, and weight monitoring.

Abdominal examination: Fundal height, fetal lie, presentation, and heart rate (via Doppler after 12 weeks).

General examination: Pallor, edema, or signs of systemic illness.

High-Risk Identification: Screening for conditions like preeclampsia, gestational diabetes, or anemia.

3. Diagnostic Tests

Routine Tests

Blood: Hemoglobin, blood group, Rh typing, anemia screening and serology (HIV, syphilis, hepatitis B).

Urine: Proteinuria, glycosuria and urinary tract infections.

Ultrasound: Dating scan (8–12 weeks), anomaly scan (18–22 weeks), and growth scans (as needed).

Specialized Tests (for high-risk cases)

Glucose tolerance test for gestational diabetes.

Thyroid function tests for hypothyroidism.

Screening for group B streptococcus (GBS) in late pregnancy.

Immunizations: Tetanus toxoid (two doses in first pregnancy, boosters in subsequent pregnancies).

Supplements

Iron and folic acid: 60 mg elemental iron and 400 μg folic acid daily to prevent anemia and neural tube defects.

Calcium: 1–2 g daily in areas with low dietary calcium intake to reduce preeclampsia risk.

Vitamin A (if deficient): Up to 10,000 IU/day in deficient populations.

Infection Prevention

Treatment of asymptomatic bacteriuria or sexually transmitted infections.

Malaria prophylaxis (e.g., intermittent preventive treatment in endemic areas).

5. Counseling and Health Education

Nutrition: Balanced diet rich in protein, iron, calcium, and micronutrients; weight gain recommendations (11–16 kg for normal BMI).

Lifestyle: Avoidance of smoking, alcohol, and illicit drugs; moderate exercise.

Danger Signs: Educate on symptoms requiring immediate care (e.g., vaginal bleeding, severe headache, reduced fetal movements).

Plan for delivery location, transport, and emergency contacts.

Postpartum Care: Breastfeeding, contraception, and newborn care.

6. Management of High-Risk Pregnancies

Monitoring for intrauterine growth restriction (IUGR) or preterm labor.

Planning for cesarean section or induction if indicated.

Impact of ANC

Maternal Outcomes: Reduced risk of maternal mortality from hemorrhage, preeclampsia and sepsis.

Fetal/Neonatal Outcomes: Lower rates of preterm birth, low birth weight, and congenital anomalies.

Challenges: Inadequate infrastructure, shortage of trained providers and cultural barriers to ANC uptake.

Minor Ailments in Pregnancy

Introduction

Minor ailments in pregnancy are common, non-life-threatening symptoms that arise due to physiological changes during pregnancy. While generally self-limiting, these ailments can cause significant discomfort and, if mismanaged, may lead to complications. Proper counseling and management are essential to improve quality of life and ensure maternal well-being.

Common Minor Ailments and Management

1. Nausea and Vomiting (Morning Sickness)

Prevalence: Affects 50–80% of pregnant women, typically in the first trimester (6-12weeks).

Cause: Elevated human chorionic gonadotropin (hCG), estrogen, and progesterone levels; altered gastric motility.

Clinical Features: Nausea, vomiting (often in the morning but can occur anytime), and food aversions.

Management

Non-Pharmacological: Small, frequent meals high in carbohydrates and low in fat. Avoid triggers (e.g., strong odors, spicy foods).

Pharmacological (if severe)

Vitamin B6 (pyridoxine) 10–25 mg every 8 hours.

Antihistamines like doxylamine (10 mg at bedtime).

If persistent, consider ondansetron (4–8 mg) under medical supervision.

2. Heartburn (Gastroesophageal Reflux)

Prevalence: Affects 30–50% of pregnant women, especially in the second and third trimesters.

Cause: Progesterone-induced relaxation of the lower esophageal sphincter; increased intra-abdominal pressure from the gravid uterus.

Clinical Features: Burning sensation in the chest, regurgitation, and epigastric discomfort.

Management

Non-Pharmacological

Small, frequent meals; avoid lying down immediately after eating.

Elevate head of bed during sleep.

Avoid spicy, fatty, or acidic foods (e.g., citrus, caffeine).

Pharmacological

Antacids (e.g., calcium carbonate, magnesium hydroxide) as first-line.

H2 receptor antagonists (e.g., ranitidine) if antacids fail.

Proton pump inhibitors (e.g., omeprazole) in refractory cases, under specialist guidance.

3. Constipation

Prevalence: Affects 10–40% of pregnant women.

Cause: Progesterone-induced reduced gut motility; pressure from the gravid uterus; iron supplementation.

Clinical Features: Infrequent, hard stools; straining; and abdominal discomfort.

Management

Non-Pharmacological

Increase dietary fiber (25–30 g/day) through fruits, vegetables, and whole grains.

Adequate hydration (8–10 glasses of water daily).

Regular physical activity (e.g., walking).

Pharmacological

Bulk-forming laxatives (e.g., psyllium husk).

Osmotic laxatives (e.g., lactulose or polyethylene glycol) if needed.

Avoid stimulant laxatives unless prescribed.

4. Hemorrhoids

Prevalence: Common in the third trimester and postpartum.

Cause: Increased pelvic pressure, constipation and straining during defecation.

Clinical Features: Painful or itchy perianal swelling, bleeding during bowel movements.

Management

Non-Pharmacological

Treat constipation (fiber, hydration, laxatives).

Sitz baths (warm water soaks) for 10–15 minutes, 2–3 times daily.

Avoid prolonged sitting or straining.

Pharmacological

Topical hydrocortisone or anesthetic creams (short-term use).

With hazel pads for soothing relief.

5. Backache

Prevalence: Affects 50–70% of pregnant women, especially in the third trimester.

Cause: Increased lumbar lordosis, weight gain and relaxin-induced ligament laxity.

Clinical Features: Lower back pain, worsened by standing, bending or lifting.

Management

Non-Pharmacological: Maintain good posture; use supportive footwear. Pelvic tilts, prenatal yoga, or physiotherapy exercises. Maternity support belts for severe cases.

Pharmacological: Acetaminophen (paracetamol) for pain relief (avoid NSAIDs).

6. Leg Cramps

Prevalence: Affects 30–50% of pregnant women, often at night in the second and third trimesters.

Cause: Uncertain; possibly due to calcium/magnesium imbalance, nerve compression, or poor circulation.

Clinical Features: Sudden, painful muscle contractions in the calves or feet.

Management

Non-Pharmacological

Stretching exercises before bed (e.g., calf stretches).

Warm compresses or massage to affected muscles.

Ensure adequate hydration and electrolyte balance.

Pharmacological

Calcium (1,000 mg/day) or magnesium supplements (300–400 mg/day) if deficient.

7. Fatigue

Prevalence: Common in the first and third trimesters.

Cause: Hormonal changes, increased metabolic demands, anemia or poor sleep quality.

Clinical Features: Excessive tiredness, difficulty concentrating.

Management

Non-Pharmacological

Adequate rest and short naps.

Balanced diet with iron-rich foods.

Light exercise to boost energy.

Pharmacological: Treat underlying anemia with iron and folic acid supplements.

8. Varicose Veins

Prevalence: Affects 10–20% of pregnant women.

Cause: Increased blood volume, venous stasis and progesterone-induced vein relaxation.

Clinical Features: Swollen, painful veins in legs or vulva; heaviness or aching.

Management

Non-Pharmacological

Compression stockings (15–20 mmHg pressure).

Elevate legs when resting.

Avoid prolonged standing or sitting.

Pharmacological: None routinely required.

9. Vaginal Discharge

Prevalence: Common throughout pregnancy.

Cause: Increased estrogen, cervical mucus production, and vaginal blood flow.

Clinical Features: Thin, white, odorless discharge (leukorrhea).

Management

Non-Pharmacological

Maintain hygiene with mild soap and water.

Wear breathable cotton underwear.

Avoid douching or scented products.

Pharmacological: None unless infection confirmed.

10. Edema

Prevalence: Affects 50–80% of pregnant women, especially in the third trimester.

Cause: Increased blood volume, sodium retention, and pressure on pelvic veins.

Clinical Features: Swelling of ankles, feet, or hands; usually mild and resolves with rest.

Management

Non-Pharmacological

Elevate legs when sitting or lying down.

Avoid tight clothing and prolonged standing.

Maintain adequate hydration.

Pharmacological: None required unless associated with preeclampsia.

General Principles for Managing Minor Ailments

Reassure women that most ailments are normal and self-limiting.

Prioritize lifestyle and dietary modifications to minimize medication use.

Monitor for Complications: Differentiate minor ailments from serious conditions (e.g., severe edema vs. preeclampsia).

Conclusion

Antenatal care is a necessary framework for promoting maternal and fetal health, preventing complications, and preparing for safe childbirth. By adhering to WHO's eight-visit and integrating with national health programs, ANC ensures comprehensive care. Minor ailments, though common, require careful assessment and management to improve maternal comfort and prevent complications.

References

World Health Organization. (2016). WHO Recommendations on Antenatal Care for a Positive Pregnancy Experience.

J'Kishore's National Health Programs of India: 14/E 2022.

Dutta, D.C. (2020). Textbook of Obstetrics.

Clinical Guidelines for Pregnancy Care (e.g., NICE, WHO).

3.8 National Health Programs in Obstetrics

(Qaumi sehatee program braye qabalat)

Introduction

National health programs in obstetrics aim to address the high burden of maternal and neonatal mortality, promote safe motherhood, and ensure healthy outcomes for mothers and newborns.

Key Objectives of National Health Programs in Obstetrics

1. Reduce Maternal Mortality and Morbidity: Address preventable causes such as hemorrhage, hypertensive disorders, sepsis, unsafe abortions and obstructed labor.
2. Reduce Neonatal and Perinatal Mortality: Focus on preterm birth, birth asphyxia, infections and congenital anomalies.
3. Promote Universal Access to Care: Ensure equitable access to antenatal, intrapartum, and postnatal care, especially for marginalized and rural populations.
4. Improve Quality of Care: Standardize clinical practices, enhance healthcare infrastructure and train healthcare providers.
5. Address Social Determinants: Tackle issues like malnutrition, gender inequality and lack of education that impact maternal and neonatal health.
6. Strengthen Emergency Obstetric Care (EmOC): Ensure availability of comprehensive and basic emergency obstetric care to manage complications.

Major National Health Programs in Obstetrics

1. Janani Suraksha Yojana (JSY)

Launched in 2005 under the National Health Mission (NHM), JSY is a conditional cash transfer scheme to promote institutional deliveries and reduce maternal and neonatal mortality, particularly in low-performing states.

Objectives

Increase institutional deliveries among low-income and rural women.

Reduce out-of-pocket expenses for childbirth.

Improve access to skilled birth attendants.

Components

Cash Incentives: Financial assistance to pregnant women for institutional deliveries (e.g., ₹1,400 for rural areas, ₹1,000 for urban areas in low-performing states; ₹700 for high-performing states).

Accredited Social Health Activist (ASHA): Community health workers facilitate access to healthcare, accompany women to facilities, and provide counseling.

Free Delivery Services: Free transport, medicines, and diagnostics in public health facilities.

Focus on Low-Performing States: Prioritizes states with high maternal mortality rates (e.g., Uttar Pradesh, Bihar).

Implementation

Partnerships with public and private health facilities.

Integration with primary health centers (PHCs), community health centers (CHCs), and district hospitals.

Monitoring through Health Management Information Systems (HMIS).

2. Janani Shishu Suraksha Karyakram (JSSK) – India

Launched in 2011, JSSK complements JSY by ensuring free maternal and neonatal care, addressing financial barriers to accessing services.

Objectives

Provide free entitlements for pregnant women and sick infants up to one year of age.

Eliminate out-of-pocket expenses for delivery, cesarean sections, and neonatal care.

Components

Free Services: Delivery (normal and cesarean), diagnostics, drugs, blood transfusions, and hospital stay.

Free Transport: Ambulance services for pregnant women and sick infants to and from facilities.

Free Diet: Nutritional support during hospital stay.

Neonatal Care: Free treatment for sick newborns, including intensive care.

Implementation

Implemented through public health facilities, with funding from the central and state governments.

Collaboration with ASHA workers for community outreach.

Regular audits to ensure compliance with free service mandates.

Impact

Increased access to emergency obstetric and neonatal care.

Reduced financial burden, particularly for rural and low-income families.

Challenges include inadequate infrastructure in some regions and supply chain issues for drugs and diagnostics.

3. Pradhan Mantri Surakshit Matritva Abhiyan (PMSMA)

Launched in 2016, PMSMA focuses on improving antenatal care (ANC) quality to detect and manage high-risk pregnancies.

Objectives

Provide free, comprehensive ANC on the 9th of every month.

Identify and manage high-risk pregnancies (e.g., preeclampsia, anemia, gestational diabetes).

Enhance private sector participation in maternal health.

Components

Special ANC Days: Designated days for free checkups, diagnostics and counseling.

High-Risk Pregnancy Identification: Use of color-coded stickers (e.g., red for high-risk cases) for tracking.

Diagnostics and Counseling: Free ultrasound, blood tests and health education.

4. LaQshya Initiative

Launched in 2017, LaQshya aims to improve the quality of care in labor rooms and maternity operation theaters to reduce preventable maternal and neonatal deaths.

Objectives

Enhance quality of intrapartum and postpartum care.

Reduce maternal and neonatal mortality due to preventable causes (e.g., postpartum hemorrhage, sepsis). Ensure respectful maternity care.

Components

Infrastructure Upgrades: Standardized labor rooms and obstetric operation theaters.

Training: Capacity building for healthcare providers in emergency obstetric care.

Quality Certification: Facilities meeting standards receive LaQshya certification.

Respectful Maternity Care: Focus on dignity, privacy, and informed consent.

Impact

Improved labor room standards and reduced infection rates.

Enhanced provider competency in managing obstetric emergencies.

Challenges include slow adoption in resource-constrained settings.

5. National Clinical Guidelines (Global Perspective, e.g., NWIHP)

National Women and Infants Health Programme (NWIHP) develops evidence-based clinical guidelines for maternity and gynecology services, which can serve as a model for national programs globally.

Objectives

Standardize clinical practices for obstetric care.

Improve outcomes through evidence-based protocols.

Components

Guidelines on reduced fetal movements, antenatal corticosteroids, domestic violence screening, and management of high-risk pregnancies.

Multidisciplinary expert advisory groups for guideline development.

Focus on conditions like preterm birth, hypertensive disorders, and obstetric emergencies.

6. WHO's Emergency Obstetric Care (EmOC) Programs

The World Health Organization promotes EmOC as a global standard for managing obstetric emergencies, adopted by many countries national health programs.

Objectives

Ensure access to basic and comprehensive EmOC services.

Reduce maternal and neonatal mortality from complications.

Components

Basic EmOC: Includes administration of antibiotics, oxytocics, anticonvulsants, manual removal of placenta, assisted vaginal delivery, and neonatal resuscitation.

Comprehensive EmOC: Includes basic EmOC plus cesarean section and blood transfusion capabilities.

Training and Infrastructure: Equipping facilities and training providers in emergency procedures.

Implementation

Establishing EmOC centers in underserved areas.

Monitoring signal functions (e.g., ability to perform cesarean sections) to assess EmOC readiness.

Integration with national health systems.

Common Strategies Across National Health Programs

1. Community Engagement: Involving community health workers (e.g., ASHA in India) to bridge gaps between communities and healthcare systems.

2. Training and Capacity Building: Continuous education for obstetricians, midwives, and nurses in evidence-based practices.

3. Infrastructure Development: Upgrading maternity wards, labor rooms, and neonatal intensive care units.

4. Monitoring and Evaluation: Using health management information systems to track maternal and neonatal outcomes.

5. Focus on Equity: Targeting underserved populations, including rural, tribal, and socioeconomically disadvantaged groups.

Conclusion

National health programs in obstetrics are pivotal in reducing maternal and neonatal mortality, improving quality of care, and promoting health equity. Programs like JSY, JSSK, PMSMA, LaQshya, and global initiatives like EmOC demonstrate the power of targeted interventions, community engagement, and evidence-based practices. However, challenges such as resource constraints, quality gaps and cultural barriers require ongoing innovation, investment and collaboration to achieve sustainable improvements in maternal and neonatal health outcomes.

References

J'Kishore's National Health Programs of India: 14/E 2022 (https://prithvibooks.com/product/jkishores-national-health-programs-of-india/)

Medical Informatics In Obstetrics And Gynecology (https:/vdoc.pub/documents/medical-informatics-in-obstetrics-and-gynecology-m24dv0n7ras0)

Clinical Guidelines - HSE.ie(https://www.hse.ie/eng/about/who/acute-hospitals-division/woman-infants/clinical-guidelines/)

World Health Organization (WHO) guidelines on Emergency Obstetric Care

Long Answer Questions (LAQs)

1. Describe physiological changes during pregnancy in detail.
2. Explain signs and symptoms of pregnancy along with diagnosis.
3. Describe antenatal care (*Haml ki Nigahdasht*) and its importance.
4. Define preconception counselling and discuss its role in maternal health.
5. Explain PNDT Act and its importance in obstetric practice.

Short Answer Questions (SAQs)

1. Define pregnancy (*Haml*).
2. What is *Haml-e-Kazib* (pseudocyesis)?
3. Mention two objectives of antenatal care.
4. Name any two minor ailments of pregnancy.
5. Write full form of PNDT Act.

Multiple Choice Questions (1 Mark Each)

1.Normal duration of pregnancy is:

A. 36 weeks B. 38 weeks

C. 40 weeks D. 42 weeks

Ans: C. 40 weeks

2. Most reliable sign of pregnancy is:

A. Amenorrhea B. Morning sickness

C. Fetal heart sound heard D. Breast tenderness

Ans: C. Fetal heart sound heard

3. Implantation occurs in:

A. Cervix B. Fundus of uterus

C. Vagina D. Ovary

Ans: B. Fundus of uterus

4. Haml-e-Kazib refers to:

A. Ectopic pregnancy B. False pregnancy

C. Multiple pregnancy D. Molar pregnancy

Ans: B. False pregnancy

5. PNDT Act is related to:

A. Abortion B. Sex determination

C. Family planning D. Infertility

Ans: B. Sex determination

6. Fetal heart sound is heard by Doppler at:

A. 4 weeks B. 6 weeks

C. 10–12 weeks D. 20 weeks

Ans: C. 10-12 weeks

7. First antenatal visit should be before:

A. 6 months B. 5 months

C. 4 months D. 7 months

Ans: C. 4 months

8. Morning sickness occurs mainly due to:

A. Progesterone B. Estrogen

C. hCG D. Prolactin

Ans: C. hCG

9. Supine hypotension syndrome is due to pressure on:

A. Aorta B. Inferior vena cava

C. Uterine artery D. Renal vein

Ans: B. Inferior vena cava

10. National programme related to maternal health is:

A. RNTCP   B. NVBDCP

C. RMNCH+A   D. NACP

Ans: C. RMNCH+A

04

Female pelvis & Fetal Skull

(Ana-i-zanan aur jumjuma -i-janin)

4.1 *Jumjuma-i-Janin aur uske aqtar* (Fetal Skull &its Diameters)
4.2 *Ana-i-zanan: aqsam aur aqtar* (Maternal pelvis: Types & Diameters)
4.3 *Ana-e-munqabiz* (Contracted Pelvis)
4.4 *Rasi Hauzi Adm-i-tanasub* (Cephalo-Pelvic disproportion/CPD)

Learning Objective (At the end of the session, the students should be able to)

Enumerate & Interpret the Fetal Skull & its Diameters along with diagram and Maternal Pelvis & its types with labelled diagram.
Define *Ana e Munqabiz* (Contracted Pelvis).
Elaborate the diagnosis of contracted pelvis.
Explain the etiology and diagnosis of Cephalopelvic disproportion.

4.1 Fetal Skull & its Diameters

(*Jumjuma-i-Janin aur uske aqtar*)

Introduction

The fetal skull is a critical anatomical structure in obstetrics due to its role as the leading part in most deliveries (cephalic presentation). Its bony structure, sutures, fontanelles and diameters influence the mechanism of labor, particularly during vaginal delivery. Understanding the fetal skull's anatomy and its measurements is essential for assessing fetal head engagement, descent and potential complications such as cephalopelvic disproportion (CPD).

Anatomy of the Fetal Skull

The fetal skull consists of bones, sutures, and fontanelles, which are adapted to withstand the compressive forces of labor while allowing for flexibility and brain growth postnatally.

1. Bones of the Fetal Skull

The fetal skull is composed of several bones, primarily

Two Frontal Bones: Form the forehead and anterior part of the cranium.

Two Parietal Bones: Form the sides and roof of the cranium.

One Occipital Bones: Forms the back and base of the skull, including the foramen magnum.

Two Temporal Bones: Contain the squamous and mastoid portions, located on the sides of the skull.

Other Bones: Sphenoid and ethmoid bones contribute to the base of the skull but are less relevant to labor dynamics.

These bones are thin, flexible, and not fully ossified at birth, allowing for molding during labor.

2. Sutures

Sutures are immovable fibrous joints that connect the skull bones, enabling slight movement (molding) during delivery to adapt to the maternal pelvis.

Sagittal Suture: Lies between the two parietal bones, running anteroposteriorly.

Coronal Suture: Separates the frontal bones from the parietal bones, running transversely.

Lambdoid Suture: Separates the occipital bone from the parietal bones, forming a lambda-shaped junction.

Frontal (Metopic) Suture: Lies between the two frontal bones (fuses postnatally).

Temporal Sutures: Connect the temporal bones to the parietal and occipital bones.

Clinical Significance: Sutures are palpable during vaginal examination and help identify the fetal head's position (e.g., occiput anterior or posterior).

3. Fontanelles

Fontanelles are membranous gaps at the junction of sutures, allowing compressibility and brain growth.

Anterior Fontanelle (Bregma)

Location: Junction of sagittal, coronal, and frontal sutures.

Shape: Diamond-shaped.

Size: Approximately 2–3 cm in diameter at term.

Closure: 18–24 months postnatally.

Clinical Relevance: Palpable during labor; helps assess position and degree of flexion.

Posterior Fontanelle

Location: Junction of sagittal and lambdoid sutures.

Shape: Triangular.

Size: Smaller, about 1–2 cm.

Closure: 2–3 months postnatally.

Clinical Relevance: Indicates the occiput's position.

Other Fontanelles: Sphenoid (anterolateral) and mastoid (posterolateral) fontanelles are less clinically significant during labor.

Clinical Significance: Fontanelles allow molding and are used to assess intracranial pressure postnatally (e.g., sunken or bulging fontanelles).

4. Regions of the Fetal Skull

Vertex: Area bounded by the anterior fontanelle, parietal bones and posterior fontanelle; the most common presenting part.

Brow: Area between the anterior fontanelle and the forehead.

Face: Area from the chin to the orbits.

Occiput: Posterior part of the skull, below the posterior fontanelle.

Clinical Relevance: The presenting region determines the fetal presentation (e.g., vertex, brow, or face) and influences labor progression.

5. Molding

Molding is the temporary reshaping of the fetal skull during labor due to the overlapping of cranial bones at sutures. This process reduces the skull's diameter to fit through the maternal pelvis.

Mechanism: Parietal bones slide over each other or under the occipital/frontal bones, facilitated by sutures and fontanelles.

Degrees of Molding

0: Sutures are separate.

+1: Sutures touch but do not overlap.

+2: Sutures overlap but are reducible.

+3: Sutures overlap and are irreducible (may indicate CPD).

Clinical Significance: Excessive molding may suggest obstructed labor, requiring intervention.

Fetal Skull Diameters

The diameters of the fetal skull are critical measurements that determine how the fetal head navigates the maternal pelvis during labor. These diameters vary depending on the degree of flexion or deflexion of the fetal head and the presentation. Below are the key diameters, their measurements and their obstetric significance, measured at term (approximately 37–40 weeks gestation).

1. Suboccipitobregmatic Diameter

Measurement: 9.5 cm (average at term).

Description: Extends from the suboccipital region (below the occipital protuberance) to the bregma (anterior fontanelle).

Presentation: Vertex, with the head fully flexed (occiput anterior or posterior).

Obstetric Significance: The smallest anteroposterior diameter, allowing optimal engagement and passage through the pelvis. It is the most favorable diameter for vaginal delivery.

2. Occipitofrontal Diameter

Measurement: 11.5 cm (average at term).

Description: Extends from the occipital protuberance to the glabella (midpoint between the eyebrows).

Presentation: Vertex, with partial deflexion (e.g., occiput posterior or military attitude).

Obstetric Significance: Larger than the suboccipitobregmatic diameter, potentially causing prolonged labor if the head remains deflexed. May require rotation or operative delivery.

3. Supraoccipitomental Diameter

Measurement: 13.5 cm (average at term).

Description:Extends from the vertex (highest point of the skull) to the chin.

Presentation: Brow presentation.

Obstetric Significance: One of the largest diameters, often incompatible with vaginal delivery due to poor fit with the maternal pelvis. Frequently necessitates cesarean section.

4. Occipitomental Diameter

Measurement: 12.5–13 cm (average at term).

Description: Extends from the occipital protuberance to the chin.

Presentation: Partial extension, between vertex and brow presentations.

Obstetric Significance: Larger diameter that may complicate labor; often requires intervention if persistent.

5. Submentobregmatic Diameter

Measurement: 9.5 cm (average at term).

Description: Extends from the junction of the neck and chin to the bregma.

Presentation: Face presentation, with the head fully extended.

Obstetric Significance: Similar in size to the suboccipitobregmatic diameter, allowing vaginal delivery in some cases, provided the pelvis is adequate and the chin is anterior (mento-anterior).

6. Biparietal Diameter

Measurement: 9.5 cm (average at term).

Description: The greatest transverse diameter, between the two parietal eminences.

Presentation: Relevant in all cephalic presentations.

Obstetric Significance: Determines the fit of the fetal head through the pelvic inlet and outlet. It is critical in assessing cephalopelvic disproportion.

7. Bitemporal Diameter

Measurement: 8.0 cm (average at term).

Description: The shortest transverse diameter, between the temporal bones.

Presentation: Relevant in all cephalic presentations.

Obstetric Significance: Facilitates passage through the pelvis, especially in the midpelvis.

8. Suboccipitofrontal Diameter

Measurement: 10.0 cm (average at term).

Description: Extends from the suboccipital region to the forehead.

Presentation: Vertex, with slight deflexion.

Obstetric Significance: Slightly larger than the suboccipitobregmatic diameter, potentially affecting labor progression if deflexion persists.

Diameter	**Measurement (cm)**	**Presentation**	**Obstetric Significance**
Suboccipitobregmatic	9.5	Vertex (fully flexed)	Most favorable for vaginal delivery
Occipitofrontal	11.5	Vertex (partially deflexed) |	May prolong labor; may require intervention
Supraoccipitomental	13.5	Brow	Often incompatible with vaginal delivery
Occipitomental	12.5-13	Partial extension	May complicate labor; often requires cesarean section
Submentobregmatic	9.5	Face (fully extended)	Possible vaginal delivery if mento-anterior
Biparietal	9.5	All cephalic presentations	Critical for pelvic fit; assesses CPD
Bitemporal	8.0	All cephalic presentations	Facilitates midpelvic passage
Suboccipitofrontal	10	Vertex (slight deflexion)	May affect labor progression if deflexion persists

Fetal Skull Diameters

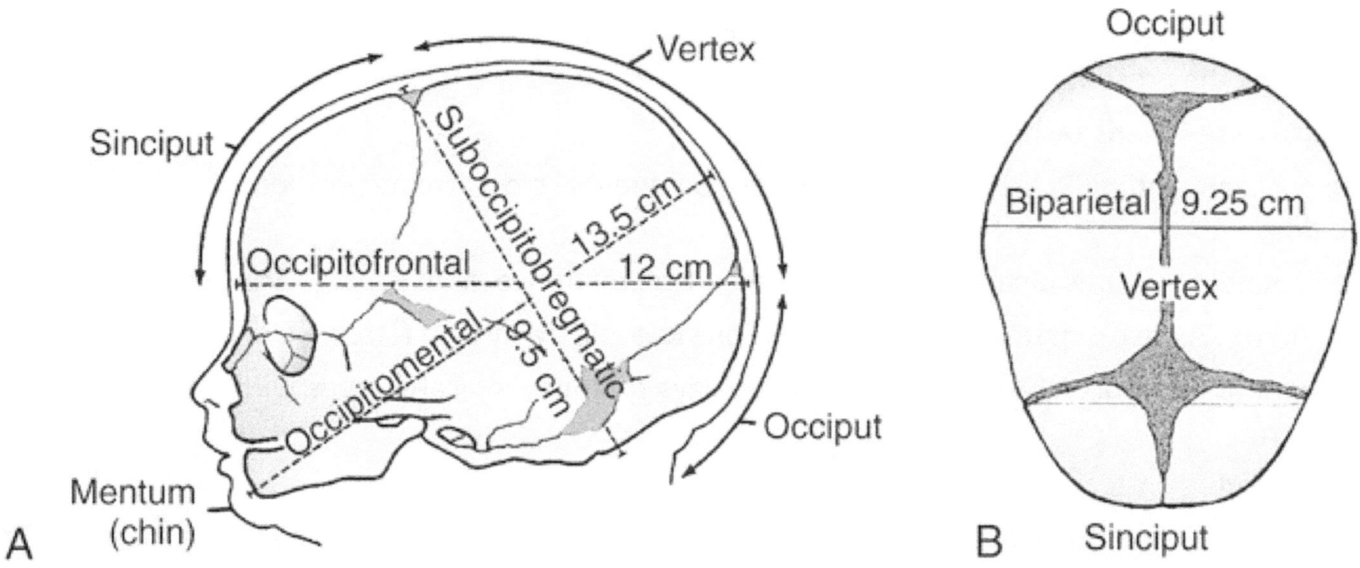

Clinical Relevance in Obstetrics

1. Mechanism of Labor

The fetal skull's diameters determine how the head engages, descends, rotates, and delivers through the maternal pelvis.

Optimal flexion (suboccipitobregmatic diameter) allows the smallest diameter to present, facilitating vaginal delivery.

Deflexed or extended presentations (e.g., brow or face) present larger diameters, increasing the risk of prolonged labor or dystocia.

2. Cephalopelvic Disproportion (CPD)

CPD occurs when the fetal skull's diameters exceed the maternal pelvic dimensions.

The biparietal diameter (9.5 cm) is compared with the pelvic inlet (anteroposterior ~11–12 cm, transverse ~13 cm) and outlet dimensions.

Clinical or radiologic pelvimetry, combined with ultrasound assessment of fetal head size, aids in diagnosing CPD.

3. Molding and Caput Succedaneum

Molding reduces the effective diameter of the fetal head, aiding passage.

Caput succedaneum (soft tissue swelling due to pressure) may obscure sutures and fontanelles, complicating position assessment.

4. Fetal Position and Presentation

Sutures and fontanelles are palpated during vaginal examination to determine the fetal head's position (e.g., occiput anterior, posterior, or transverse).

For example, palpating the posterior fontanelle in the anterior position indicates optimal flexion.

5. Operative Interventions

Larger diameters (e.g., supraoccipitomental in brow presentation) often necessitate cesarean section. In vertex presentations with prolonged labor, forceps or vacuum extraction may be used, guided by the presenting diameter.

Clinical Assessment Techniques

Vaginal Examination: Palpation of sutures and fontanelles to determine position, presentation, and molding.

Ultrasound: Measures biparietal diameter, head circumference, and assesses presentation.

Pelvimetry: Assesses maternal pelvic dimensions to evaluate fit with fetal skull diameters.

Partogram: Monitors labor progress, noting delays that may indicate issues with fetal skull size or position.

Conclusion

The fetal skull's anatomy and diameters are fundamental to understanding the mechanics of labor and delivery. The suboccipitobregmatic and biparietal diameters are critical for successful vaginal delivery, while larger diameters (e.g., supraoccipitomental) may necessitate operative intervention. Knowledge of sutures, fontanelles and molding enables obstetricians to assess fetal position and progress, diagnose complications like CPD, and make informed clinical decisions.

References

Dutta, D.C. (2020). Textbook of Obstetrics.

Cunningham, F.G., et al. (2022). Williams Obstetrics.

World Health Organization. (2006). Managing Complications in Pregnancy and Childbirth.

Gabbe, S.G., et al. (2017). Obstetrics: Normal and Problem Pregnancies.

4.2 Maternal pelvis: Types & Diameters

(Ana-i-zanan: aqsam aur aqtar)

Introduction

The maternal pelvis is a bony structure that plays a pivotal role in childbirth, as it forms the birth canal through which the fetus passes during vaginal delivery. Its size, shape, and dimensions influence the mechanism of labor, the likelihood of successful vaginal delivery, and the risk of complications such as cephalopelvic disproportion (CPD).

Anatomy of the Maternal Pelvis

The maternal pelvis is composed of four bones: two innominate (hip) bones, the sacrum, and the coccyx. These are connected by joints and ligaments, forming a rigid yet slightly flexible structure. The pelvis is divided into two regions:

1. False Pelvis (Pelvis Major)

Located above the pelvic brim (linea terminalis).

Supports the gravid uterus but is not directly involved in labor.

Formed by the iliac wings and upper sacrum.

2. True Pelvis (Pelvis Minor)

Located below the pelvic brim.

Forms the birth canal, critical for fetal passage during labor.

Consists of three planes: inlet, midpelvis, and outlet.

Bones of the Pelvis

Innominate Bones (2): Each comprises the ilium, ischium, and pubis, fused at the acetabulum.

Sacrum: A wedge-shaped bone with five fused vertebrae, forming the posterior wall of the pelvis.

Coccyx: A small, mobile bone that can tilt backward during labor to facilitate delivery.

Joints and Ligaments

Symphysis Pubis: A cartilaginous joint connecting the pubic bones, allowing slight movement during labore.

Sacroiliac Joints: Connect the sacrum to the ilium, stabilized by strong ligaments.

Sacrococcygeal Joint: Allows coccyx mobility, aiding feta passage.

Ligaments: Sacrospinous, sacrotuberus, and anterior longitudinal ligaments provide stability.

Planes of the True Pelvis

1. Pelvic Inlet: The upper boundary of the true pelvis, defined by the linear terminalis (iliac crests, iliopectineal line, and sacral promontory).

2. Midpelvis: The narrowest part, at the level of the ischial spines.

3. Pelvic Outlet: The lower boundary, formed by the pubic arch, ischial tuberosities and coccyx.

Types of Maternal Pelvis

The maternal pelvis is classified into four main types based on its shape, as described by Caldwell and Moloy (1933). These types influence the ease of fetal passage during labor. The classification is based on the shape of the pelvic inlet, with variations in the midpelvis and outlet also considered.

1. Gynecoid Pelvis

Prevalence: Most common (50–60% of women).

Shape

Inlet: Oval, with a slightly wider transverse diameter.

Midpelvis: Wide and shallow.

Outlet: Wide pubic arch (80–90°).

Obstetric Significance

Ideal for vaginal delivery due to its rounded shape and adequate diameters.

Facilitates fetal engagement, descent and rotation.

Associated with the lowest risk of CPD.

2. Android Pelvis

Prevalence: More common in men, but found in 20–30% of women.

Shape

Inlet: Heart-shaped or triangular, with a narrower transverse diameter.

Midpelvis: Convergent sidewalls, narrow ischial spines.

Outlet: Narrow pubic arch (<70°).

Obstetric Significance

Associated with a higher risk of CPD due to narrower dimensions.

May lead to prolonged labor, posterior positions, or need for operative delivery (e.g., cesarean section).

3. Anthropoid Pelvis

Prevalence: Found in 20–30% of women, more common in certain populations (e.g., African descent).

Shape

Inlet: Oval, with a wider anteroposterior diameter than transverse.

Midpelvis: Long and narrow.

Outlet: Adequate but elongated.

Obstetric Significance

Favorable for vaginal delivery, especially in occiput posterior or anterior positions.

May prolong labor due to the need for more rotation.

4. Platypelloid Pelvis

Prevalence: Rare (2–5% of women).

Shape

Inlet: Flattened, with a wide transverse diameter and short anteroposterior diameter.

Midpelvis: Wide but shallow.

Outlet: Wide pubic arch.

Obstetric Significance

May cause difficulty in fetal engagement due to the short anteroposterior diameter.

Increased risk of transverse arrest, requiring operative intervention.

Mixed Pelvic Types

In clinical practice, many women have mixed pelvic types (e.g., gynecoid with anthropoid features). The Caldwell-Moloy classification provides a framework, but individual variations require clinical assessment.

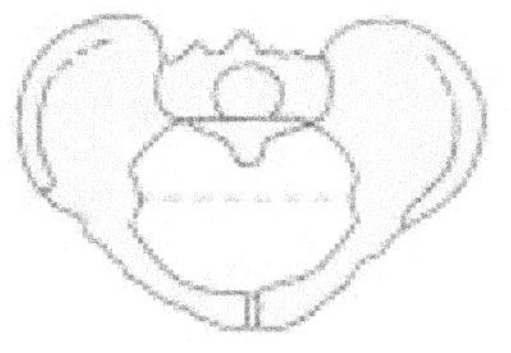	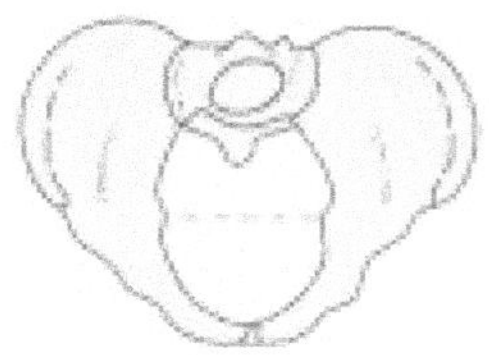	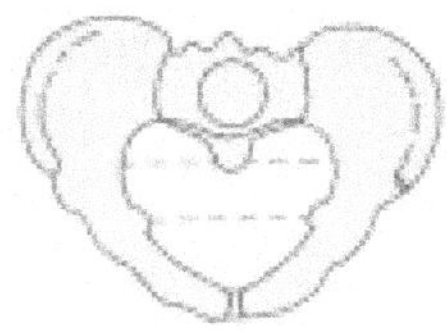	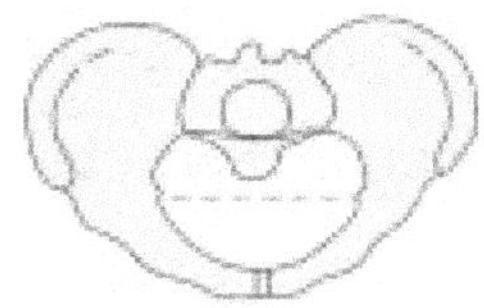
Gynecoid or female type pelvis	Anthropoid or ape type pelvis	Android or male type pelvis	Platypelloid or flat type pelvis

Diameters of the Maternal Pelvis

The diameters of the true pelvis at the inlet, midpelvis and outlet are critical for assessing the feasibility of vaginal delivery. These measurements are compared with fetal skull diameters (e.g., biparietal diameter of 9.5 cm) to evaluate cephalopelvic fit.

1. Pelvic Inlet Diameters

The pelvic inlet is the entry point for the fetal head into the true pelvis.

Anteroposterior (True Conjugate)

Measurement: 11.0–11.5 cm.

Description: From the sacral promontory to the upper inner margin of the symphysis pubis.

Clinical Significance: Determines whether the fetal head can engage. A true conjugate <10 cm suggests inlet contraction.

Obstetric Conjugate

Measurement: 10.5–11.0 cm.

Description: From the sacral promontory to the thickest part of the symphysis pubis (shortest anteroposterior diameter).

Clinical Significance: Most important for engagement; measured indirectly via diagonal conjugate (subtract 1.5–2 cm).

Diagonal Conjugate

Measurement: 12.5–13.0 cm.

Description: From the sacral promontory to the lower inner margin of the symphysis pubis.

Clinical Significance: Measured during vaginal examination (clinically) to estimate obstetric conjugate.

Transverse Diameter

Measurement: 13.0–13.5 cm.

Description: The widest distance between the iliopectineal lines.

Clinical Significance: Accommodates the biparietal diameter of the fetal head (9.5 cm).

Oblique Diameters (Right and Left)

Measurement: ~12.0 cm.

Description: From the sacroiliac joint on one side to the iliopectineal eminence on the opposite side.

Clinical Significance: Facilitates fetal rotation during labor.

2. Midpelvis Diameters

The midpelvis is the narrowest part of the birth canal, at the level of the ischial spines.

Anteroposterior Diameter

Measurement: ~11.5 cm.

Description: From the lower sacrum to the symphysis pubis.

Clinical Significance: Must accommodate the fetal head during descent.

Transverse (Interspinous) Diameter

Measurement: 10.0–10.5 cm.

Description: Distance between the ischial spines.

Clinical Significance: The narrowest pelvic diameter; a measurement <9.5 cm suggests midpelvic contraction, increasing CPD risk.

Posterior Sagittal Diameter

Measurement: ~4.5–5.0 cm.

Description: From the midpoint of the interspinous diameter to the sacrum.

Clinical Significance: Contributes to space for fetal head rotation.

3. Pelvic Outlet Diameters

The pelvic outlet is the exit point of the birth canal.

Anteroposterior Diameter

Measurement: 9.5–11.5 cm.

Description: From the tip of the coccyx to the lower margin of the symphysis pubis (increases with coccyx mobility).

Clinical Significance: Must accommodate the fetal head during delivery; coccyx movement can add 1–2 cm.

Transverse (Intertuberous) Diameter

Measurement: 10.0–11.0 cm.

Description: Distance between the ischial tuberosities.

Clinical Significance: Accommodates the biparietal diameter; <9 cm suggests outlet contraction.

Pubic Arch Angle

Measurement: 80–90° (gynecoid pelvis).

Description: Angle formed by the pubic bones at the symphysis.

Clinical Significance: A narrow angle (<70°) may impede delivery, common in android pelvis.

Table of Maternal Pelvic Diameters

Plane	Diameter	Measurement (cm)	Clinical Significance
Inlet	Anteroposterior (True Conjugate)	11.0–11.5	Determines engagement; <10 cm suggests contraction
	Obstetric Conjugate	10.5–11.0	Shortest AP diameter; critical for head entry
	Diagonal Conjugate	12.5–13.0	Measured clinically to estimate obstetric conjugate
	Transverse	13.0–13.5	Widest diameter; accommodates biparietal diameter
	Oblique	~12.0	Facilitates fetal rotation
Midpelvis	Anteroposterior	~11.5	Accommodates descent
	Transverse (Interspinous)	10.0–10.5	Narrowest diameter; <9.5 cm risks CPD
	Posterior Sagittal	4.5–5.0	Aids rotation and descent
Outlet	Anteroposterior	9.5–11.5	Accommodates delivery; coccyx mobility adds space
	Transverse (Intertuberous)	10.0–11.0	Must fit biparietal diameter; <9 cm risks obstruction
	Pubic Arch Angle	80–90°	Narrow angle may impede delivery

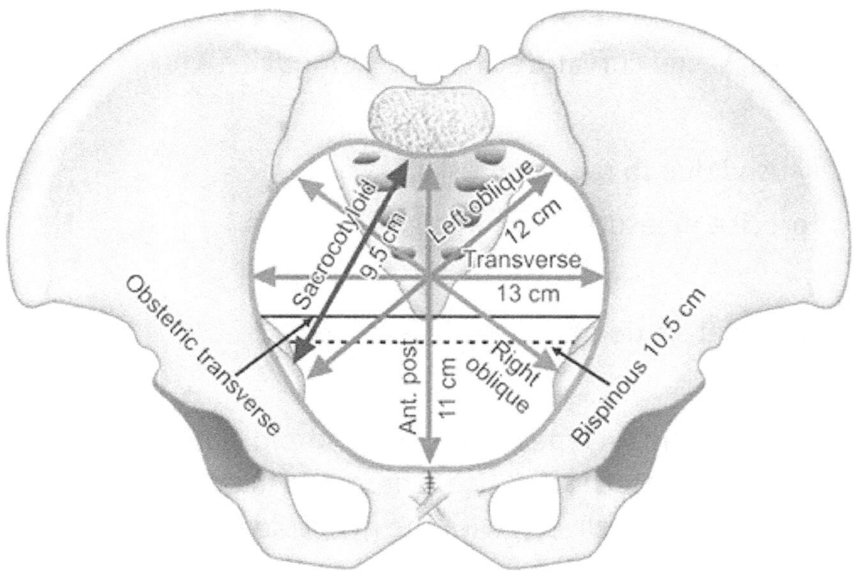

Ant. post, anteroposterior.

Clinical Relevance in Obstetrics

1. Mechanism of Labor

The fetal head must navigate the pelvic inlet, midpelvis and outlet, aligning its diameters (e.g.,suboccipitobregmatic, 9.5 cm) with the maternal pelvic diameters. The gynecoid pelvis is most favorable, while android or platypelloid pelvises may complicate labor.

2. Cephalopelvic Disproportion (CPD)

CPD occurs when fetal skull diameters (e.g., biparietal, 9.5 cm) exceed pelvic diameters, particularly at the midpelvis (interspinous <9.5 cm). Assessed clinically via vaginal examination (e.g., diagonal conjugate) or imaging (e.g., pelvimetry).

3. Fetal Head Engagement

Engagement occurs when the widest part of the fetal head (biparietal diameter) passes the pelvic inlet. A transverse diameter <12 cm or obstetric conjugate <10 cm may prevent engagement.

4. Labor Progression

The midpelvis (interspinous diameter) is critical for fetal descent and rotation. A narrow pubic arch or contracted outlet may cause arrest at delivery.

5. Operative Interventions

Narrow pelvic diameters (e.g., android pelvis) may necessitate cesarean section. Assisted vaginal delivery (forceps or vacuum) may be considered if the outlet is adequate but labor is prolonged.

Clinical Assessment Techniques

Vaginal Examination

Measure the diagonal conjugate to estimate the obstetric conjugate.

Assess ischial spine prominence and pubic arch angle.

Clinical Pelvimetry

Evaluate inlet, midpelvis and outlet dimensions manually.

Note sidewall convergence, sacral curvature and coccyx mobility.

Imaging

X-ray pelvimetry (rarely used due to radiation risks).

Ultrasound or MRI for precise measurements in high-risk cases.

Partogram

Monitors labor progress to detect delays suggestive of CPD.

Conclusion

The maternal pelvis, with its four main types (gynecoid, android, anthropoid, platypelloid) and critical diameters, is a cornerstone of obstetric practice. The pelvic inlet, midpelvis and outlet dimensions determine the feasibility of vaginal delivery, with the gynecoid pelvis being the most favorable.

References

Dutta, D.C. (2020). Textbook of Obstetrics.

Cunningham, F.G., et al. (2022). Williams Obstetrics.

World Health Organization. (2006). Managing Complications in Pregnancy and Childbirth.

Caldwell, W.E., & Moloy, H.C. (1933). Anatomical variations in the female pelvis and their effect on labor.

4.3 Contracted Pelvis

(*Ana-e-munqabiz*)

Introduction

A contracted pelvis is defined as a pelvis with one or more dimensions (inlet, midpelvis, or outlet) significantly smaller than normal, potentially impeding vaginal delivery. It is a major cause of cephalopelvic disproportion (CPD), where the fetal head cannot pass through the maternal pelvis due to size mismatch. The condition is particularly significant in regions with high prevalence of nutritional deficiencies or pelvic deformities.

Definition

A contracted pelvis is characterized by pelvic measurements that are below the normal range, compromising the birth canal's capacity to allow passage of the fetal head. Clinically, it is identified when key pelvic diameters (e.g., obstetric conjugate, interspinous diameter) are reduced, leading to potential obstruction during labor. The threshold for a contracted pelvis varies by population but is generally defined as:

Obstetric conjugate <10 cm (normal: 10.5–11 cm).

Interspinous diameter <9.5 cm (normal: 10–10.5 cm).

Transverse diameter of inlet <12 cm (normal: 13–13.5 cm).

Causes of Contracted Pelvis

The contracted pelvis results from congenital, developmental, or acquired factors that alter pelvic shape or size. Common causes include:

1. Congenital Causes

Developmental Anomalies: Abnormal pelvic shapes (e.g., platypelloid or android pelvis) due to genetic or intrauterine factors.

Congenital Malformations: Conditions like congenital hip dislocation or spinal deformities (e.g., kyphoscoliosis).

Osteogenesis Imperfecta: Rare genetic disorders affecting bone development.

2. Developmental Causes

Nutritional Deficiencies: Rickets or osteomalacia in childhood, leading to pelvic flattening or deformity (common in low-resource settings).

Vitamin D Deficiency: Causes softening of pelvic bones, resulting in a contracted inlet or outlet.

Malnutrition: Stunted pelvic growth due to chronic undernutrition.

3. Acquired Causes

Trauma: Pelvic fractures from accidents, leading to asymmetry or narrowing.

Infection: Tuberculosis or osteomyelitis affecting pelvic bones.

Tumors or Masses: Bone tumors or soft tissue masses compressing the pelvis.

Metabolic Disorders: Conditions like hyperparathyroidism causing bone resorption.

4. Iatrogenic Causes

Surgical Interventions: Previous pelvic surgeries (e.g., fixation of fractures) altering pelvic architecture.

Radiation: Pelvic irradiation in childhood affecting bone growth.

5. Cultural and Environmental Factors

Early Childbearing: Pregnancy before pelvic growth completion (common in adolescent mothers).

Chronic Labor: Prolonged labor in previous pregnancies causing pelvic deformity.

Classification of Contracted Pelvis

The contracted pelvis is classified based on the anatomical plane affected or the underlying cause. The Caldwell-Moloy classification of pelvic shapes (gynecoid, android, anthropoid, platypelloid) is often used to describe associated deformities, with android and platypelloid pelvises more likely to be contracted.

1. By Anatomical Plane

Inlet Contraction

Obstetric conjugate <10 cm or transverse diameter <12 cm.

Common in platypelloid pelvis or rickets.

Prevents fetal head engagement.

Midpelvis Contraction

Interspinous diameter <9.5 cm or convergent sidewalls.

Common in android pelvis or post-traumatic deformities.

Causes arrest of fetal descent or rotation.

Outlet Contraction

Intertuberous diameter <9 cm or pubic arch angle <70°.

Common in android pelvis or sacral deformities.

Impedes delivery of the fetal head.

Combined Contraction: Involvement of two or more planes, often due to severe rickets or trauma.

2. By Cause

Congenital: Deformities like Naegele's pelvis (unilateral sacroiliac joint absence) or Robert's pelvis (bilateral sacroiliac joint absence).

Acquired: Rickets, osteomalacia, or traumatic deformities.

Mixed: Combination of congenital and acquired factors.

3. By Severity

Mild: Slight reduction in diameters, often manageable with vaginal delivery.

Moderate: Significant reduction requiring careful monitoring or trial of labor.

Severe: Grossly contracted pelvis, usually necessitating cesarean section.

Diameters of the Contracted Pelvis

The normal pelvic diameters (described in detail in the maternal pelvis section) are compared with those in a contracted pelvis to assess the degree of obstruction. Key measurements include:

Pelvic Inlet

Obstetric Conjugate: <10 cm (normal: 10.5–11 cm).

Transverse Diameter: <12 cm (normal: 13–13.5 cm).

Diagonal Conjugate: <11.5 cm (normal: 12.5–13 cm).

Midpelvis

Interspinous Diameter: <9.5 cm (normal: 10–10.5 cm).

Posterior Sagittal Diameter: <4 cm (normal: 4.5–5 cm).

Pelvic Outlet

Intertuberous Diameter: <9 cm (normal: 10–11 cm).

Anteroposterior Diameter: <9 cm (normal: 9.5–11.5 cm).

Diagnosis of Contracted Pelvis

Accurate diagnosis is essential to plan delivery and prevent complications. Diagnosis involves clinical, imaging and labor-based assessments.

1. Clinical Assessment

History

Past obstetric history: Previous prolonged labor, operative delivery, or CPD.

Medical history: Rickets, pelvic trauma, or congenital deformities.

Anthropometric factors: Short stature (<150 cm), limping, or spinal deformities.

Physical Examination

External Pelvimetry: Measure intertuberous diameter (normal: 10–11 cm) using a pelvimeter or knuckles. Assess pubic arch angle (normal: 80–90°).

Vaginal Examination

Measure diagonal conjugate (normal: 12.5–13 cm) by reaching the sacral promontory.

Assess ischial spine prominence, sidewall convergence, and sacral curvature.

Note coccyx mobility and pubic arch width.

General Examination: Look for signs of rickets (e.g., bowlegs, kyphosis) or short stature.

2. Imaging

Ultrasound: Measures fetal head size (e.g., biparietal diameter, 9.5 cm) to assess cephalopelvic fit.

X-ray Pelvimetry (rarely used due to radiation risks): Provides precise measurements of inlet, midpelvis, and outlet.

MRI or CT: Used in complex cases to assess pelvic dimensions and deformities (e.g., post-traumatic pelvis).

3D Imaging: Emerging tool for accurate pelvic and fetal measurements.

3. Labor-Based Assessment

Trial of Labor: In cases of borderline contraction, labor progress is monitored using a partogram to assess descent, rotation, and molding.

Signs of CP: Failure of descent, excessive molding, caput succedaneum, or prolonged labor.

Obstetric Implications

A contracted pelvis significantly impacts labor and delivery, increasing the risk of complications for both mother and fetus.

1. Maternal Complications

Prolonged or Obstructed Labor: Due to failure of fetal head engagement or descent.

Uterine Rupture: From prolonged labor or excessive force in severe contraction.

Fistula Formation: Prolonged pressure on pelvic tissues leading to vesicovaginal or rectovaginal fistulae.

Infections: Increased risk of postpartum endometritis or sepsis.

Pelvic Trauma: Soft tissue injuries or pubic symphysis separation.

2. Fetal Complications

Fetal Distress: Due to prolonged labor or cord compression.

Intracranial Hemorrhage: From excessive molding or trauma.

Asphyxia: Resulting from delayed delivery.

Stillbirth or Neonatal Death: In severe cases of obstructed labor.

3. Labor

Inlet Contraction: Prevents engagement, leading to failure to progress in the first stage.

Midpelvis Contraction: Causes arrest of descent or rotation, often in the second stage.

Outlet Contraction: Impedes delivery, leading to deep transverse arrest or posterior positions.

Management of Contracted Pelvis

Management depends on the degree of contraction, fetal size, presentation and labor progress. The goal is to ensure safe delivery while minimizing maternal and fetal risks.

1. Antenatal Management

Screening and Risk Assessment

Identify high-risk women (e.g., short stature, history of rickets, or previous CPD) during antenatal care (ANC). Use clinical pelvimetry and ultrasound to assess pelvic dimensions and fetal size.

Counseling

Educate women about the potential need for cesarean section.

Discuss birth, including hospital delivery and access to emergency obstetric care.

Nutritional Support

Address deficiencies (e.g., vitamin D, calcium) to optimize pelvic health in future pregnancies.

2. Intrapartum Management

Trial of Labor

Indicated in mild or borderline contraction with a favorable fetal presentation (e.g., vertex, occiput anterior).

Monitor labor progress with a partogram, noting cervical dilatation, fetal descent, and molding.

Ensure access to operative facilities in case of failure to progress.

Cesarean Section

Indicated for severe contraction, significant CPD, or failed trial of labor.

Preferred in cases of inlet contraction (<10 cm obstetric conjugate) or midpelvis contraction (<9.5 cm interspinous).

Assisted Vaginal Delivery

Forceps or vacuum extraction may be considered in outlet contraction with adequate descent and rotation. Requires skilled personnel and careful assessment to avoid trauma.

Symphysiotomy (rare)

Used in resource-limited settings for outlet contraction when cesarean section is unavailable. Involves dividing the symphysis pubis to increase pelvic diameter (risks include instability and infection).

3. Postpartum Management

Monitoring: Assess for postpartum hemorrhage, infections, or fistulae.

Rehabilitation: Physiotherapy for pelvic injuries or deformities.

Counseling: Discuss future pregnancies, emphasizing planned cesarean section for severe cases.

Prevention

Nutritional Interventions: Address vitamin D and calcium deficiencies in childhood to prevent rickets and osteomalacia.

Health Education: Promote ANC attendance to identify high-risk cases early.

Public Health Programs: Strengthen maternal health programs to provide access to imaging and skilled care.

Adolescent Health: Delay early pregnancies to allow complete pelvic growth.

Conclusion

The contracted pelvis is a significant obstetric challenge that increases the risk of CPD and complications during labor. Its causes range from congenital deformities to acquired conditions like rickets or trauma. Accurate diagnosis through clinical pelvimetry, imaging, and labor monitoring is crucial for planning delivery. Management strategies, including trial of labor, cesarean section, or assisted delivery, depend on the degree of contraction and fetal factors.

References

Dutta, D.C. (2020). Textbook of Obstetrics.

Cunningham, F.G., et al. (2022). Williams Obstetrics.

World Health Organization. (2006). Managing Complications in Pregnancy and Childbirth.

4.4 Cephalo-Pelvic Disproportion/CPD

(*Rasi Hauzi Adm-i-tanasub*)

Introduction

Cephalopelvic disproportion (CPD) is a condition in which the fetal head is too large or the maternal pelvis is too small to allow for vaginal delivery, leading to potential obstruction during labor. CPD is a leading cause of dystocia (difficult labor) and is associated with significant maternal and fetal complications if not managed appropriately. It requires careful assessment and decision-making to determine the safest mode of delivery, often necessitating operative interventions such as cesarean section.

Definition

CPD is defined as a mismatch between the size or position of the fetal head and the maternal pelvic dimensions, preventing the fetus from passing through the birth canal. It can be absolute (no possibility of vaginal delivery due to significant disproportion) or relative (dependent on fetal position, molding, or labor dynamics). CPD is typically diagnosed when labor fails to progress despite adequate uterine contractions, or when clinical or imaging assessments confirm incompatible fetal and pelvic measurements.

Causes of Cephalopelvic Disproportion

CPD results from factors related to the fetus, the maternal pelvis or both. These can be categorized as follows

1. Fetal Factors

Macrosomia: Fetal weight >4,000 g, increasing biparietal diameter (BPD, normal: 9.5 cm) or head circumference.

Abnormal Fetal Presentation

Deflexed presentations (e.g., occipitofrontal diameter, 11.5 cm, or supraoccipitomental, 13.5 cm) increase the presenting diameter.

Brow or face presentations present larger diameters, complicating passage.

Fetal Anomalies: Hydrocephalus or other conditions enlarging the fetal head.

Post-term Pregnancy: Prolonged gestation leading to larger fetal size.

Multiple Gestation: Increased fetal head size or malpresentation in twins.

2. Maternal Pelvic Factors

Contracted Pelvis

Inlet contraction: Obstetric conjugate <10 cm or transverse diameter <12 cm.

Midpelvis contraction: Interspinous diameter <9.5 cm.

Outlet contraction: Intertuberous diameter <9 cm or narrow pubic arch (<70°).

Pelvic Deformities

Congenital: Naegele's pelvis, Robert's pelvis, or kyphoscoliosis.

Acquired: Rickets, osteomalacia, or pelvic fractures.

Pelvic Shape: Android or platypelloid pelvises, less favorable than gynecoid.

Soft Tissue Obstruction: Pelvic tumors, fibroids, or ovarian cysts narrowing the birth canal.

3. Combined Factors

Relative CPD occurs when a borderline pelvis meets a large fetus or suboptimal presentation. Dynamic factors, such as inadequate fetal head molding or poor uterine contractions, exacerbate disproportion.

Risk Factors

Maternal short stature, obesity, or diabetes (increasing macrosomia risk).

Fetal anomalies or post-term pregnancy.

Classification of CPD

CPD is classified based on its severity and clinical implications:

1. Absolute CPD

Severe mismatch (e.g., obstetric conjugate <8 cm with normal fetal head size).

Vaginal delivery is impossible, requiring cesarean section.

Common in severe pelvic deformities or extreme macrosomia.

2. Relative CPD

Borderline mismatch that may allow vaginal delivery with optimal conditions (e.g., good fetal head flexion, adequate molding).

May resolve with labor progression or require operative intervention if labor stalls.

3. Dynamic CPD

Arises during labor due to malposition (e.g., occiput posterior) or failure of head molding. May be managed with positional changes or assisted delivery.

Diagnosis of Cephalopelvic Disproportion

Accurate diagnosis of CPD is critical to guide delivery planning. It involves antenatal screening, intrapartum monitoring, and clinical or imaging assessments.

1. Antenatal Diagnosis

History: Previous CPD, prolonged labor, or cesarean section for dystocia.

Risk factors: Short stature (<150 cm), history of rickets, pelvic trauma, or macrosomia.

Clinical Pelvimetry

Vaginal Examination: Measure diagonal conjugate (<11.5 cm suggests inlet contraction). Assess ischial spine prominence, sidewall convergence, sacral curvature, and pubic arch angle.

External Pelvimetry: Measure intertuberous diameter (<9 cm indicates outlet contraction).

Ultrasound: Measure fetal head dimensions (BPD, head circumference) and estimated fetal weight (EFW). Compare with pelvic dimensions to predict fit.

2. Intrapartum Diagnosis

Monitor using a partogram to assess cervical dilatation, fetal descent, and station.

Signs of CPD include:

Failure of descent despite adequate contractions.

Arrest of dilatation in the active phase (e.g., <1 cm/hour in nulliparas).

Excessive molding (+2 or +3) or caput succedaneum.

Vaginal Examination

Palpate sutures and fontanelles to assess fetal position (e.g., occiput posterior, deflexed head).

Note lack of engagement or high station after rupture of membranes.

Clinical Signs

Prolonged first or second stage of labor.

Fetal distress (e.g., abnormal heart rate patterns).

Maternal exhaustion or signs of obstruction (e.g., Bandl's ring).

3. Trial of Labor

Indicated in suspected relative CPD to assess whether vaginal delivery is possible. Requires close monitoring with a partogram, fetal heart rate assessment, and access to emergency obstetric care.

Contraindicated in absolute CPD or high-risk cases (e.g., severe inlet contraction).

Complications

1. Maternal Complications

Prolonged Labor: Increases risk of maternal exhaustion, dehydration, and infection.

Uterine Rupture: Rare but serious, especially in multiparous women with obstructed labor.

Vesicovaginal/Rectovaginal Fistulae: From prolonged pressure on pelvic tissues.

Postpartum Hemorrhage: Due to uterine atony or trauma.

Pelvic Trauma: Soft tissue injuries or pubic symphysis separation.

2. Fetal Complications

Fetal Distress: Due to cord compression or reduced placental perfusion.

Intracranial Hemorrhage: From excessive molding or trauma during prolonged labor.

Birth Asphyxia: Resulting from delayed delivery.

Stillbirth or Neonatal Death: In severe, untreated cases.

3. Labor

Inlet CPD: Prevents engagement, leading to failure to progress in the first stage.

Midpelvis CPD: Causes arrest of descent or rotation, often in the second stage.

Outlet CPD: Impedes delivery, leading to deep transverse arrest or persistent posterior positions.

Management of Cephalopelvic Disproportion

Management depends on the severity of CPD, fetal condition and labor progress. The goal is to ensure safe delivery while minimizing maternal and fetal risks.

1. Antenatal Management

Screening and Risk Assessment: Identify high-risk women during antenatal care (ANC) using clinical pelvimetry and ultrasound. Assess fetal size, presentation and maternal pelvic dimensions.

Counseling: Educate women about the possibility of cesarean section or assisted delivery. Discuss birth preparedness, including hospital delivery and access to emergency obstetric care (EmOC).

Preventive Measures: Manage maternal conditions like diabetes to reduce macrosomia risk. Optimize nutrition to prevent pelvic deformities .

2. Intrapartum Management

Trial of Labor: Indicated for relative or borderline CPD with favorable conditions (e.g., vertex presentation, good contractions). Monitor labor with a partogram, fetal heart rate, and vaginal examinations. Use oxytocin augmentation cautiously if contractions are inadequate, ensuring no absolute CPD. Discontinue if no progress after 2–4 hours in the active phase or if fetal distress occurs.

Cesarean Section: Indicated for absolute CPD, failed trial of labor or fetal distress. Ensures safe delivery but carries risks (e.g., infection, bleeding).

Preferred in cases of:

Severe inlet contraction (<10 cm obstetric conjugate).

Midpelvis contraction (<9.5 cm interspinous diameter).

Macrosomia with EFW >4,500 g or abnormal presentation (e.g., brow).

Assisted Vaginal Delivery: Forceps or vacuum extraction may be considered in relative CPD with adequate descent and rotation (e.g., second stage arrest at outlet). Requires skilled personnel, proper fetal positioning (e.g., occiput anterior), and no significant pelvic contraction. Contraindicated in midpelvis arrest or absolute CPD.

Symphysiotomy (rare): Used in resource-limited settings for outlet CPD when cesarean section is unavailable. Involves dividing the symphysis pubis to increase pelvic diameter (risks include pelvic instability and infection).

3. Postpartum Management

Monitoring: Assess for postpartum hemorrhage, infection or fistulae, especially after prolonged labor. Monitor neonatal condition for signs of asphyxia or trauma.

Rehabilitation: Physiotherapy for pelvic or perineal injuries. Psychological support for women experiencing traumatic labor.

Counseling: Discuss future pregnancies, emphasizing planned cesarean section for absolute CPD. Provide contraception advice to space pregnancies.

Prevention

Antenatal Screening: Routine ANC to identify risk factors (e.g., short stature, macrosomia) using ultrasound and pelvimetry.

Nutritional Interventions: Address childhood malnutrition, rickets, or vitamin D deficiency to prevent pelvic deformities.

Maternal Health Management: Control diabetes to reduce macrosomia risk. Promote healthy weight gain during pregnancy.

Health Education: Encourage early ANC visits and institutional deliveries. Raise awareness about CPD risks and the importance of skilled care.

Public Health Programs: Strengthen maternal health infrastructure to ensure access to CEmOC.

Conclusion

Cephalopelvic disproportion is a critical obstetric condition that arises from a mismatch between the fetal head and maternal pelvis, leading to potential labor obstruction. It is caused by fetal factors (e.g., macrosomia, abnormal presentation) or maternal factors (e.g., contracted pelvis, deformities). Diagnosis involves antenatal screening, clinical pelvimetry, ultrasound, and intrapartum monitoring. Management ranges from trial of labor in relative CPD to cesarean section in absolute cases.

References

Dutta, D.C. (2020). Textbook of Obstetrics.

Cunningham, F.G., et al. (2022). Williams Obstetrics.

World Health Organization. (2006). Managing Complications in Pregnancy and Childbirth.

J'Kishore's National Health Programs of India: 14/E 2022.

Long Answer Questions (LAQs)

1. Describe the female pelvis with its types and diameters.
2. Describe the fetal skull including sutures and fontanelles.
3. Explain the diameters of fetal skull and their obstetric importance.
4. Define contracted pelvis and discuss its types.
5. Explain cephalo-pelvic disproportion (CPD) and its significance in labour.

Short Answer Questions (SAQs)

1. Define female pelvis.
2. Name the bones forming fetal skull.
3. What is contracted pelvis?
4. Define CPD.
5. Name any two pelvic diameters.

Multiple Choice Questions (1 Mark Each)

1. Female pelvis is adapted mainly for:

A. Walking B. Sitting

C. Childbirth D. Running

Ans: C. Childbirth

2. The widest transverse diameter of fetal skull is:

A. Biparietal diameter B. Suboccipito-bregmatic

C. Occipito-frontal D. Mento-vertical

Ans: A. Biparietal diameter

3. Normal biparietal diameter is about:

A. 7 cm B. 8 cm

C. 9.5 cm D. 11 cm

Ans: C. 9.5 cm

4. Pelvis with reduced inlet is called:

A. Gynecoid B. Android

C. Contracted pelvis D. Anthropoid

Ans: C. Contracted pelvis

5. CPD means:

A. Large fetus B. Small pelvis

C. Disproportion between head & pelvis D. Breech presentation

Ans: C. Disproportion between head & pelvis

4. Which suture lies between parietal bones?

A. Sagittal suture B. Coronal

C. Lambdoid D. Frontal

Ans: A. Sagittal suture

5. The most favorable pelvis for labour is:

A. Android B. Gynecoid

C. Platypelloid D. Anthropoid

Ans: B. Gynecoid

6. Largest AP diameter of fetal skull is:

A. Suboccipito-bregmatic. B. Occipito-frontal

C. Mento-vertical D. Biparietal

Ans: C. Mento-vertical

7. Contracted pelvis mainly causes:

A. Preterm labour B. Obstructed labour

C. Postpartum hemorrhage D. Abortion

Ans: B. Obstructed labour

8. Fontanelle felt in normal labour is:

A. Posterior B. Anterior

C. Mastoid D. Temporal

Ans: B. Anterior

05

Fetopelvic Relationship & Fetus in Utero

(Rahim-wa-Ana se janin ka Rishta aur Rahim me janin ka irteqa)

5.1 *Wid-ah* (Lie)
5.2 *Maji* (Presentation)
5.3 *Juz-ul-maji* (Presenting part)
5.4 *Wad-ah/mauqif* (Attitude)
5.5 *Makam* (Denominator)
5.6 *Wad-yeeyah* (Position)
5.7 *Qabalati imtehan ke tareeqe: Batini wa mahbili* (Methods of Obstetrical examination: Abdominal & Vaginal)

Learning Objective (At the end of the session, the students should be able to)

Describe the Lie, Presentation, Presenting Part, Attitude, Denominator & Position of the fetus

Demonstrate the Methods of Obstetrical examination including Leopold maneuvers (Abdominal) and Pelvic (Internal) examination

5. Fetopelvic Relationship and Fetus in Utero

(*Rahim-wa-Ana se janin ka Rishta aur Rahim me janin ka irteqa*)

Introduction

The fetopelvic relationship describes the dynamic interaction between the fetus and the maternal pelvis, which determines the feasibility of vaginal delivery and influences labor outcomes. It involves assessing the fetus's orientation, size, and position relative to the maternal pelvic dimensions and shape. The fetus in utero refers to the developing fetus within the amniotic cavity, and its characteristics —lie, presentation, presenting part, attitude, denominator, and position - are critical for understanding labor dynamics and diagnosing complications such as cephalopelvic disproportion (CPD).

Fetus in Utero

The fetus's orientation within the uterus is described using specific obstetric terms that reflect its relationship to the maternal pelvis. These terms are assessed antenatally and intrapartum to predict labor progression and potential complications.

5.1 Lie (*Wid-ah*)

Definition: The relationship of the fetal long axis (spine or longitudinal axis) to the maternal long axis (spine or longitudinal axis of the uterus).

Types

1. Longitudinal Lie

The fetal spine is parallel to the maternal spine. Prevalence: ~95–97% of term pregnancies.

Subtypes

Cephalic: Head is the presenting part (most common).

Breech: Buttocks or feet are the presenting part.

Clinical Significance: Optimal for vaginal delivery, as it aligns the fetus with the birth canal.

2. Transverse Lie

The fetal spine is perpendicular to the maternal spine. Prevalence: ~0.5–1% at term.

Often associated with shoulder presentation or placenta previa.

Clinical Significance: Usually incompatible with vaginal delivery; requires cesarean section or external cephalic version (ECV) to convert to longitudinal lie.

3. Oblique Lie

The fetal spine is at an angle (neither parallel nor perpendicular) to the maternal spine.

Prevalence: Rare, often unstable, and may convert to longitudinal or transverse lie as labor progresses.

Clinical Significance: May resolve spontaneously or require ECV; persistent oblique lie often necessitates cesarean section.

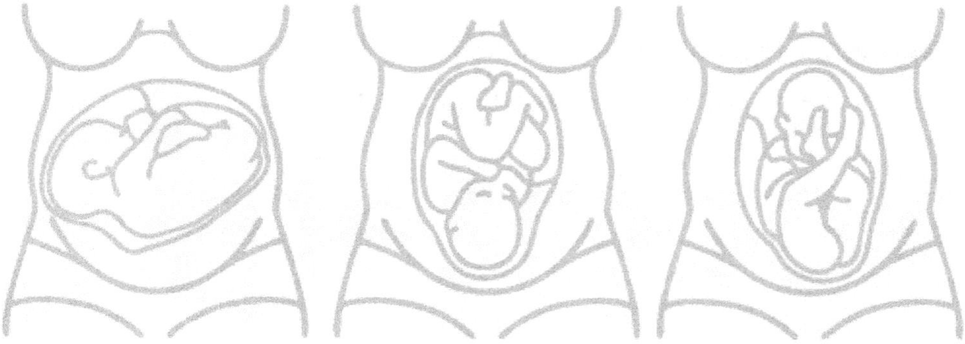

Assessment

Antenatal: Leopold's maneuvers or ultrasound to confirm fetal spine orientation.

Intrapartum: Vaginal examination to assess presenting part and lie.

Clinical Implications

Longitudinal lie facilitates engagement and descent. Transverse or oblique lie increases risks of cord prolapse, obstructed labor, or uterine rupture, requiring prompt intervention.

5.2 Presentation (*Maji*)

Definition: The fetal body part that lies closest to or engages with the maternal pelvic inlet, entering the birth canal first.

Types

1. Cephalic Presentation (~95% at term)

Vertex: Fetal head flexed, presenting the suboccipitobregmatic diameter (9.5 cm).

Brow: Head partially extended, presenting the supraoccipitomental diameter (13.5 cm).

Face: Head fully extended, presenting the submentobregmatic diameter (9.5 cm).

Clinical Significance: Vertex is most favorable for vaginal delivery; brow and face presentations increase CPD risk due to larger diameters.

2. Breech Presentation (~3–4% at term)

Complete: Hips and knees flexed, buttocks presenting.

Frank: Hips flexed, knees extended, buttocks presenting.

Footling: One or both feet presenting.

Clinical Significance: Breech delivery is riskier due to potential head entrapment or cord prolapse; often managed with ECV or cesarean section.

3. Shoulder Presentation (~0.5%)

Shoulder, arm, or trunk presents, associated with transverse lie.

Clinical Significance: Incompatible with vaginal delivery; requires cesarean section.

4. Compound Presentation (rare)

Multiple fetal parts present (e.g., hand alongside head).

Clinical Significance: Increases risk of labor obstruction or trauma.

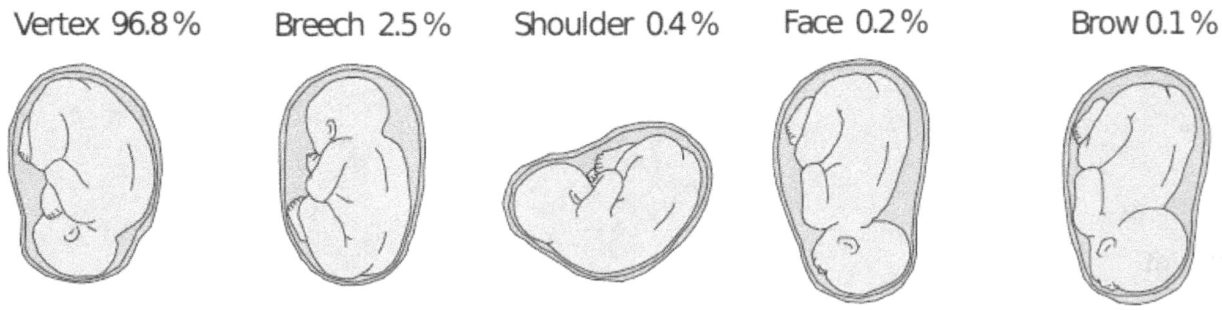

Assessment

Antenatal: Ultrasound or Leopold's maneuvers to identify the presenting part.

Intrapartum: Vaginal examination to palpate presenting part (e.g., sutures/fontanelles for cephalic, sacrum for breech).

Clinical Implications

Vertex presentation optimizes fetopelvic fit.

Non-vertex presentations (breech, shoulder, brow) increase complications, often requiring operative delivery.

5.3 Presenting part (*Juz-ul-maji*)

Definition: The specific portion of the fetus that is foremost in the birth canal and engages with the maternal pelvis during labor.

Cephalic

Vertex: Occipital region (suboccipitobregmatic diameter).

Brow: Forehead (supraoccipitomental diameter).

Face: Chin (submentobregmatic diameter).

Breech

Complete/Frank: Buttocks.

Footling: Foot or feet.

Shoulder: Scapula, arm, or trunk.

Compound: Combination (e.g., head and hand).

Measurement of Presenting Diameters

Vertex (flexed): Suboccipitobregmatic (9.5 cm).

Vertex (deflexed): Occipitofrontal (11.5 cm).

Brow: Supraoccipitomental (13.5 cm).

Face: Submentobregmatic (9.5 cm).

Clinical Significance

The presenting part determines the diameter entering the pelvis, affecting labor progression.

Smaller diameters (e.g., suboccipitobregmatic) facilitate vaginal delivery, while larger diameters (e.g., supraoccipitomental) increase CPD risk.

Assessment

Antenatal: Ultrasound to confirm presenting part.

Intrapartum: Vaginal examination to palpate landmarks (e.g., fontanelles, sacrum).

Clinical Implications

Optimal presenting part (vertex, flexed) aligns with pelvic dimensions.

Non-optimal parts (e.g., brow, footling breech) may require cesarean section.

5.4 Attitude (*Wad-ah/mauqif*)

Definition: The relationship of fetal body parts to one another, particularly the degree of flexion or extension of the fetal head and limbs.

Types

Full Flexion

Head flexed, chin on chest, presenting suboccipitobregmatic diameter (9.5 cm).

Common in vertex presentation.

Clinical Significance: Optimal for vaginal delivery, presenting the smallest diameter.

Partial Flexion

Head neutral, presenting occipitofrontal diameter (11.5 cm).

Clinical Significance: May prolong labor; may require rotation or intervention.

Partial Extension

Head partially extended, presenting occipitomental diameter (12.5–13 cm).

Common in brow presentation.

Clinical Significance: Often incompatible with vaginal delivery due to large diameter.

Full Extension

Head fully extended, presenting submentobregmatic diameter (9.5 cm).

Common in face presentation.

Clinical Significance: Vaginal delivery possible if mento-anterior, but mento-posterior often requires cesarean section.

Breech

Complete: Hips and knees flexed.

Frank: Hips flexed, knees extended.

Footling: Hips and knees extended.

Assessment

Antenatal: Ultrasound to visualize head and limb posture.

Intrapartum: Vaginal examination to palpate sutures/fontanelles (e.g., anterior fontanelle in deflexed positions).

Clinical Implications

Full flexion optimizes fetopelvic fit.

Deflexion or extension increases presenting diameter, raising CPD risk.

5.5 Denominator (*Makam*)

Definition: The specific fetal anatomical landmark used as a reference point to describe the position of the presenting part relative to the maternal pelvis.

The denominators of various presentation are:

Cephalic (Vertex): Occiput (O).

Cephalic (Face): Mentum (chin, M).

Breech: Sacrum (S).

Shoulder: Scapula (Sc).

Clinical Significance

The denominator helps identify the fetal position (e.g., occiput anterior, mento-posterior).

Assessment

Antenatal: Ultrasound to identify the denominator.

Intrapartum: Vaginal examination to palpate landmarks (e.g., occiput via sutures, mentum in face presentation).

Clinical Implications

Accurate identification of the denominator is essential for diagnosing malpositions and planning interventions.

5.6 Position (Wad-yeeyah)

Definition: The relationship of the denominator (reference point of the presenting part) to the maternal pelvis, described as anterior, posterior, or transverse, and right or left.

Cephalic (Vertex)

Occiput Anterior (OA): Occiput faces maternal pubis (e.g., left occiput anterior, LOA; right occiput anterior, ROA).

Occiput Posterior (OP): Occiput faces maternal sacrum (e.g., LOP, ROP).

Occiput Transverse (OT): Occiput faces maternal side (e.g., LOT, ROT).

Cephalic (Face)

Mento-Anterior (MA): Chin faces maternal pubis (e.g., LMA, RMA).

Mento-Posterior (MP): Chin faces maternal sacrum (e.g., LMP, RMP).

Breech

Sacrum Anterior (SA): Sacrum faces maternal pubis (e.g., LSA, RSA).

Sacrum Posterior (SP): Sacrum faces maternal sacrum.

Sacrum Transverse (ST): Sacrum faces maternal side.

Shoulder

Scapula anterior, posterior, or transverse.

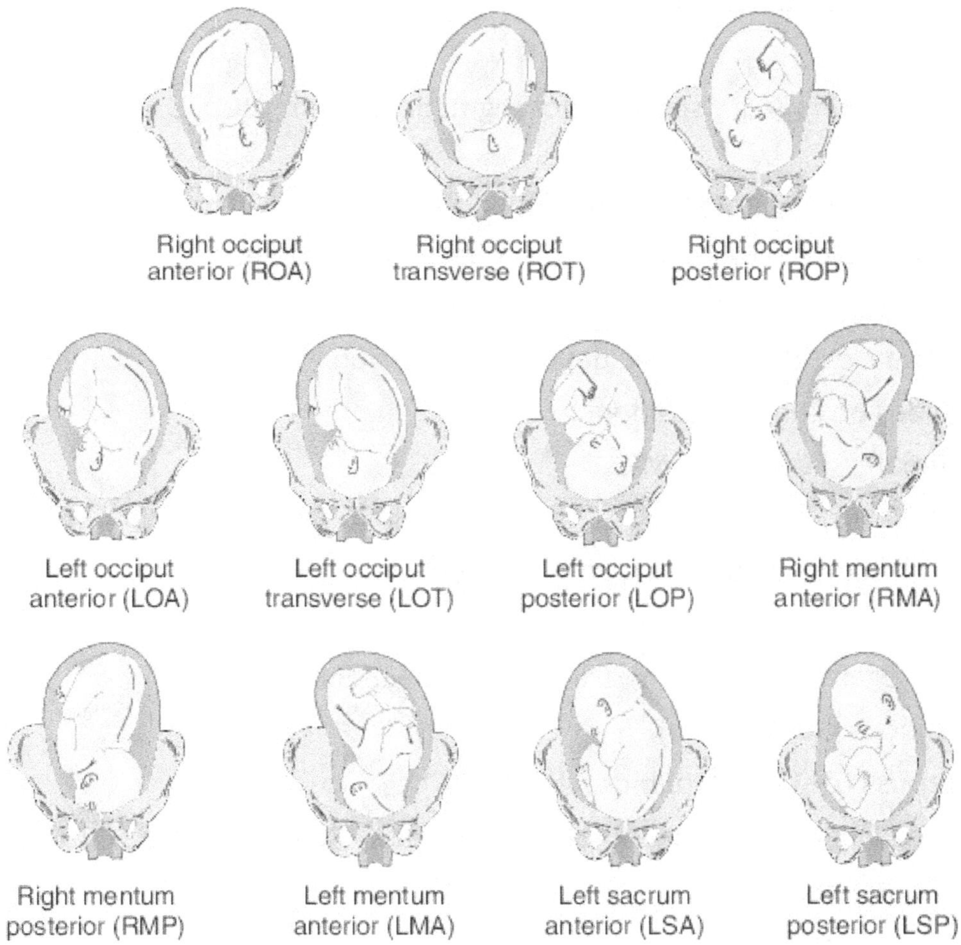

Clinical Significance

OA: Most favorable for vaginal delivery, aligning with pelvic outlet.

OP: May prolong labor, cause back pain, or require rotation (manual or spontaneous) to OA.

OT: Often transient; persistent OT may lead to transverse arrest.

MA: Allows vaginal delivery in face presentation if pelvic dimensions are adequate.

MP: Often incompatible with vaginal delivery due to inability to rotate.

Assessment

Antenatal: Ultrasound to visualize denominator orientation.

Intrapartum: Vaginal examination to palpate sutures/fontanelles (e.g., anterior fontanelle in OP, posterior fontanelle in OA).

Clinical Implications

Malpositions (e.g., OP, MP) increase labor duration and CPD risk.

Accurate position assessment guides maneuvers (e.g., manual rotation) or operative decisions.

Fetopelvic Relationship

The fetopelvic relationship integrates the above fetal characteristics with the maternal pelvis to determine labor feasibility and outcomes.

1. Components of the Fetopelvic Relationship

Passenger (Fetus)

Size: Fetal head diameters (e.g., suboccipitobregmatic, 9.5 cm; BPD, 9.5 cm) compared to pelvic diameters.

Lie: Longitudinal (optimal) vs. transverse/oblique.

Presentation: Vertex (favorable) vs. breech, brow, face, or shoulder.

Presenting Part: Affects diameter entering the pelvis.

Attitude: Flexion (smallest diameter) vs. deflexion/extension.

Denominator: Guides position assessment.

Position: OA (optimal) vs. OP, OT, or MP.

Passage (Maternal Pelvis)

Types: Gynecoid (ideal), android, anthropoid, platypelloid.

Diameters

Inlet: Obstetric conjugate (10.5–11 cm), transverse (13–13.5 cm).

Midpelvis: Interspinous (10–10.5 cm).

Outlet: Intertuberous (10–11 cm), pubic arch (80–90°).

Contraction: Reduced diameters (e.g., obstetric conjugate <10 cm) increase CPD risk.

Powers (Uterine Contractions)

Adequate contractions facilitate descent and rotation.

Inadequate contractions exacerbate relative CPD.Psyche (Maternal Psychological State)

Anxiety or exhaustion can impair labor progress.

Supportive care enhances cooperation.

2. Interactions in Labor

Engagement: Occurs when the widest fetal head diameter (BPD, 9.5 cm) passes the pelvic inlet. Requires obstetric conjugate >10 cm and favorable presentation (vertex, flexed).

Descent: Fetal head moves through the midpelvis (interspinous >9.5 cm), aided by flexion and holding.

Rotation: Fetal head rotates to align with the pelvic axis (e.g., OA in gynecoid pelvis).

OP or OT positions may require manual or spontaneous rotation.

Expulsion: Fetal head passes the outlet (intertuberous >9 cm), facilitated by coccyx mobility.

Molding: Cranial bones overlap at sutures, reducing head diameter to fit the pelvis.

Excessive molding (+3, irreducible) indicates CPD.

3. Optimal Fetopelvic Relationship

Fetal Characteristics: Longitudinal lie, vertex presentation, full flexion, occiput anterior, BPD 9.5 cm.

Pelvic Characteristics: Gynecoid pelvis, obstetric conjugate >10.5 cm, interspinous >10 cm, intertuberous >10 cm.

Outcome: Smooth engagement, descent, rotation, and vaginal delivery.

Clinical Assessment

Accurate assessment of the fetopelvic relationship and fetal orientation is critical for diagnosing complications and planning delivery.

1. Antenatal Assessment

History

Previous CPD, prolonged labor, or cesarean section.

Risk factors: Short stature, macrosomia, or pelvic deformities.

Leopold's Maneuvers: Palpate fundus (lie), lower pole (presentation), and sides (position).

Ultrasound

Confirm lie, presentation, attitude, position, and denominator.

Measure BPD, head circumference, and EFW to assess fetopelvic fit.

Clinical Pelvimetry

Measure diagonal conjugate, ischial spines, and pubic arch to assess pelvic adequacy.

2. Intrapartum Assessment

Vaginal Examination: Palpate sutures/fontanelles to determine presentation, attitude, position, and denominator.

Assess station (e.g., 0 at ischial spines) and molding.

Partogram: Monitor cervical dilatation, descent, and contractions. Signs of CPD: Arrest of dilatation or descent, excessive molding (+3).

Fetal Heart Rate Monitoring: Detect distress (e.g., decelerations) indicating obstruction or malposition.

Obstetric Implications

An unfavorable fetopelvic relationship increases the risk of complications:

1. Cephalopelvic Disproportion (CPD)

Occurs when fetal head diameters (e.g., BPD 9.5 cm) exceed pelvic dimensions (e.g., interspinous <9.5 cm).

Absolute CPD (severe mismatch) requires cesarean section.

Relative CPD (e.g., deflexed head) may resolve with optimal positioning or molding.

2. Prolonged or Obstructed Labor

Malpositions (e.g., OP, OT) or malpresentations (e.g., brow) prolong labor.

Increases maternal risks (e.g., exhaustion, fistula) and fetal risks (e.g., asphyxia, trauma).

3. Fetal Distress

Cord compression or prolonged labor may cause abnormal heart rate patterns.

Requires urgent intervention (e.g., cesarean section).

4. Maternal and Fetal Trauma

Excessive molding or caput indicates obstruction.

Maternal risks include perineal tears or pelvic injury.

Management

Management aims to optimize the fetopelvic relationship and ensure safe delivery.

1. Antenatal Management

Screening: Routine ANC to assess lie, presentation, position, and fetopelvic fit via ultrasound and pelvimetry.

Interventions: ECV for breech or transverse lie at 36–37 weeks (success rate ~50%). Manage macrosomia (e.g., control maternal diabetes).

2. Intrapartum Management

Optimizing Fetopelvic Relationship: Maternal positions (e.g., hands-and-knees for OP) to facilitate rotation. Ensure adequate contractions with oxytocin if indicated (avoid in absolute CPD).

Trial of Labor: For relative CPD, vertex presentation, and favorable position (e.g., OA). Monitor with partogram and fetal heart rate. Discontinue if no progress or distress occurs.

Cesarean Section: Indicated for absolute CPD, persistent malpresentation (e.g., brow, MP), or failed trial of labor.

Assisted Vaginal Delivery: Forceps or vacuum for second-stage arrest with OA position and adequate descent. Contraindicated in midpelvis CPD or high station.

Manual Rotation: For OP or OT positions to convert to OA, performed by skilled providers.

3. Postpartum Management

Monitoring: Assess for hemorrhage, infection, or neonatal trauma.

Counseling: Discuss future pregnancies, especially if CPD or malpresentation persists.

Rehabilitation: Physiotherapy for maternal injuries.

Prevention

Antenatal Care: Early ultrasound to detect malpresentations or macrosomia.

Nutritional Interventions: Prevent pelvic deformities or macrosomia.

Education: Promote ANC and institutional delivery.

Advanced Imaging: 3D ultrasound/MRI for precise fetopelvic assessment.

Conclusion

The fetal lie, presentation, presenting part, attitude, denominator, and position determine how the fetus navigates the maternal pelvis. Optimal relationships (longitudinal lie, vertex presentation, OA position, full flexion) facilitate vaginal delivery, while malpresentations or malpositions increase CPD risk.

5.7 Methods of Obstetrical examination: Abdominal & Vaginal

(*Qabalati imtehan ke tareeqe: Batini wa mahbili*)

Introduction

Obstetrical examination is a cornerstone of maternal and fetal assessment during pregnancy and labor. It involves systematic evaluation to monitor maternal health, assess fetal well-being, and determine the fetopelvic relationship, which is critical for planning delivery and identifying complications such as cephalopelvic disproportion (CPD), malpresentation, or fetal distress. The two primary methods—abdominal examination and vaginal examination—provide complementary information about fetal lie, presentation, position, attitude, and pelvic adequacy. These techniques are integral to antenatal care (ANC) and intrapartum management, guiding clinical decisions to ensure safe maternal and fetal outcomes.

Abdominal Examination

Abdominal examination is a non-invasive method used to assess the fetus's orientation, size, and well-being, as well as maternal uterine and abdominal characteristics. It is performed routinely during ANC visits and intrapartum to monitor labor progress.

1. Objectives

Determine fetal lie, presentation, position, attitude, and station.

Assess fetal size, growth, and heart rate.

Evaluate uterine size, tone, and contractions.

Identify maternal or fetal abnormalities (e.g., polyhydramnios, fetal distress).

Monitor labor progress and fetopelvic relationship.

2. Preparation

Informed Consent: Explain the procedure to the patient, ensuring comfort and privacy.

Positioning: The patient lies supine with knees slightly flexed or in a semi-recumbent position (to avoid supine hypotension syndrome in late pregnancy).

Environment: Warm, private room with adequate lighting.

Equipment: Measuring tape, stethoscope or Doppler for fetal heart rate (FHR), and ultrasound (if needed).

Hygiene: Wash hands and wear gloves if palpating near the perineum.

3. Technique: **Leopold's Maneuvers**

Leopold's maneuvers are a systematic four-step abdominal palpation technique to assess fetal orientation and engagement. Performed after 28 weeks gestation when fetal parts are more distinguishable.

First Maneuver (Fundal Palpation)

Purpose: Determine the fetal part in the uterine fundus (lie and presentation).

Technique: Stand at the patient's side, facing her head. Place both hands on the fundus and gently palpate.

Findings

Hard, round mass (fetal head) suggests breech presentation.

Soft, irregular mass (buttocks) suggests cephalic presentation.

No distinct part suggests transverse or oblique lie.

Clinical Significance: Confirms longitudinal (head or breech) vs. transverse/oblique lie.

Second Maneuver (Lateral Palpation)

Purpose: Identify the fetal back and limbs to determine position and lie.

Technique: Place one hand on each side of the uterus, applying gentle pressure to palpate the fetal back (smooth, firm) and limbs (small, irregular parts).

Findings

Fetal back on one side (e.g., left or right) indicates position (e.g., left occiput anterior, LOA).

Limbs on the opposite side confirm longitudinal lie.

Back across the abdomen suggests transverse lie.

Clinical Significance: Helps identify occiput or sacrum orientation relative to the maternal pelvis.

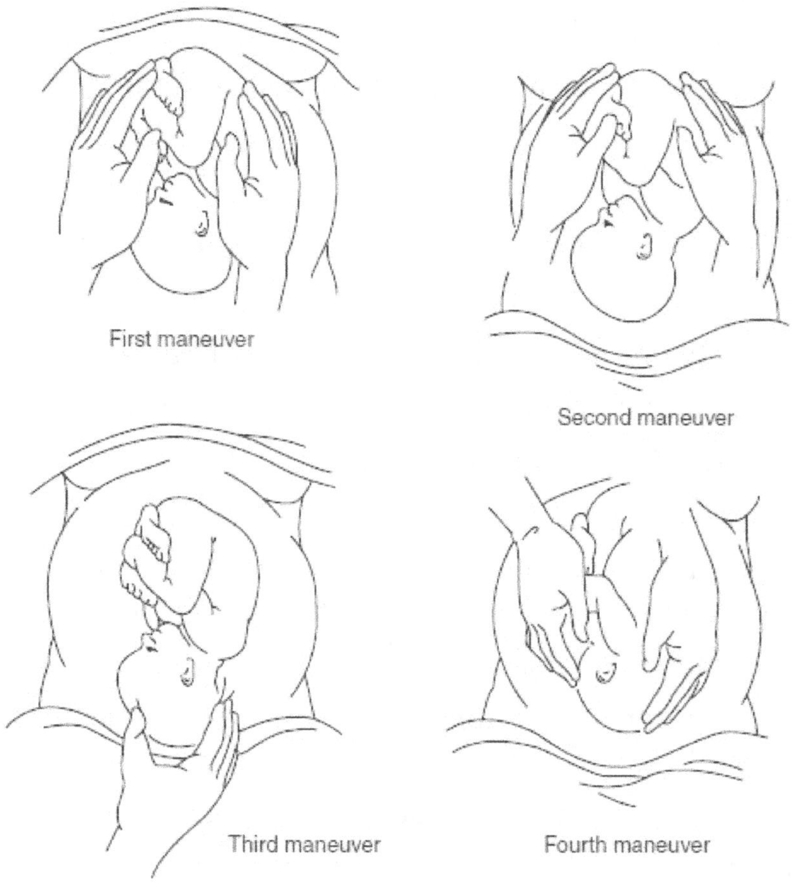

Third Maneuver (Pawlik's Grip)

Purpose: Confirm the presenting part and assess engagement.

Technique: Face the patient's feet. Use the thumb and fingers of one hand to grasp the lower uterine pole just above the symphysis pubis.

Findings

Hard, round mass (head) confirms cephalic presentation.

Soft, irregular mass confirms breech.

Movable (floating) vs. fixed (engaged) head indicates station.

Clinical Significance: Assesses whether the presenting part has entered the pelvic inlet.

Fourth Maneuver (Pelvic Palpation)

Purpose: Determine the attitude (flexion/extension) and station of the presenting part.

Technique: Face the patient's feet. Place both hands on the lower uterus, sliding fingers toward the pelvic inlet to palpate the presenting part.

Findings

In cephalic presentation, palpate the occiput (posterior) and forehead (anterior).

If occiput is lower, the head is flexed (favorable, suboccipitobregmatic diameter, 9.5 cm).

If forehead is prominent, the head is deflexed (e.g., occipitofrontal, 11.5 cm).Depth of the head indicates station (floating or engaged).

Clinical Significance: Confirms attitude and engagement, critical for fetopelvic fit.

4. Additional Components

Fundal Height Measurement

Technique: Use a measuring tape from the symphysis pubis to the top of the fundus.

Findings

After 20 weeks, fundal height (in cm) approximates gestational age (±2 cm).

Discrepancies suggest intrauterine growth restriction (IUGR), macrosomia, or poly/oligohydramnios.

Clinical Significance: Monitors fetal growth and amniotic fluid volume.

Fetal Heart Rate (FHR)

Technique: Use a stethoscope, Pinard fetoscope, or Doppler to auscultate FHR (normal: 110–160 bpm). Location: Heard best over the fetal back (e.g., left lower quadrant in LOA).

Clinical Significance: Confirms fetal viability and detects distress (e.g., bradycardia, tachycardia).

Uterine Assessment: Palpate for uterine tone, tenderness, or contractions (frequency, duration, intensity).

Clinical Significance: Identifies preterm labor, placental abruption, or uterine rupture.

Maternal Signs: Assess for edema, abdominal scars, or signs of preeclampsia (e.g., epigastric pain).

5. Clinical Significance

Fetopelvic Relationship: Determines lie, presentation, position, attitude, and station, guiding labor planning.

Fetal Well-Being: Monitors growth and heart rate to detect distress or anomalies.

Labor Progress: Assesses engagement and descent, predicting vaginal delivery feasibility.

Complications: Identifies malpresentation (e.g., breech, transverse lie) or CPD risk.

Vaginal Examination

Vaginal examination is an invasive method used to assess the cervix, fetal presenting part, and pelvic adequacy. It is performed primarily during labor but may be used antenatally in specific cases (e.g., suspected preterm labor or membrane rupture).

1. Objectives

Assess cervical dilatation, effacement, and position.

Confirm fetal presentation, position, attitude, station, and molding

Evaluate pelvic dimensions (pelvimetry) for adequacy.

Detect abnormalities (e.g., cord prolapse, placental previa).

Monitor labor progress and fetopelvic relationship.

2. Preparation

Informed Consent: Explain the procedure, purpose, and potential discomfort.

Positioning: Patient in lithotomy or dorsal position with knees flexed and legs apart. Environment: Private, sterile setting with adequate lighting.

Hygiene: Wash hands, wear sterile gloves, and use antiseptic solution (e.g., chlorhexidine) for cleaning the perineum.

Equipment: Sterile gloves, lubricant, speculum (if needed), and antiseptic solution.

Contraindications

Active vaginal bleeding (suspected placenta previa or abruption).

Premature rupture of membranes (PROM) without labor (risk of infection).

Patient refusal or discomfort.

3. Technique

Inspection

Observe the perineum for lesions, discharge, or signs of infection.

Note membrane status (intact, ruptured, or bulging).

Digital Examination

Insert two lubricated fingers (index and middle) into the vagina, avoiding excessive pressure.

Cervical Assessment

Dilatation: Measure cervical opening (0–10 cm; 10 cm = fully dilated).

Effacement: Assess cervical thinning (0–100%; 100% = fully effaced).

Position: Note if posterior, mid, or anterior (anterior indicates labor progress).

Consistency: Soft, medium, or firm (soft indicates ripening).

Application: Presenting part's pressure on cervix (applied or not).

Fetal Assessment

Presenting Part: Identify by palpating landmarks:

Cephalic: Sutures (sagittal, coronal, lambdoid) and fontanelles (anterior, posterior).

Breech: Sacrum, buttocks, or feet.

Shoulder: Scapula or arm.

Position: Determine denominator orientation:

Occiput (vertex): Anterior (OA), posterior (OP), or transverse (OT).

Mentum (face): Mento-anterior (MA) or mento-posterior (MP).

Sacrum (breech): Anterior (SA), posterior (SP), or transverse (ST).

Attitude: Assess head flexion/extension:

Flexed: Posterior fontanelle lower (suboccipitobregmatic, 9.5 cm).

Deflexed: Anterior fontanelle prominent (occipitofrontal, 11.5 cm).

Extended: Mentum prominent (submentobregmatic, 9.5 cm).

Station: Measure presenting part relative to ischial spines (–5 to +5 cm).

Molding: Assess suture overlap (0 to +3; +3 indicates CPD risk).

Caput Succedaneum: Note soft tissue swelling (may obscure sutures).

Pelvic Assessment (Clinical Pelvimetry)

Diagonal Conjugate: Distance from sacral promontory to lower symphysis pubis (normal: 12.5–13 cm; <11.5 cm suggests inlet contraction).

Ischial Spines: Prominence and interspinous diameter (normal: 10–10.5 cm; <9.5 cm suggests midpelvis contraction).

Sidewalls: Convergent or straight (convergent suggests android pelvis).

Sacral Curvature: Flat, curved, or prominent (flat suggests contraction).

Pubic Arch: Angle (normal: 80–90°; <70° suggests outlet contraction).

Intertuberous Diameter: Distance between ischial tuberosities (normal: 10–11 cm; <9 cm suggests outlet contraction).

Coccyx Mobility: Assess flexibility (increases outlet diameter).

Membranes and Amniotic Fluid

Intact, bulging, or ruptured.

Note fluid color (clear, meconium-stained, or bloody).

Other Findings

Cord prolapse, vaginal masses, or abnormal discharge.

Frequency

Every 4 hours in early labor, every 1–2 hours in active labor, or as needed (e.g., suspected distress).

Minimize examinations to reduce infection risk.

Clinical Significance

Cervical Changes: Indicate labor stage (latent vs. active) and progress.

Fetopelvic Relationship: Confirms lie, presentation, position, attitude, and station, assessing CPD risk.

Pelvic Adequacy: Identifies contracted pelvis (e.g., interspinous <9.5 cm).

Fetal Well-Being: Detects distress via cord prolapse or meconium.

Labor Complications: Identifies arrest, malposition, or obstruction.

Limitations

Infection Risk: Repeated examinations increase endometritis risk.

Discomfort: May cause pain, especially in early labor or with posterior cervix. Subjectivity: Accuracy depends on examiner skill.

Contraindications: Avoid in bleeding or PROM without labor.

Clinical Applications

1. Antenatal Care

Abdominal examination monitors fetal growth, lie, and presentation during routine ANC visits.

Vaginal examination used selectively (e.g., suspected preterm labor or PROM).

Supported by programs like India's Pradhan Mantri Surakshit Matritva Abhiyan (PMSMA) for free screening.

2. Intrapartum Management

Abdominal examination assesses labor progress and fetal heart rate.

Vaginal examination monitors cervical dilatation, station, and fetopelvic fit, guiding decisions (e.g., trial of labor, cesarean section).

3. Complication Detection

Identifies CPD (e.g., arrest of descent, excessive molding).

Detects malpresentation (e.g., breech, shoulder) or malposition (e.g., OP, mento-posterior).

Guides interventions like external cephalic version (ECV) or cesarean section.

Conclusion

Abdominal and vaginal examinations are essential methods of obstetrical assessment, providing critical data on fetal lie, presentation, position, attitude, station, and pelvic adequacy. Abdominal examination (e.g., Leopold's maneuvers) is non-invasive and ideal for routine ANC, while vaginal examination offers precise intrapartum insights into cervical changes and fetopelvic fit.

References

Dutta, D.C. (2020). Textbook of Obstetrics.

Cunningham, F.G., et al. (2022). Williams Obstetrics.

World Health Organization. (2006). Managing Complications in Pregnancy and Childbirth.

Long Answer Questions (LAQs)

1. Define lie of the fetus (Wad-an) and describe its types.
2. Explain presentation (Maji) and classify its types with examples.
3. Describe attitude (Wad-ah/Mauqif) of the fetus and its obstetric importance.
4. Define position (Wad-yeeyah) and explain fetal positions in vertex presentation.
5. Explain fetopelvic relationship and its importance in labour.

Short Answer Questions (SAQs)

1. Define fetal lie.
2. What is presenting part?
3. Define denominator.
4. Name types of fetal presentation.
5. What is longitudinal lie?

Multiple Choice Questions (1 Mark Each)

1. Normal lie of the fetus at term is:

A. Transverse B. Oblique

C. Longitudinal D. Variable

An: C. Longitudinal

2. Most common presentation is:

A. Breech B. Shoulder

C. Vertex D. Face

Ans: C. Vertex

3. Presenting part in vertex presentation is:

A. Face B. Brow

C. Occiput D. Chin

Ans: C. Occiput

4. Attitude of fetus normally is:

A. Extension B. Partial flexion

C. Complete flexion D. Hyperextension

Ans: C. Complete flexion

5. Denominator in vertex presentation is:

A. Chin B. Sacrum

C. Occiput D. Forehead

Ans: C. Occiput

6. Transverse lie commonly results in:

A. Normal delivery B. Breech delivery

C. Shoulder presentation D. Face presentation

Ans: C. Shoulder presentation

7. In breech presentation, denominator is:

A. Occiput B. Sacrum

C. Chin D. Shoulder

Ans: B. Sacrum

8. Position refers to relationship of:

A. Fetal back to uterus B. Denominator to pelvic quadrants

C. Head to cervix D. Pelvis to uterus

Ans: B. Denomiator to pelvic quadrants

9. Left occipito-anterior (LOA) is:

A. Abnormal position B. Most favorable position

C. Transverse position D. Posterior position

Ans: B. Most favourable position

10. Oblique lie is seen commonly:

A. At term B. During labour

C. Early pregnancy D. After delivery

Ans: C. Early pregnancy

06

Normal Labor

(Taba -i wada -e haml)

6.1 *Taba-i-wada-e-haml: Mikania wa Mu'alaja* (Normal Labor, its mechanism & Management)
6.2 *Tahreez-ul-makhaz* (Induction of Labor)
6.3 *Nauzayedah ki nigahdast* (Essential Newborn Care)

Learning Objective (At the end of the session, the students should be able to)

Describe Normal Labor, causes of the onset of labor, and stages, and demonstrate its Mechanism & Management)
Demonstrate the principles of IM/IV injections/NS/RL Techniques
Demonstrate Normal Labor on Manikins & Simulators
Demonstrate the technique of Catheterization on the Simulator
Observe & Chart Partograph
Observe and describe Amniotomy
Document the normal delivery notes
Explain the immediate care of newborn *(Nauzaida Ki Nighahdasht*)
Define Induction of Labor, its indications & contraindications, and enlist the methods of Cervical ripening & Induction of labor

6.1 Normal Labor, its mechanism & Management

(*Taba-i-wada-e-haml: Mikania wa Mu'alaja*)

Introduction

Normal labour, also known as spontaneous vaginal delivery, is a physiological process by which a fetus is expelled from the uterus through the birth canal without complications, typically at term (37–42 weeks gestation). It involves coordinated uterine contractions, cervical dilatation and fetal descent, culminating in the delivery of the fetus and placenta. Normal labour reflects an optimal fetopelvic relationship, adequate uterine activity, and maternal well-being, minimizing the need for operative interventions.

Definition

Normal labour is characterized by

Spontaneous onset at term (37–42 weeks).

Vertex presentation with the fetal head flexed (suboccipitobregmatic diameter, 9.5 cm).

Progressive cervical dilatation and fetal descent.

Vaginal delivery within 12–18 hours (primigravida) or 6–12 hours (multigravida) without complications.

No need for operative intervention (e.g., cesarean section, forceps).

Favorable fetopelvic relationship: Fetal head fits through the maternal pelvis (e.g., gynecoid pelvis, obstetric conjugate >10.5 cm).

Physiology of Labour

Labour is initiated and sustained by a complex interplay of hormonal, mechanical, and neural factors:

Hormonal Changes

Progesterone withdrawal: Decreased progesterone activity enhances uterine contractility.

Estrogen surge: Increases oxytocin receptors and prostaglandin synthesis.

Oxytocin release: Stimulates uterine contractions via the posterior pituitary.

Prostaglandins: Produced by the amnion and decidua, soften the cervix and augment contractions.

Fetal cortisol: Triggers placental corticotropin-releasing hormone (CRH), promoting labour onset.

Mechanical Factors

Uterine stretch from the growing fetus stimulates contractions.

Cervical ripening (softening and effacement) facilitates dilatation.

Myometrial Activity

Coordinated contractions originate from uterine pacemakers (near tubal ostia).

Contractions are involuntary, rhythmic, and increase in frequency, duration, and intensity.

Stages of Labour

Normal labour is divided into three stages, each with distinct physiological and clinical features

1. First Stage: Cervical Dilatation

Definition: From the onset of true labour contractions to full cervical dilatation (10 cm).

Duration

Primigravida: 8–12 hours.

Multigravida: 6–8 hours.

Phases

Latent Phase

Cervical dilatation: 0–3 cm.

Duration: 6–8 hours (primigravida), 4–6 hours (multigravida).

Contractions: Irregular, mild (15–20 mmHg), every 5–10 minutes.

Clinical Features: Cervical effacement (0–100%), mild discomfort.

Active Phase

Cervical dilatation: 4–10 cm.

Duration: 4–6 hours (primigravida), 2–4 hours (multigravida).

Contractions: Regular, strong (30–50 mmHg), every 2–3 minutes, lasting 40–60 seconds.

Rate of Dilatation: ≥1 cm/hour (primigravida), ≥1.2 cm/hour (multigravida).

Clinical Features: Increased pain, fetal descent begins.

Physiology

Uterine contractions cause cervical effacement and dilatation.

Fetal head pressure aids cervical stretching.

Amniotic sac may rupture (spontaneous rupture of membranes, SROM), releasing prostaglandins.

Clinical Significance

Monitors labour progression via cervical changes.

Prolonged latent phase (>20 hours primigravida, >14 hours multigravida) or active phase (<1 cm/hour) suggests dystocia.

2. Second Stage: Fetal Expulsion

Definition: From full cervical dilatation (10 cm) to delivery of the fetus.

Duration

Primigravida: 30 minutes–2 hours.

Multigravida: 15–60 minutes.

Physiology

Strong uterine contractions (50–80 mmHg) every 1–2 minutes.

Maternal voluntary pushing (Valsalva maneuver) augments expulsion.

Fetal head descends, rotates, and delivers through the birth canal.

Clinical Features

Intense contractions and urge to push.

Crowning (fetal head visible at introitus).

Delivery of head, shoulders, and body.

Clinical Significance

Assesses fetal descent and maternal effort.

Prolonged second stage (>2 hours primigravida, >1 hour multigravida without epidural) may indicate CPD or malposition.

3. Third Stage: Placental Delivery

Definition: From delivery of the fetus to expulsion of the placenta and membranes.

Duration: 5–30 minutes (average 10–15 minutes).

Physiology

Uterine contractions shear the placenta from the decidua basalis.

Placental separation signs: Gush of blood, uterine fundal rise, cord lengthening.

Oxytocin release or exogenous administration promotes uterine contraction.

Clinical Features

Controlled cord traction (Brandt-Andrews maneuver) aids placental delivery.

Inspection of placenta for completeness to prevent retained fragments.

Clinical Significance

Prevents postpartum hemorrhage (PPH) via uterine contraction.

Retained placenta (>30 minutes) requires manual removal.

Mechanism of Labour

The mechanism of labour refers to the series of movements the fetus undergoes to navigate the maternal pelvis during vaginal delivery. It is influenced by the fetopelvic relationship, including fetal lie, presentation, position, attitude and pelvic shape (ideally gynecoid). The mechanism is described for the most common scenario: vertex presentation, occiput anterior (OA) position, left occiput anterior (LOA).

1. Fetal and Pelvic Factors

Fetal Head Diameters

Suboccipitobregmatic (9.5 cm, flexed vertex, optimal).

Biparietal diameter (BPD, 9.5 cm, transverse).

Pelvic Diameters

Inlet: Obstetric conjugate (10.5–11 cm), transverse (13–13.5 cm).

Midpelvis: Interspinous (10–10.5 cm).

Outlet: Intertuberous (10–11 cm), pubic arch (80–90°).

Fetopelvic Relationship: Favorable when fetal head aligns with pelvic dimensions, allowing molding (suture overlap) and flexion.

2. Cardinal Movements of Labour

The fetus undergoes seven cardinal movements to adapt to the maternal pelvis:

Engagement

Fetal head enters the pelvic inlet with BPD aligned with the transverse diameter.

Occurs in late pregnancy or early labour.

Station: –2 to 0 (ischial spines).

Descent

Fetal head moves through the pelvis, driven by uterine contractions and maternal pushing.

Influenced by pelvic shape and fetal flexion.

Flexion

Fetal head flexes (chin to chest), presenting the suboccipitobregmatic diameter (9.5 cm).

Occurs as the head encounters pelvic resistance.

Enhances fetopelvic fit.

Internal Rotation

Fetal head rotates 90° from occiput transverse (OT) to occiput anterior (OA).

Aligns the head with the anteroposterior diameter of the pelvic outlet.

Occurs in the midpelvis, facilitated by the levator ani muscles.

Extension

Fetal head extends under the symphysis pubis, delivering the occiput, forehead, and face.

Occurs during crowning and delivery of the head.

Restitution and External Rotation

Restitution: Head rotates 45° to align with shoulders (undoing internal rotation).

External Rotation: Head rotates further (45°) as shoulders rotate to the anteroposterior diameter for delivery.

Expulsion

Anterior shoulder delivers under the symphysis pubis, followed by the posterior shoulder and body.

3. Clinical Significance

Ensures efficient passage through the birth canal.

Deviations (e.g., persistent occiput posterior, OP) may prolong labour or require intervention.

Molding and caput succedaneum (soft tissue swelling) facilitate passage but excessive molding (+3) suggests CPD.

Management of Normal Labour

The management of normal labour focuses on supporting physiological processes, monitoring progress, and ensuring maternal and fetal well-being.

1. Antenatal Preparation

Antenatal Care (ANC)

Regular visits to confirm vertex presentation, assess fetal growth, and screen for risk factors (e.g., macrosomia, contracted pelvis).

Supported by programs like India's Pradhan Mantri Surakshit Matritva Abhiyan (PMSMA) for free screening.

Education

Counsel on labour signs (contractions, rupture of membranes, bloody show).

Discuss birth plan, pain relief options, and institutional delivery benefits.

Promote Janani Suraksha Yojana (JSY) for incentivized hospital births.

Nutrition and Exercise

Ensure adequate maternal nutrition to support labour energy demands.

Encourage light exercise (e.g., walking) to promote pelvic flexibility.

2. Intrapartum Management

Management is tailored to each stage of labour, emphasizing supportive care and vigilant monitoring.

First Stage

Admission Assessment

History: Onset of contractions, membrane status, bleeding, or fetal movements.

Examination

Abdominal: Leopold's maneuvers to confirm lie (longitudinal), presentation (vertex), position (OA), and engagement.

Vaginal: Assess cervical dilatation, effacement, station, and membrane status.

Vital Signs: Maternal pulse, blood pressure, temperature; fetal heart rate (FHR, 110–160 bpm).

Diagnosis of Labour: Regular contractions (2–3 every 10 minutes, lasting 40–60 seconds) with cervical dilatation ≥4 cm or effacement.

Monitoring

Partogram: WHO-recommended tool to track cervical dilatation, fetal descent, FHR, contractions, and maternal vitals.

Latent phase: Dilatation <4 cm, slow progress. Active phase: Dilatation ≥4 cm, ≥1 cm/hour (primigravida).

Alert line: Indicates normal progress; crossing suggests dystocia.

FHR: Auscultate every 15–30 minutes in active phase (every 5 minutes in second stage) using Doppler or fetoscope.

Contractions: Assess frequency, duration, and intensity every 30 minutes.

Maternal Vitals: Monitor every 4 hours (pulse, BP, temperature).

Supportive Care

Positioning: Encourage upright positions (walking, sitting) or left lateral to enhance contractions and fetal descent.

Hydration and Nutrition: Oral fluids or light snacks in early labour; IV fluids if dehydrated.

Pain Relief

Non-pharmacological: Breathing exercises, massage, warm compresses.

Pharmacological: Nitrous oxide, parenteral opioids (e.g., pethidine), or epidural analgesia (if available).

Emotional Support: Continuous presence of a birth companion (e.g., family member) reduces stress and improves outcomes.

Interventions

Amniotomy: Artificial rupture of membranes (ARM) if labour is slow but cervix ≥4 cm and head engaged (controversial; risks cord prolapse).

Oxytocin: Augment contractions if inadequate (e.g., <3 contractions/10 minutes), titrated carefully (4–8 mU/min).

Antibiotics: For prolonged rupture of membranes (>18 hours) to prevent infection.

Second Stage

Assessment

Vaginal Examination: Confirm full dilatation (10 cm), station (+1 to +3), position (OA), and molding.

Abdominal Palpation: Monitor descent and contractions.

FHR: Auscultate every 5 minutes to detect distress.

Supportive Care

Positioning: Upright (squatting, kneeling) or semi-recumbent to aid descent; avoid prolonged supine position.

Pushing: Encourage coordinated pushing with contractions once the urge is felt (avoid directed pushing in early second stage).

Pain Relief: Continue epidural if in place; local perineal anesthesia (e.g., lidocaine) for episiotomy if needed.

Delivery Technique

Head Delivery: Support perineum to prevent tears (hands-on technique).Control head extension to avoid rapid expulsion and trauma. Check for nuchal cord; slip over head or clamp if tight.

Shoulder Delivery: Gentle downward traction for anterior shoulder under symphysis pubis.Upward traction for posterior shoulder.

Body Delivery: Support torso and legs as they deliver.

Episiotomy: Selective use (e.g., rigid perineum, fetal distress); mediolateral preferred to midline to reduce anal sphincter injury.

Interventions

Assisted Delivery: Forceps or vacuum if prolonged second stage (>2 hours primigravida) or fetal distress, provided station is +2 or lower.

Cesarean Section: If arrest of descent, CPD, or fetal distress.

Third Stage

Active Management (recommended to reduce PPH):

Oxytocin: Administer 10 IU IM or IV bolus within 1 minute of delivery to promote uterine contraction.

Controlled Cord Traction (CCT): Apply gentle traction on the cord with counterpressure on the uterus (Brandt-Andrews maneuver) after signs of placental separation.

Uterine Massage: Post-delivery to ensure uterine tone.

Expectant Management (alternative)

Allow spontaneous placental delivery without oxytocin or CCT.

Higher PPH risk; used in low-resource settings or per maternal preference.

Inspection

Examine placenta and membranes for completeness (cotyledons, vessels).

Check for retained fragments (risk of PPH).

Interventions

Manual Removal: If placenta retained >30 minutes, under anesthesia.

Uterotonics: Additional oxytocin, ergometrine, or misoprostol for PPH.

3. Postpartum Management

Monitoring

Maternal: Vitals every 15 minutes for 2 hours, assess uterine tone, bleeding, and perineal condition.

Neonatal: Apgar scores at 1 and 5 minutes, warmth, breastfeeding initiation, and vitamin K administration.

Laceration Repair: Suture perineal tears or episiotomy under local anesthesia.

Breastfeeding: Initiate within 1 hour to promote bonding and oxytocin release.

Pain Management: Analgesics (e.g., paracetamol, ibuprofen) for perineal or uterine pain.

Discuss postpartum care, contraception, and warning signs (e.g., heavy bleeding, fever).

Discharge: Typically 24–48 hours post-delivery, with follow-up at 1–2 weeks.

Monitoring and Assessment Tools

Partogram: Tracks cervical dilatation, fetal descent, FHR, contractions, and maternal vitals. Alert and action lines guide intervention for slow progress.

Fetal Heart Rate Monitoring: Intermittent auscultation (preferred in low-risk labour) or continuous cardiotocography (CTG) if high-risk. Abnormal patterns (e.g., late decelerations) indicate distress.

Vaginal Examination: Every 4 hours in latent phase, every 2 hours in active phase to assess dilatation, station, and position.Minimize to reduce infection risk.

Abdominal Examination: Leopold's maneuvers to confirm presentation and position. Palpate contractions for intensity and frequency.

Complications and Deviations

While normal labour is physiological, deviations may occur, requiring vigilance:

Prolonged Labour: Arrest of dilatation or descent, often due to CPD or malposition.

Fetal Distress: Abnormal FHR (bradycardia <110 bpm, tachycardia >160 bpm).

Postpartum Hemorrhage: Excessive bleeding (>500 mL) due to uterine atony or retained placenta.

Perineal Trauma: Severe tears (third/fourth-degree) involving anal sphincter.

Infection: Endometritis or sepsis from prolonged labour or PROM.

Conclusion

Normal labour is a physiological process involving coordinated uterine contractions, cervical dilatation, and fetal descent through the birth canal, typically resulting in spontaneous vaginal delivery. Its mechanism includes engagement, descent, flexion, internal rotation, extension, external rotation, and expulsion, optimized by a favorable fetopelvic relationship. Management emphasizes supportive care, vigilant monitoring (e.g., partogram, FHR), and timely interventions (e.g., oxytocin, episiotomy), with active third-stage management to prevent PPH.

References

Dutta, D.C. (2020). Textbook of Obstetrics.

Cunningham, F.G., et al. (2022). Williams Obstetrics.

World Health Organization. (2018). WHO Recommendations: Intrapartum Care for a Positive Childbirth Experience.

6.2 Induction of Labor

(*Tahreez-ul-makhaz)*

Introduction

Induction of labor (IOL) is the artificial initiation of labor before its spontaneous onset to achieve vaginal delivery. It is a common obstetric procedure performed when continuing the pregnancy poses risks to the mother or fetus, or when specific medical, obstetric, or social factors necessitate delivery. IOL involves pharmacological or mechanical methods to stimulate uterine contractions and cervical ripening, mimicking the physiological processes of spontaneous labor.

Definition

Induction of labor is the deliberate stimulation of uterine contractions to initiate labor before spontaneous onset, typically at term (37–41 weeks gestation), but occasionally preterm, with the goal of vaginal delivery. It differs from augmentation of labor, which enhances contractions in already established labor, and elective induction, which is performed without medical or obstetric indications.

Indications

IOL is indicated when the benefits of delivery outweigh the risks of continuing the pregnancy. Indications are categorized as medical, obstetric, or social, with evidence-based guidelines supporting their use.

1. Maternal Indications

Hypertensive Disorders

Preeclampsia, eclampsia, or gestational hypertension (≥37 weeks; earlier if severe).

Chronic hypertension with superimposed complications.

Diabetes Mellitus

Gestational or pre-existing diabetes with poor glycemic control or fetal compromise (e.g., macrosomia, polyhydramnios).

Typically induced at 37–39 weeks to prevent stillbirth or shoulder dystocia.

Medical Conditions

Renal disease, cardiac disease, or autoimmune disorders (e.g., systemic lupus erythematosus) worsening with pregnancy.

Intrahepatic cholestasis of pregnancy (ICP) with severe symptoms (induced at 36–37 weeks due to stillbirth risk).

Infections

Chorioamnionitis or maternal infections (e.g., HIV with high viral load) requiring delivery.

Prolonged Pregnancy

Post-term pregnancy (>41 weeks) due to increased risks of placental insufficiency, stillbirth, and meconium aspiration.

WHO and ACOG recommend IOL at 41–42 weeks.

2. Fetal Indications

Fetal Growth Restriction (FGR)

Severe FGR with abnormal Doppler studies (e.g., absent/reversed umbilical artery flow).

Induced at 37 weeks or earlier if compromised.

Oligohydramnios

Amniotic fluid index (AFI) <5 cm or maximum vertical pocket <2 cm, indicating fetal distress risk.

Fetal Anomalies

Anomalies requiring postnatal intervention (e.g., congenital heart defects).

Intrauterine Fetal Death (IUFD)

To expedite delivery and reduce maternal psychological distress or coagulopathy risk.

Non-Reassuring Fetal Status

Abnormal fetal heart rate (FHR) patterns or biophysical profile (BPP) score ≤4–6.

Multiple Gestation

Twin pregnancies often induced at 37–38 weeks to reduce complications.

3. Obstetric Indications

Premature Rupture of Membranes (PROM)

Term PROM (>37 weeks) if labor does not start within 12–24 hours (reduces infection risk).

Preterm PROM (PPROM) may require IOL if fetal maturity is confirmed (≥34 weeks).

Placental Abnormalities

Placenta previa (marginal) or abruption with stable maternal/fetal status.

History of Rapid Labor

To ensure delivery in a controlled hospital setting.

4. Elective Indications

Maternal Request: After 39 weeks, if informed of risks/benefits (controversial; ACOG recommends shared decision-making).

Psychosocial Factors: Severe maternal anxiety or history of stillbirth (after counseling).

Note: Elective IOL before 39 weeks is discouraged due to increased neonatal morbidity (e.g., respiratory distress).

Contraindications

IOL is contraindicated when vaginal delivery is unsafe or infeasible. Contraindications are absolute or relative, based on maternal and fetal risks.

1. Absolute Contraindications

Maternal: Active genital herpes with lesions (risk of neonatal transmission). Previous classical cesarean section or high-risk uterine surgery (e.g., myomectomy with endometrial entry) due to rupture risk. Severe maternal pelvic deformity (e.g., contracted pelvis with obstetric conjugate <8 cm).

Fetal: Transverse lie or unstable presentation (e.g., shoulder presentation). Severe feta anomalies incompatible with vaginal delivery (e.g., large sacrococcygeal teratoma).

Obstetric: Complete placenta previa or vasa previa. Cord prolapse or presentation. Prior uterine rupture.

2. Relative Contraindications

Maternal: Previous low transverse cesarean section (requires trial of labore after cesarean, TOLAC, assessment). Grand multiparity (≥5 deliveries) due to increased uterine atony risk.

Fetal: Breech presentation (external cephalic version, ECV, or cesarean preferred). Macrosomia (estimated feta weight, EFW >4,500 g) with borderline pelvis.

Obstetric: Unfavorable cervix (Bishop score <6) unless ripening methods are feasible. Fetal distress requiring immediate delivery (cesarean preferred).

Pre-Induction Assessment

Successful IOL depends on thorough evaluation of maternal, fetal and cervical status to determine appropriateness and method.

1. Maternal Assessment

History

Indication for IOL, obstetric history (e.g., previous cesarean, rapid labore).

Medical comorbidities (e.g., diabetes, hypertension).

Contraindications (e.g., placenta previa, prior uterine surgery).

Physical Examination

Vital signs (pulse, blood pressure, temperature).

Abdominal examination (Leopold's maneuvers) for lie, presentation, and engagement.

Pelvimetry to assess pelvic adequacy (e.g., diagonal conjugate >11.5 cm).

2. Fetal Assessment

Ultrasound

Confirm gestational age, lie (longitudinal), presentation (vertex), and position (e.g., occiput anterior, OA).

Measure EFW, biparietal diameter (BPD, ~9.5 cm), and amniotic fluid index (AFI).

Assess placental location and feta anomalies.

Fetal Heart Rate (FHR)

Non-stress test (NST) or biophysical profile (BPP) to confirm feta well-being (reactive NST: ≥2 accelerations in 20 minutes).

Presentation Confirmation

Vertex presentation is ideal; breech or transverse lie may require ECV or cesarean.

3. Cervical Assessment: Bishop Score

The Bishop score evaluates cervical readiness for labore, guiding method selection and predicting IOL success. Components (scored 0–3 each, total 0–13):

Dilatation (cm)	0 (closed)	1 (1–2)	2 (3–4)	3 (≥5).
Effacement (%)	0 (0–30)	1 (40–50)	2 (60–70)	3 (≥80).
Station	0 (–3)	1 (–2)	2 (–1/0)	3 (+1/+2).
Consistency	0 (firm)	1 (medium)	2 (soft).	
Position	0 (posterior)	1 (mid)	2 (anterior).	

Interpretation

Favorable Cervix: Score ≥6; higher likelihood of successful vaginal delivery.

Unfavorable Cervix: Score <6; requires cervical ripening.

Clinical Significance

Score ≥8 predicts spontaneous labore-like success.

Score <6 indicates need for prostaglandins or mechanical methods.

4. Informed Consent

Discuss indications, methods, risks (e.g., cesarean, hyperstimulation), benefits and alternatives (e.g., expectant management).

Ensure patient understanding and agreement, respecting autonomy.

Methods of Induction

IOL methods are pharmacological, mechanical, or surgical, chosen based on cervical status, parity, and clinical context. They aim to ripen the cervix and stimulate contractions.

1. Pharmacological Methods

Prostaglandins

1. Misoprostol (PGE1)

Route: Oral, sublingual, or vaginal (25–50 mcg every 4–6 hours).

Indication: Cervical ripening and contraction stimulation (unfavorable cervix).

Advantages: Inexpensive, effective, stable at room temperature.

Risks: Uterine hyperstimulation (tachysystole, >5 contractions/10 minutes), feta distress.

Contraindications: Previous cesarean (relative, due to rupture risk).

2. Dinoprostone (PGE2)

Route: Vaginal gel (0.5 mg) or insert (10 mg, removed after 12 hours).

Indication: Cervical ripening.

Advantages: Controlled release (insert), reversible.

Risks: Hyperstimulation, higher cost than misoprostol.

Oxytocin

Route: Intravenous infusion, titrated (start at 2–4 MU/min, increase by 1–2 MU/min every 15–30 minutes).

Indication: Stimulate contractions in favorable cervix (Bishop score ≥6) or after ripening.

Advantages: Precise dosing, rapid cessation if hyperstimulation.

Risks: Hyperstimulation, water intoxication (rare, with high doses).

Protocol: Aim for 3–5 contractions every 10 minutes, lasting 40–60 seconds.

Mifepristone (RU-486)

Route: Oral (200 mg single dose).

Indication: Cervical ripening, often in IUFD or preterm IOL.

Mechanism: Progesterone antagonist, softens cervix.

Risks: Limited use in viable pregnancies due to teratogenicity concerns.

2. Mechanical Methods

Foley Catheter

Technique: Insert a single- or double-balloon catheter through the cervix, inflate with 30–80 mL saline, and apply gentle traction.

Indication: Cervical ripening (unfavorable cervix).

Mechanism: Mechanical dilatation releases endogenous prostaglandins.

Advantages: Low risk of hyperstimulation, safe in previous cesarean.

Risks: Infection, discomfort, balloon displacement.

Hygroscopic Dilators (e.g., Laminaria, Dilapan)

Technique: Insert osmotic dilators into the cervix, which expand by absorbing moisture.

Indication: Cervical ripening (rarely used).

Risks: Infection, cervical trauma.

3. Surgical Methods

Amniotomy (Artificial Rupture of Membranes, ARM)

Technique: Use an amnihook to rupture membranes during vaginal examination (cervix ≥3 cm, head engaged).

Indication: Augment labore in favorable cervix or after ripening.

Mechanism: Releases prostaglandins, enhances contractions.

Advantages: Accelerates labore, allows meconium assessment.

Risks: Cord prolapse, infection (if prolonged rupture >18 hours).

Contraindications: High presenting part, polyhydramnios.

4. Non-Pharmacological Methods (Limited Evidence)

Membrane Sweeping

Technique: Digital separation of membranes from the lower uterine segment during vaginal examination (≥37 weeks).

Indication: Promote spontaneous labore, reduce need for formal IOL.

Advantages: Safe, outpatient procedure.

Risks: Discomfort, minor bleeding.

Other: Nipple stimulation.

5. Combined Methods

Often used sequentially or concurrently (e.g., Foley catheter followed by oxytocin, or misoprostol then amniotomy).

Tailored to Bishop score and response (e.g., ripening with prostaglandins for score <6, then oxytocin for contractions).

Monitoring During Induction

IOL requires continuous monitoring to ensure maternal and feta safety and assess labore progress.

1. Maternal Monitoring

Vital Signs: Pulse, blood pressure, temperature every 4 hours (more frequent if high-risk).

Contractions

Assess frequency, duration, and intensity every 15–30 minutes (manual palpation or tocodynamometry).

Goal: 3–5 contractions/10 minutes, lasting 40–60 seconds.

Tachysystole (>5 contractions/10 minutes) requires intervention (e.g., stop oxytocin, tocolytics).

Pain Management

Non-pharmacological: Breathing, massage, hydrotherapy.

Pharmacological: Epidural, nitrous oxide, or opioids (e.g., pethidine).

Fluid Balance: Monitor intake/output to prevent dehydration or overhydration (oxytocin-related).

2. Fetal Monitoring

FHR

Continuous cardiotocography (CTG) or intermittent auscultation (every 15 minutes in active phase, every 5 minutes in second stage).

Normal: 110–160 bpm, reactive with accelerations.

Abnormal: Late decelerations, bradycardia (<110 bpm), or reduced variability indicate distress.

Amniotic Fluid

Post-amniotomy, note color (clear, meconium-stained, bloody).

Meconium suggests feta stress, requiring closer monitoring.

3. Labor Progress

Partogram (WHO-recommended)

Tracks cervical dilatation (≥1 cm/hour in active phase), feta descent, station, and contractions.

Alert line: Normal progress; crossing indicates slow labore.

Action line: Triggers intervention (e.g., oxytocin, cesarean).

Vaginal Examination

Every 2–4 hours to assess dilatation, effacement, station, position, and molding.

Minimize to reduce infection risk.

Complications of Induction

IOL increases certain risks compared to spontaneous labor, requiring prompt recognition and management.

1. Maternal Complications

Uterine Hyperstimulation

Tachysystole or hypertonus (>5 contractions/10 minutes or lasting >2 minutes).

Management: Stop oxytocin/prostaglandins, administer tocolytics (e.g., terbutaline 0.25 mg IV), left lateral position.

Uterine Rupture

Rare (0.5–1% in TOLAC with prostaglandins), but life-threatening.

Signs: Sudden FHR abnormalities, abdominal pain, vaginal bleeding, or loss of contractions.

Management: Emergency cesarean, uterine repair, or hysterectomy.

Postpartum Hemorrhage (PPH)

Increased due to prolonged labor or atony from oxytocin overuse.

Management: Uterotonics (oxytocin, ergometrine, misoprostol), uterine massage.

Infection

Chorioamnionitis from prolonged rupture or frequent vaginal examinations.

Management: Antibiotics (e.g., ampicillin, gentamicin).

Failed Induction

No progress (dilatation <4 cm) after 12–24 hours of oxytocin and ripening.

Management: Cesarean section or rest/retry (if maternal/fetal status allows).

2. Fetal Complications

Fetal Distress

Caused by hyperstimulation, cord compression, or placental insufficiency.

Management: Intrauterine resuscitation (left lateral position, oxygen, IV fluids, stop oxytocin), or cesarean.

Meconium Aspiration Syndrome

Increased with post-term IOL or distress.

Management: Pediatric support at delivery, suction if needed.

Neonatal Morbidity

Preterm IOL (<39 weeks) increases respiratory distress or NICU admission.

Management: Confirm gestational age before IOL.

3. Increased Cesarean Risk

IOL with unfavorable cervix (Bishop score <6) increases cesarean rate (20–30% vs. 10–15% spontaneous labore).

Nulliparity, obesity, or macrosomia further elevate risk.

Management: Optimize cervical ripening, monitor progress, and counsel patients.

Management of Failed Induction

Definition: No active labore (dilatation <4 cm) after adequate ripening (e.g., 12–24 hours of prostaglandins) and oxytocin (12–18 hours at maximum dose).

Confirm indication, fetal status (NST/BPP), and cervical response.

Options

Cesarean Section: If urgent delivery needed (e.g., feta distress, preeclampsia).

Rest and Retry: Stop induction for 12–24 hours, then resume ripening (if stable).

Expectant Management: Rarely used if non-urgent (e.g., elective IOL).

Counseling: Discuss risks of prolonged induction (infection, cesarean) vs. benefits.

Special cases

1. Trial of Labor After Cesarean (TOLAC)

IOL increases uterine rupture risk (0.5–1% with oxytocin, higher with prostaglandins).

Use low-dose oxytocin or Foley catheter; avoid misoprostol in most cases.

Monitor closely with CTG and surgical backup.

2. Preterm Induction

Indicated for severe maternal/feta conditions (e.g., preeclampsia, FGR).

Requires corticosteroids (betamethasone 12 mg IM, 2 doses 24 hours apart) for fetal lung maturity (<34 weeks).

Higher cesarean risk due to immature cervix.

3. Outpatient Induction

Feasible with membrane sweeping or Foley catheter in low-risk women (≥39 weeks).

Requires reliable follow-up and rapid hospital access.

4. Low-Resource Settings

Misoprostol and Foley catheter are cost-effective and stable.

Conclusion

Induction of labor is a critical obstetric intervention to expedite delivery when medically indicated, balancing maternal and fetal risks. It requires careful patient selection based on indications (e.g., post-term pregnancy, preeclampsia), cervical assessment (Bishop score), and contraindications (e.g., placenta previa). Methods include prostaglandins, oxytocin, Foley catheter, and amniotomy, according to cervical status and clinical context.

6.3 Essential Newborn Care

(*Nauzayedah ki nigahdast*)

Introduction

Essential newborn care (ENC) encompasses a set of interventions provided immediately after birth and during the first 28 days of life (neonatal period) to ensure the survival, health, and well-being of the newborn. ENC aims to prevent and manage common neonatal complications, promote early bonding, and establish a foundation for long-term development. It is a critical component of obstetric and neonatal practice, as the first hours and days of life are the most vulnerable, with approximately 2.4 million neonatal deaths occurring globally each year, primarily in low- and middle-income countries (LMICs).

Definition

Essential newborn care refers to a standardized package of interventions delivered at birth and during the early neonatal period to:

Ensure immediate survival by maintaining thermoregulation, airway, and circulation.

Prevent infections through clean delivery and cord care.

Promote early initiation of breastfeeding for nutrition and immunity.

Identify and manage neonatal complications (e.g., asphyxia, sepsis).

Support maternal-newborn bonding and caregiver education.

Principles of Essential Newborn Care

1. Timeliness: Interventions are most effective when provided immediately after birth (within the first hour, the "golden hour").
2. Universality: Applicable to all newborns, regardless of gestational age, birth weight, or setting.
3. Simplicity: Practices are low-cost, feasible in resource-limited settings, and require minimal equipment.
4. Integration: Links with maternal care, family education, and community health systems.
5. Evidence-Based: Supported by WHO, AAP, and national guidelines to reduce neonatal mortality.
6. Respectful Care: Promotes dignity, cultural sensitivity, and family involvement.

Components of Essential Newborn Care

ENC includes a series of interventions categorized by timing (immediate, early, and ongoing) and focus (physiological support, infection prevention, nutrition, and monitoring).

1. Immediate Newborn Care (First Hour After Birth)

These interventions are performed in the delivery room to stabilize the newborn and prevent complications.

Thermal Care

Objective: Prevent hypothermia, as newborns lose heat rapidly due to high surface area, wet skin, and limited thermoregulatory capacity (normal axillary temperature: 36.5–37.5°C).

Procedure

Dry Immediately: Wipe the newborn with a clean, dry cloth within seconds of birth to remove amniotic fluid and blood, reducing evaporative heat loss.

Skin-to-Skin Contact (SSC): Place the newborn prone on the mother's bare chest, covered with a warm, dry blanket, within 1–2 minutes of birth.

Maintains temperature, promotes bonding, and stimulates early breastfeeding.

Continue SSC for at least 1 hour or until the first breastfeed.

Delay Bathing: Postpone bathing for at least 24 hours (or 6 hours in high-infection settings) to preserve vernix caseosa (natural thermal and antimicrobial barrier).

Warm Environment: Keep delivery room temperature at 25–28°C; use radiant warmers or incubators for preterm/low-birth-weight (LBW) infants (<2,500 g).

Clinical Significance

Hypothermia increases risk of hypoglycemia, respiratory distress, and mortality (e.g., 10% mortality increase per 1°C drop below 36°C).

SSC reduces hypothermia by 50–70% and enhances breastfeeding success.

Monitoring: Check axillary temperature every 30 minutes for 2 hours; rewarm if <36.5°C using SSC or warmer.

Airway and Breathing

Objective: Ensure a patent airway and adequate ventilation to prevent or manage birth asphyxia (failure to initiate spontaneous breathing at birth).

Procedure

Clear Airway: If the newborn is not crying or breathing, gently suction mouth and nose with a bulb syringe or suction catheter (only if secretions obstruct airway).

Positioning: Place the newborn in a neutral head position (sniffing position) to maintain airway patency.

Stimulation: Rub the back or soles of feet gently to stimulate breathing if no spontaneous respiration within 30 seconds.

Neonatal Resuscitation (if needed, per AAP guidelines)

Positive Pressure Ventilation (PPV): Use a self-inflating bag and mask (40–60 breaths/min) if no breathing after stimulation.

Oxygen: Administer 21% (room air) initially; titrate to 30–40% if preterm (<32 weeks).

Chest Compressions: If heart rate <60 bpm after 30 seconds of PPV, compress at 120/min (3:1 ratio with ventilations).

Cord Clamping: Delay umbilical cord clamping for 1–3 minutes in vigorous term newborns to improve hemoglobin and iron stores; clamp immediately if resuscitation is needed.

Clinical Significance

Birth asphyxia accounts for ~23% of neonatal deaths globally.

Effective resuscitation within 1 minute (golden minute) reduces mortality by 30–50%.

Monitoring: Assess respiratory rate (30–60 breaths/min), heart rate (100–160 bpm), and color (pink lips/tongue) at 1 and 5 minutes (Apgar scoring).

Apgar Scoring

Objective: Evaluate newborn condition and need for resuscitation.

Components (scored 0–2 each, total 0–10):

Appearance: Color (pale, cyanotic, pink).

Pulse: Heart rate (absent, <100 bpm, >100 bpm).

Grimace: Reflex irritability (none, grimace, cry).

Activity: Muscle tone (flaccid, some flexion, active).

Respiration: Breathing effort (absent, weak, strong).

Timing: Performed at 1 and 5 minutes; repeat at 10 minutes if score <7.

Interpretation

7–10: Normal, routine care.

4–6: Moderate distress, provide oxygen/stimulation.

0–3: Severe distress, initiate full resuscitation.

Clinical Significance: Guides immediate intervention and predicts short-term outcomes.

Clean Cord Care

Objective: Prevent umbilical cord infection (e.g., omphalitis, neonatal sepsis).

Procedure

Clamp cord with a sterile plastic clamp or tie 2–3 cm from the base after delayed clamping.

Cut with a sterile blade or scissors 1 cm beyond the clamp.

Apply no antiseptics in high-resource settings (dry cord care); in LMICs, apply 7.1% chlorhexidine digluconate daily for 7 days if high infection risk.

Keep cord clean and dry, exposed to air, and avoid tight diapers.

Clinical Significance

Chlorhexidine reduces omphalitis by 50% and neonatal mortality by 12% in high-risk settings.

Sepsis accounts for ~15% of neonatal deaths in LMICs.

Monitoring: Inspect cord daily for redness, discharge, or foul odor.

2. Early Newborn Care (First 24 Hours)

These interventions establish feeding, prevent complications, and promote maternal-newborn bonding.

Breastfeeding

Objective: Provide nutrition, immunity (colostrum), and bonding within the first hour (golden hour).

Procedure

Encourage breastfeeding during SSC, allowing the newborn to crawl to the breast and latch spontaneously (breast crawl).

Support proper latch: Mouth wide, lips everted, areola mostly in mouth, chin touching breast.

Feed on demand (8–12 times/24 hours), ensuring 10–15 minutes per breast.

Avoid prelacteal feeds (e.g., water, formula) unless medically indicated (e.g., hypoglycemia in diabetic mothers' infants).

Clinical Significance

Early breastfeeding reduces neonatal mortality by 22% (WHO).

Colostrum provides immunoglobulins (IgA), growth factors, and nutrients.

Enhances uterine involution via oxytocin release, reducing postpartum hemorrhage (PPH).

Monitoring: Observe latch, swallow sounds, and urine/stool output (≥1 wet diaper, meconium by 24 hours).

Vitamin K Prophylaxis

Objective: Prevent vitamin K deficiency bleeding (VKDB), as newborns have low vitamin K stores and immature liver function.

Procedure

Administer 1 mg vitamin K1 (phytonadione) intramuscularly (IM) in the anterolateral thigh within 6 hours of birth (term infants).

Preterm (<1,000 g): 0.3–0.5 mg IM.

Oral doses (2 mg at birth, repeated at 1–2 weeks) less effective, used if IM refused.

Clinical Significance

VKDB occurs in 0.25–1.7% of untreated newborns, causing intracranial or gastrointestinal bleeding.

IM vitamin K reduces VKDB risk to <0.01%.

Monitoring: Watch for bleeding (e.g., bruising, hematemesis) in first 2–4 weeks.

Eye Prophylaxis

Objective: Prevent ophthalmia neonatorum (neonatal conjunctivitis) from gonorrhea or chlamydia.

Procedure

Apply 0.5% erythromycin or 1% tetracycline ointment to both eyes within 1–2 hours of birth.

In LMICs, 2.5% povidone-iodine drops may be used if erythromycin unavailable.

Clean eyes before application to remove debris.

Clinical Significance

Reduces gonococcal conjunctivitis risk, which can lead to blindness.

Chlamydia conjunctivitis requires systemic antibiotics if infection occurs.

Monitoring: Check for eye discharge or redness in first week.

Immunizations

Objective: Protect against early infections.

Procedure

Hepatitis B Vaccine: Administer 0.5 mL IM within 24 hours if mother is hepatitis B surface antigen (HBsAg) negative; combine with hepatitis B immunoglobulin (HBIG, 0.5 mL IM) if HBsAg positive.

BCG Vaccine: In high-tuberculosis settings (e.g., India), give 0.1 mL intradermally within 24 hours or before discharge.

Oral Polio Vaccine (OPV): In endemic areas, administer 2 drops at birth (India's National Immunization Schedule).

Clinical Significance

Hepatitis B vaccination prevents vertical transmission (90% risk without prophylaxis).

BCG reduces severe tuberculosis risk in infancy.

Monitoring: Observe for local reactions (e.g., BCG nodule) or fever.

3. Newborn Care (First 28 Days)

These interventions ensure continued health, growth, and early detection of complications.

Exclusive Breastfeeding

Objective: Provide optimal nutrition and immunity for the first 6 months.

Procedure

Continue on-demand feeding (8–12 feeds/day).

Counsel mothers on breastfeeding challenges (e.g., sore nipples, engorgement).

Supplement with expressed breast milk or formula only if medically indicated (e.g., severe jaundice, LBW <1,500 g).

Clinical Significance

Reduces risk of diarrhea, pneumonia and malnutrition.

Improves cognitive development and maternal health (e.g., reduced breast cancer risk).

Monitoring: Assess weight gain (20–30 g/day after day 3), urine (≥6 wet diapers/day), and stools (yellow, seedy by day 4–5).

Cord Care Monitoring

Objective: Ensure cord healing and prevent infection.

Procedure: Keep cord dry and clean; avoid dressings or traditional substances (e.g., ash, cow dung). Cord typically detaches by 5–15 days.

Clinical Significance: Omphalitis can progress to sepsis, with 20–40% mortality in untreated cases.

Monitoring: Refer if redness extends >1 cm, pus, or fever.

Thermoregulation

Objective: Maintain normal body temperature beyond the first hour.

Procedure

Dress newborn in layers (hat, socks, blanket) appropriate for ambient temperature.

Use kangaroo mother care (KMC) for preterm/LBW infants: Continuous SSC with mother or caregiver, supporting breastfeeding and warmth.

Avoid drafts or cold surfaces during examinations.

Clinical Significance: KMC reduces mortality in preterm infants by 40% (WHO).

Monitoring: Check temperature daily; rewarm if <36.5°C.

Screening for Congenital Conditions

Objective: Detect treatable disorders early to prevent disability or death.

Procedure

Physical Examination (within 24–48 hours)

Check for anomalies (e.g., cleft palate, clubfoot, imperforate anus).

Assess hips for developmental dysplasia (Ortolani/Barlow maneuvers).

Evaluate heart (murmurs), lungs, and abdomen.

Metabolic Screening (48–72 hours, before discharge)

Heel-prick blood test for conditions like congenital hypothyroidism, phenylketonuria (PKU), and galactosemia (varies by region).

Hearing Screening: Otoacoustic emissions (OAE) or automated auditory brainstem response (AABR) to detect congenital deafness.

Pulse Oximetry: Screen for critical congenital heart disease (CCHD) by measuring pre- and post-ductal oxygen saturation (≥95%, <3% difference).

Clinical Significance

Early treatment of hypothyroidism prevents intellectual disability.

CCHD screening reduces undiagnosed cardiac mortality by 33%.

Monitoring for Danger Signs

Objective: Identify and manage neonatal complications promptly.

Danger Signs (WHO Integrated Management of Childhood Illness, IMCI):

Not feeding well or refusing feeds.

Convulsions or lethargy.

Fast breathing (>60 breaths/min) or chest indrawing.

Fever (>37.5°C) or hypothermia (<36.5°C).

Jaundice (yellow skin/eyes) within 24 hours or severe (palms/soles).

Umbilical redness, pus, or foul odor.

Procedure

Educate caregivers to recognize and seek care for danger signs.

Perform daily assessments in hospital (or at home visits in LMICs).

Clinical Significance

Sepsis, jaundice, and respiratory distress account for 50–60% of neonatal deaths.

Early referral reduces mortality by 20–30%.

Management

Refer to neonatal intensive care unit (NICU) or pediatrician.

Administer antibiotics (e.g., ampicillin, gentamicin) for suspected sepsis.

Phototherapy for jaundice (bilirubin >15–20 mg/dL, depending on age).

Special Cases

1. Preterm and Low-Birth-Weight Infants

Require intensive ENC: KMC, frequent feeding (every 2 hours), and respiratory support (e.g., CPAP for preterm <32 weeks).

Administer antenatal corticosteroids (betamethasone) to mothers at risk of preterm delivery (<34 weeks) to enhance lung maturity.

Monitor for apnea, necrotizing enterocolitis (NEC), and retinopathy of prematurity (ROP).

2. Small for Gestational Age (SGA)

Increased risk of hypoglycemia and hypothermia.

Monitor blood glucose (normal: >45 mg/dL) and feed frequently.

3. Neonates of High-Risk Mothers

HIV-Positive: Administer nevirapine/zidovudine prophylaxis within 72 hours; encourage breastfeeding with antiretroviral therapy (ART).

Diabetic Mothers: Check glucose within 1–2 hours; treat hypoglycemia (<45 mg/dL) with oral glucose or IV dextrose.

Substance Use: Monitor for neonatal abstinence syndrome (NAS); manage with non-pharmacological care or morphine if severe.

Conclusion

Essential newborn care is a vital intervention to reduce neonatal mortality and morbidity, focusing on immediate stabilization, infection prevention, nutrition and early complication detection. Key components include thermal care, airway management, breastfeeding initiation, vitamin K prophylaxis and danger sign monitoring, delivered within the first hour and continued for 28 days. Special attention to preterm, LBW and high-risk infants enhances outcomes.

References

Dutta, D.C. (2020). Textbook of Obstetrics.

World Health Organization. (2017). WHO Recommendations on Newborn Health.

American Academy of Pediatrics. (2021). Textbook of Neonatal Resuscitation, 8th Edition.

UNICEF/WHO. (2020). Every Newborn Action Plan.

Long Answer Questions (LAQs)

1. Define normal labor and describe its stages in detail.
2. Explain the mechanism of normal labor with cardinal movements.
3. Describe the management of first stage of normal labor.
4. Discuss the management of second and third stages of labor.
5. Describe maternal and fetal monitoring during normal labor.

Short Answer Questions (SAQs)

1. Define normal labor.
2. List the cardinal movements of labor.
3. What is engagement?
4. Define parturition.
5. Mention signs of onset of true labor.

Multiple Choice Questions (1 Mark Each)

1. Normal labor usually occurs between:

A. 34–36 weeks B. 36–38 weeks

C. 37–42 weeks D. After 42 weeks

Answer: C

2. The first stage of labor ends with:

A. Onset of contractions B. Rupture of membranes

C. Full cervical dilatation D. Delivery of placenta

Answer: C

3. Engagement means:

A. Descent of head below ischial spines B. Biparietal diameter passing pelvic inlet

C. Flexion of fetal head D. Internal rotation

Answer: B

4. Which is NOT a cardinal movement of labor?

A. Flexion B. Extension

C. Circumduction D. Internal rotation

Answer: C

5. Duration of first stage of labor in primigravida is approximately:

A. 4–6 hours B. 6–8 hours

C. 10–12 hours D. 18–20 hours

Answer: C

6. The strongest uterine contractions occur in:

A. Latent phase B. First stage

C. Second stage D. Third stage

Answer: C

7. Delivery of placenta occurs in which stage of labor?

A. First B. Second

C. Third D. Fourth

Answer: C

8. Normal presentation in labor is:

A. Breech B. Face

C. Shoulder D. Vertex

Answer: D

9. The normal mechanism of labor applies best to:

A. Breech presentation B. Face presentation

C. Vertex presentation D. Transverse lie

Answer: C

10. Controlled cord traction is used in:

A. First stage B. Second stage

C. Third stage of labor D. Fourth stage

Answer: C

07

Abnormal labour & Abnormal Presentations

(Ghaiyr Tabi'l Wada -e-Haml wa Ghaiyr Tabi'l taqdeemat)

7.1 *Wiladat-e-matau-wala* (Prolonged Labor)
7.2 *Wiladat-e-muar-qla* (Obstructed Labor)
7.3 *Wazyeeya qazaliya khalfiya* (Occipito Posterior Position)
7.4 *Twaq-quf-e-mustariz ameeq* (Deep Transverse Arrest)
7.5 *Maji-e-maqadee* (Breech Presentation)
7.6 *Maji-e-wajhee* (Face Presentation)
7.7 *Maji-e-jabhee* (Brow Presentation)
7.8 *Vijah mustariza* (Transverse lie)
7.9 *Maji-e-murakkab* (Compound Presentation)
7.10 *Maji-e-ktafi aur Usr-al-Wilada* (Shoulder Presentation & Dystocia)
7.11 *Maji-e-surri aur tadalliy-e-habl-us-surrah* (Cord Presentation & Cord Prolapse)

Learning Objective (At the end of the session, the students should be able to)

Identify Prolonged labor & Obstructed Labor, its causes, diagnosis & complications
Define Occipito Posterior Position (OP), its diagnosis, mechanism of labor & complications
Define Deep Transverse Arrest (DTA)
Outline Breech Face & Brow presentation, its varieties, etiology, diagnosis and complications
Define Transverse lie & also Outline Shoulder presentation
Define Compound Presentation & Cord presentation & Identify Cord Prolapse

7.1 Prolonged Labor

(*Wiladat-e-matau-wala*)

Introduction

Abnormal labour, or dystocia, refers to a labour process that deviates from the normal progression of cervical dilatation, fetal descent, or delivery due to abnormalities in the powers (uterine contractions), passenger (fetus), passage (maternal pelvis), or psyche (maternal psychological state). Prolonged labour, a subset of abnormal labour, is characterized by an extended duration of the first or second stage of labour, leading to increased maternal and fetal risks. It is a significant cause of maternal morbidity (e.g., postpartum hemorrhage, fistulae) and neonatal complications (e.g., asphyxia, sepsis).

Definition

Prolonged labour is defined as labour that exceeds the expected duration for the first or second stage, based on parity and labour phase, as assessed by a partogram or clinical evaluation.

First Stage

Latent Phase: Primigravida: >20 hours and Multigravida: >14 hours.

Active Phase: Cervical dilatation rate <1 cm/hour (primigravida) or <1.2 cm/hour (multigravida) after 4 cm dilatation. Total active phase duration >12 hours (primigravida) or >10 hours (multigravida).

Second Stage

Primigravida: >2 hours without epidural, >3 hours with epidural.

Multigravida: >1 hour without epidural, >2 hours with epidural.

Third Stage: >30 minutes (prolonged placental delivery, often managed separately).

Prolonged labour is classified as

Primary Prolonged Labour: Slow progress from the outset due to inefficient contractions, cephalopelvic disproportion (CPD), or malposition.

Secondary Arrest: Normal initial progress followed by cessation of dilatation (arrest of dilatation) or descent (arrest of descent), often due to obstruction or exhaustion.

Causes of Prolonged Labour

Prolonged labour results from abnormalities in the four Ps of labour: powers, passenger, passage, and psyche.

1. Powers (Uterine Contractions)

a. Inefficient Uterine Action: Hypotonic contractions: Weak, infrequent (<3 contractions/10 minutes), or short (<40 seconds). Causes: Uterine overdistension (e.g., twins, polyhydramnios), maternal exhaustion, dehydration, or grand multiparity.
b. Incoordinate Uterine Action: Irregular or asynchronous contractions, reducing cervical dilatation efficiency. Causes: Primigravidity, anxiety, or epidural analgesia (reduces oxytocin release).
c. Hypertonic Uterus (rare): Excessive, painful contractions without cervical progress, often due to oxytocin overuse or abruptio placentae.

2. Passenger (Fetus)

Fetal Size: Macrosomia (estimated fetal weight, EFW >4,000 g) increases biparietal diameter (BPD, ~9.5 cm), causing CPD.

Malpresentation: Brow (supraoccipitomental diameter, 13.5 cm) or face (submentobregmatic, 9.5 cm, if mento-posterior). Breech or shoulder presentation.

Malposition: Occiput posterior (OP) or occiput transverse (OT), requiring rotation to occiput anterior (OA) for delivery. Persistent OP leads to prolonged second stage or deep transverse arrest.

Feta Anomalies: Hydrocephalus or tumors enlarging the presenting part.

Lack of Molding: Failure of cranial sutures to overlap, reducing head diameter adaptability.

3. Passage (Maternal Pelvis)

Cephalopelvic Disproportion (CPD)

Absolute CPD: Severe mismatch (e.g., obstetric conjugate <8 cm vs. BPD 9.5 cm), preventing vaginal delivery.

Relative CPD: Borderline mismatch exacerbated by malposition or macrosomia.

Contracted Pelvis

Inlet: Obstetric conjugate <10 cm or transverse diameter <12 cm.

Midpelvis: Interspinous diameter <9.5 cm.

Outlet: Intertuberous diameter <9 cm or pubic arch <70°.

Pelvic Deformities

Congenital (e.g., Naegele's pelvis, kyphoscoliosis).

Acquired (e.g., rickets, osteomalacia, pelvic fractures).

Soft Tissue Obstruction: Cervical fibroids, ovarian cysts, or vaginal septa narrowing the birth canal.

Pelvic Shape: Android or platypelloid pelvis less favorable than gynecoid.

4. Psyche (Maternal Psychological State)

Anxiety or Fear: Increases catecholamine release, reducing uterine contractility. Common in primigravidas or those with prior traumatic births.

Exhaustion: Prolonged labour depletes maternal energy, reducing pushing efficacy.

Lack of Support: Absence of a birth companion increases stress and labour duration.

5. Other Factors

Iatrogenic: Premature amniotomy (ARM) with unengaged head, causing cord prolapse. Overuse of epidural analgesia, slowing second stage.

Maternal Conditions: Obesity (BMI >30 kg/m^2) increases labour duration and CPD risk. Diabetes mellitus (increases macrosomia).

Fetal Distress: Reduced contractions due to placental insufficiency.

Diagnosis of Prolonged Labour

Accurate diagnosis relies on systematic assessment using clinical tools and examinations to identify the cause and guide management.

1. Maternal History:

Parity, previous prolonged labour, or cansarean section.

Risk factors: Short stature (<150 cm), obesity, or diabetes.

Onset, frequency, and intensity of contractions.

Membrane status (intact, ruptured, duration of rupture).

Symptoms

Severe pain (suggests obstruction or hypertonus).

Exhaustion, dehydration, or fever (indicates prolonged labour or infection).

2. Physical Examination

General- Maternal vitals: Tachycardia, fever (>38°C), or hypotension (suggests sepsis or dehydration). Signs of exhaustion: Pallor, dry mucous membranes.

Abdominal Examination

Leopold's maneuwers: Confirm lie (longitudinal), presentation (vertex), position (e.g., OP, OT), and engagement.

Fundal Height: Assess for polyhydramnios or macrosomia.

Contractions: Palpate frequency (<3/10 minutes suggests hypotonic), duration, and intensity.

Bandl's Ring: Pathological retraction ring (oblique ridge between upper and lower uterus) indicates obstruction.

Vaginal Examination

Cervical Status: Dilatation (<1 cm/hour in active phase), effacement, and position (posterior suggests slow progress).

Presenting Part: Confirm vertex, brow, face, or breech. Palpate sutures/fontanelles for position (e.g., anterior fontanelle in OP). Assess station (e.g., 0 at ischial spines, +2 below).

Holding: Degree of suture overlap (0 to +3; +3 suggests CPD).

Caput Succedaneum: Soft tissue swelling (large caput indicates obstruction).

Pelvimetry: Measure diagonal conjugate (<11.5 cm suggests inlet contraction), ischial spines, and pubic arch.

Membranes: Intact, bulging, or ruptured (note amniotic fluid colour: meconium suggests distress).

Fetal Heart Rate (FHR): Auscultate every 15 minutes in active phase (normal: 110–160 bpm). Abnormal: Bradycardia (<110 bpm), tachycardia (>160 bpm), or late decelerations indicate distress.

3. Partogram

WHO-recommended tool to monitor labour progress:

Cervical Dilatation: Plotted against time (alert line: 1 cm/hour from 4 cm; action line: 4 hours beyond alert).

Fetal Descent: Station relative to ischial spines.

Contractions: Frequency, duration, and intensity.

FHR: Abnormal patterns trigger intervention.

Maternal Vitals: Detects fever or tachycardia.

Findings: Crossing alert line suggests prolonged labour. Crossing action line indicates need for intervention (e.g., oxytocin, cesarean).

4. Additional Tests

Ultrasound: Confirm presentation, position, and EFW. Assess amniotic fluid index (AFI <5 cm suggests oligohydramnios).

Cardiotocography (CTG): Continuous FHR monitoring in high-risk cases. Non-reassuring patterns (e.g., variable decelerations) indicate distress.

Blood Tests: Complete blood count (CBC) for infection (leukocytosis) or anemia. Blood grouping and cross-match for potential cesarean or hemorrhage.

Complications of Prolonged Labour

Prolonged labour increases maternal and fetal risks, necessitating vigilant monitoring and timely intervention.

1. Maternal Complications

a. Postpartum Hemorrhage (PPH): Uterine atony from prolonged contractions or exhaustion. Incidence: 10–20% in prolonged labour.
b. Obstetric Fistulae: Vesicovaginal or rectovaginal fistulae from prolonged pressure on pelvic tissues. Common in LMICs with delayed access to CEmOC.
c. Infection: Chorioamnionitis or endometritis, especially after prolonged rupture of membranes (>18 hours). Signs: Fever, foul-smelling lochia, uterine tenderness.
d. Uterine RuptureRare (0.5–1%), but life-threatening, especially in multiparous women or obstructed labour. Signs: Sudden pain, FHR abnormalities, vaginal bleeding.
e. Maternal Exhaustion: Dehydration, ketoacidosis, or psychological trauma.

Pelvic Trauma: Perineal tears (third/fourth-degree) or pubic symphysis separation.

2. Fetal Complications

a. Birth Asphyxia: Reduced placental perfusion from prolonged contractions or cord compression. Incidence: 5–10% in prolonged labour.
b. Neonatal Sepsis: From prolonged rupture of membranes or maternal infection.
c. Intracranial Hemorrhage: From excessive moldings or trauma during prolonged second stage.
d. Meconium Aspiration Syndrome: Meconium-stained amniotic fluid increases risk in post-term or distressed fetuses.
e. Stillbirth or Neonatal Death: Risk increases with severe obstruction or untreated distress.

Management of Prolonged Labour

Management aims to identify the cause, correct reversible factors, and expedite delivery to minimize complications. It involves supportive care, medical interventions, and operative delivery when indicated.

1. General Management

Supportive Care: Hydration: IV fluids (e.g., Ringer's lactate, 125 mL/hour) to correct dehydration. Nutrition: Light oral intake in early labour; avoid heavy meals to reduce aspiration risk.

Pain Relief: Non-pharmacological: Breathing exercises, massage, warm compresses Pharmacological: Epidural analgesia (monitor for prolonged second stage), nitrous oxide, or opioids (e.g., pethidine).

Positioning: Encourage upright (walking, squatting) or left lateral positions to enhance contractions and fetal descent.

Infection Prevention: Antibiotics (e.g., ampicillin 2 g IV every 6 hours) for prolonged rupture of membranes (>18 hours) or fever. Minimize vaginal examinations to reduce endometritis risk.

2. Specific Management by Cause

a. Inefficient Uterine Contractions

Amniotomy (ARM): Perform if membranes intact, cervix ≥4 cm, and head engaged. Releases prostaglandins, enhancing contractions. Risks: Cord prolapse, infection (monitor FHR post-ARM).

Oxytocin Augmentation

Indication: Hypotonic contractions (<3/10 minutes or weak).

Protocol: IV oxytocin starting at 2–4 MU/min, increase by 1–2 MU/min every 15–30 minutes (maximum 20–40 MU/min).

Goal: 3–5 contractions/10 minutes, lasting 40–60 seconds.

Risks: Hyperstimulation (>5 contractions/10 minutes), requiring tocolytics (e.g., terbutaline 0.25 mg IV). Contraindications: Obstruction, feta distress, or previous cesarean (relative).

Monitoring: Continuous CTG or intermittent auscultation; reassess cervix every 2–4 hours.

b. Cephalopelvic Disproportion (CPD)

Trial of Labour: Indicated for relative CPD with vertex presentation and borderline pelvis. Monitor with partogram; proceed to cesarean if no progress after 2–4 hours in active phase.

Cesarean Section: Indicated for absolute CPD (e.g., obstetric conjugate <10 cm), failed trial of labour, or fetal distress. Preferred for severe inlet/midpelvis contraction or macrosomia (EFW >4,500 g).

c. Malposition/Malpresentation

Manual Rotation: For OP or OT positions, rotate to OA under anesthesia by skilled providers. Success rate: 60–80%.

Assisted Vaginal Delivery: Forceps or vacuum extraction for second-stage arrest with OA position and station ≥+2. Requires skilled operator, maternal consent, and no CPD.

Cesarean Section: Indicated for persistent OP, brow, mento-posterior face, or breech with failed external cephalic version (ECV).

d. Maternal Exhaustion

Provide IV fluids, glucose (e.g., 5% dextrose), and rest (short-term epidural if feasible). Reassess after 1–2 hours; proceed to assisted delivery or cesarean if no progress.

e. Obstruction (Soft Tissue or Bandl's Ring)

Immediate cesarean section for tumors, fibroids, or pathological retraction ring. Manage Bandl's ring with tocolytics (e.g., nitroglycerin) to relax uterus before surgery.

3. Management of Complications

Fetal Distress: Intrauterine Resuscitation: Left lateral position, oxygen (10 L/min via mask), IV fluids, stop oxytocin. Expedited Delivery: Cesarean or assisted vaginal delivery based on station and cervical dilatation.

Maternal Infection: Broad-spectrum antibiotics (e.g., ampicillin + gentamicin). Monitor for sepsis (e.g., lactate, blood cultures).

PPH: Administer uterotonics (oxytocin 10 IU IM, misoprostol 600 mcg oral), uterine massage, and bimanual compression. Prepare for blood transfusion or surgical intervention (e.g., uterine artery ligation).

Uterine Rupture: Emergency laparotomy, uterine repair, or hysterectomy. Stabilize with IV fluids, blood transfusion, and broad-spectrum antibiotics.

4. Postpartum Care

Monitoring:: Maternal: Vitals, uterine tone, bleeding, and perineal condition every 15 minutes for 2 hours. Neonatal: Apgar scores, warmth, breastfeeding, and signs of asphyxia or sepsis.

Management: Repair perineal tears or episiotomy under local anesthesia. Initiate breastfeeding within 1 hour. Administer antibiotics for infection and uterotonics for PPH prevention.

Follow-Up: Schedule postpartum visits at 1–2 weeks to assess recovery and neonatal health.

Prevention

Antenatal Care: Routine ultrasound to assess feta size, presentation, and pelvic adequacy. Clinical pelvimetry to identify contracted pelvis early. Manage diabetes to reduce macrosomia risk.

Education: Counsel on labour signs, hospital delivery, and risks of prolonged labour. Promote birth preparedness via ASHA workers.

Nutrition: Address childhood malnutrition to prevent pelvic deformities (e.g., rickets). Ensure adequate maternal weight gain to support labour stamina.

Conclusion

Prolonged labour, a form of abnormal labour, is characterized by delayed cervical dilatation or feta descent, often due to inefficient contractions, CPD, or malposition. It increases risks of maternal complications (e.g., PPH, fistulae) and feta morbidity (e.g., asphyxia, sepsis). Diagnosis involves partogram monitoring, abdominal/vaginal examinations, and ultrasound to identify causes.

Management includes supportive care (hydration, pain relief), oxytocin augmentation, assisted delivery, or cesarean section, tailored to the underlying issue.

References

Dutta, D.C. (2020). Textbook of Obstetrics.

Cunningham, F.G., et al. (2022). Williams Obstetrics.

World Health Organization. (2018). WHO Recommendations: Intrapartum Care for a Positive Childbirth Experience.

American College of Obstetricians and Gynecologists. (2020). ACOG Practice Bulletin No. 49: Dystocia and Augmentation of Labor.

7.2 Obstructed Labor

(*Wiladat-e-muar-qla*)

Introduction

Obstructed labor is a severe form of abnormal labor characterized by the failure of the fetus to progress through the birth canal despite adequate uterine contractions, due to a mechanical obstruction. It is a life-threatening obstetric emergency that significantly contributes to maternal and neonatal morbidity and mortality, particularly in low- and middle-income countries (LMICs).

Definition

Obstructed labor is defined as the arrest of labor progression due to a mechanical impediment that prevents vaginal delivery, despite strong and coordinated uterine contractions. It is diagnosed when:

a. Cervical dilatation or fetal descent stucks in the active phase of labor (first stage) or second stage, as evidenced by a partogram.

b. Clinical signs of obstruction are present, such as excessive holding, caput succedaneum, or Bandl's ring.

c. The fetus cannot be delivered vaginally without operative intervention (e.g., cesarean section).

Obstructed labor typically occurs in the context of

Cephalopelvic disproportion (CPD): The fetal head is too large or misaligned relative to the maternal pelvis.

Malpresentation or malposition: Non-vertex presentation or unfavorable position (e.g., persistent occiput posterior).

Soft tissue or pelvic abnormalities: Obstructing tumours or contracted pelvis.

Causes of Obstructed Labor

Obstructed labor results from abnormalities in the three Ps of labor (passenger, passage, powers) and occasionally maternal psychological factors (psyche). These causes often interact, complicating diagnosis and management.

1. Passenger (Fetus)

Fetal Size -Macrosomia: Estimated fetal weight (EFW) >4,000 g (or >4,500 g in diabetic mothers) increases biparietal diameter (BPD, ~9.5 cm), causing CPD. Common in gestational diabetes or post-term pregnancy (>41 weeks).

Malpresentation

Brow Presentation: Supraoccipitomental diameter (13.5 cm) is too large for most pelves.

Face Presentation: Mento-posterior position prevents rotation and delivery.

Breech Presentation: Frank, complete, or footling breech may obstruct, especially with an extended head.

Shoulder Presentation: Associated with transverse lie, incompatible with vaginal delivery.

Compound Presentation: Multiple parts (e.g., hand and head) obstruct the pelvis.

Malposition

Occiput Posterior (OP): Persistent OP increases the presenting diameter (occipitofrontal, 11.5 cm vs. suboccipitobregmatic, 9.5 cm), leading to deep transverse arrest.

Occiput Transverse (OT): Failure to rotate to occiput anterior (OA) causes midpelvis obstruction.

Fetal Anomalies

Hydrocephalus: Enlarged head (BPD >10 cm) causes absolute obstruction.

Tumors: Sacrococcygeal teratomas or meningoceles block the pelvis.

Lack of Molding: Failure of cranial sutures to overlap, preventing head diameter reduction.

2. Passage (Maternal Pelvis and Soft Tissues)

Cephalopelvic Disproportion (CPD)

Absolute CPD: Severe mismatch (e.g., obstetric conjugate <8 cm vs. BPD 9.5 cm), preventing vaginal delivery.

Relative CPD: Borderline mismatch exacerbated by macrosomia, malposition, or deflexed attitude (e.g., occipitofrontal diameter, 11.5 cm).

Contracted Pelvis

Inlet: Obstetric conjugate <10 cm or transverse diameter <12 cm (normal: 10.5–11 cm, 13–13.5 cm). Midpelvis: Interspinous diameter <9.5 cm (normal: 10–10.5 cm) Outlet: Intertuberous diameter <9 cm or pubic arch angle <70° (normal: 10–11 cm, 80–90°).

Pelvic Deformities

Congenital: Asymmetrical pelvis (e.g., Naegele's or Robert's pelvis), kyphoscoliosis, or dwarfism.

Acquired: Rickets, osteomalacia, tuberculosis, or pelvic fractures (e.g., road traffic accidents).

Pelvic Shape

Android Pelvis: Narrow anteroposterior diameter and convergent sidewalls.

Platypelloid Pelvis: Flattened inlet, reducing obstetric conjugate.

Anthropoid Pelvis: Narrow transverse diameter, favoring OP positions.

Soft Tissue Obstruction

Uterine or Cervical: Fibroids, cervical stenosis, or scarring (e.g., post-conization).

Vaginal: Septa, cysts, or tumors (e.g., ovarian cysts).

Perineal: Rigid perineum or previous severe scarring.

Other: Distended bladder or rectum impeding descent.

3. Powers (Uterine Contractions)

Inefficient Contractions: Hypotonic contractions (weak, <3/10 minutes, or short, <40 seconds) fail to overcome obstruction.Causes: Uterine overdistension (e.g., twins, polyhydramnios), maternal exhaustion, or grand multiparity.

Incoordinate Contractions: Irregular or asynchronous contractions reduce dilatation efficiency. Causes: Primigravidity, anxiety, or epidural analgesia.

Hypertonic Contractions: Excessive contractions (tachysystole, >5/10 minutes) from oxytocin misuse or obstruction, leading to Bandl's ring (pathological retraction ring).

Secondary Uterine Inertia: Contractions weaken after prolonged obstruction due to myometrial fatigue.

Diagnosis of Obstructed Labor

Prompt diagnosis is critical to prevent complications. It relies on clinical assessment, partogram monitoring and targeted investigations to confirm obstruction and identify its cause.

1. History

Maternal: Parity, previous obstructed labor, cesarean section, or pelvic trauma.

Risk factors: Short stature (<150 cm), obesity (BMI >30 kg/m^2), or diabetes (macrosomia). Duration of labor, contraction pattern, and membrane status (ruptured >18 hours increases infection risk). Symptoms: Severe, constant pain (suggests obstruction or rupture), reduced fetal movements, or fever.

Obstetric: Antenatal ultrasound findings (e.g., macrosomia, hydrocephalus). Onset of strong contractions without progress.

2. Physical Examination

Vital Signs: Tachycardia, fever (>38°C), or hypotension (indicates sepsis, dehydration, or rupture) . Signs of Exhaustion: Pallor, dry mucous membranes, ketotic breath.

Abdominal Examination: Leopold's Maneuvers: Confirm lie (longitudinal vs. transverse), presentation (vertex, breech, shoulder), position (OP, OT), and engagement.

Fundal Height: Assess for macrosomia, twins, or polyhydramnios.

Contractions: Palpate frequency, duration, and intensity (hypertonic suggests obstruction).

Bandl's Ring: Visible or palpable ridge between upper and lower uterus, indicating severe obstruction (emergency).

Uterine Tenderness: Suggests rupture or infection.

Vaginal Examination (sterile, minimize to reduce infection)

Cervical Status

Dilatation: Arrested (<1 cm/hour in active phase).

Effacement: Incomplete in early obstruction.

Position: Posterior, indicating poor progress.

Presenting Part: Identify vertex, brow, face, breech, or shoulder. Palpate sutures/fontanelles for position (e.g., anterior fontanelle in OP, posterior in OA). Assess station (e.g., –1 or 0, indicating no descent). Holding: Excessive (grade +3, irreducible overlap) suggests CPD.

Caput Succedaneum: Large, boggy swelling obscuring sutures indicates prolonged pressure.

Pelvimetry

Diagonal conjugate (<11.5 cm suggests inlet contraction).

Ischial spines prominence (interspinous <9.5 cm).

Sidewall convergence (android pelvis).

Pubic arch angle (<70° suggests outlet contraction).

Coccyx mobility (fixed coccyx reduces outlet).

Amniotic Fluid: Meconium-stained (thick, green) indicates fetal distress; foul odor suggests infection.

Soft Tissues: Palpate for fibroids, cysts, or vaginal septa.

Fetal Heart Rate (FHR): Auscultate every 15 minutes in active phase (normal: 110–160 bpm). Abnormal: Bradycardia (<110 bpm), tachycardia (>160 bpm), or late/variable decelerations indicate distress or cord compression.

3. Partogram

WHO-recommended tool to monitor labor progress.

Cervical Dilatation: Plotted against time (alert line: 1 cm/hour from 4 cm; action line: 4 hours beyond alert).

Fetal Descent: Station relative to ischial spines (arrest at 0 or above suggests obstruction).

Contractions: Frequency, duration, and intensity (adequate but no progress confirms obstruction).

FHR: Non-reassuring patterns trigger intervention.

Maternal Vitals: Fever or tachycardia indicates complications.

Findings: Crossing action line with no dilatation/descent confirms obstruction.

Prolonged active phase (>12 hours) or second stage (>2 hours primigravida) suggests CPD or malposition.

4. Additional Investigations

Ultrasound: Confirm presentation, position (e.g., OP, brow), and EFW (macrosomia >4,000 g). Assess amniotic fluid index (AFI <5 cm suggests oligohydramnios, increasing distress risk). Detect anomalies (e.g., hydrocephalus).

Cardiotocography (CTG): Continuous FHR monitoring in high-risk cases.

Non-reassuring patterns (e.g., late decelerations, reduced variability) indicate urgent delivery.

Blood Tests: Complete blood count (CBC): Leukocytosis (>15,000/mm^3) suggests infection; anemias (Hb <7 g/dL) increases PPH risk. Blood grouping and cross-match Prepare for transfusion in cesarean or rupture. C-reactive protein (CRP) or blood cultures: Confirm sepsis if fever present.

Imaging (rare): X-ray or MRI pelvimetry for suspected deformities (e.g., post-traumatic pelvis), used antenatally in high-resource settings.

Complications of Obstructed Labor

Obstructed labor is a medical emergency with severe consequences if untreated, particularly in LMICs

1. Maternal Complications

Uterine Rupture: Incidence: 0.5–2% in obstructed labore, higher in multiparous women or previous cesarean. Signs: Sudden severe pain, FHR abnormalities, vaginal bleeding, loss of contractions, or shock. Outcomes: Maternal mortality (5–10%), hysterectomy, or massive hemorrhage.

Obstetric Fistulae: Vesicovaginal or rectovaginal fistulae from prolonged pressure necrosis of pelvic tissues. Incidence: 1–2% in LMICs; causes urinary/fecal incontinence, social stigma.

Postpartum Hemorrhage (PPH): Uterine atony from prolonged contractions or rupture. Incidence: 10–20%; exacerbated by anemia or exhaustion.

Infection: Chorioamnionitis or endometritis from prolonged rupture of membranes (>18 hours) or frequent vaginal examinations.

Sepsis: Mortality 20–40% if untreated; signs include fever, tachycardia, and foul lochia.

Maternal Exhaustion: Dehydration, ketoacidosis, or psychological trauma from prolonged pain.

Pelvic Trauma: Third/fourth-degree perineal tears, pubic symphysis diastasis, or bladder injury.

Long-Term: Chronic pelvic pain, infertility, or dyspareunia from scarring or fistulae.

2. Fetal Complications

Birth Asphyxia: Reduced placental perfusion from prolonged compression or cord prolapse. Incidence: 10–20%; leads to hypoxic-ischemic encephalopathy (HIE).

Neonatal Sepsis: From maternal infection or prolonged rupture of membranes. Incidence: 5–10%; mortality 15–30% in LMICs.

Intracranial Hemorrhage: From excessive holding or trauma during prolonged pressure.

Meconium Aspiration Syndrome: Thick meconium from fetal distress increases respiratory complications.

Stillbirth or Neonatal Death: Incidence: 10–30% in untreated obstruction, highest with uterine rupture or severe asphyxia.

Long-Term: Cerebral palsy or developmental delays from HIE.

Management of Obstructed Labor

Management aims to relieve the obstruction, expedite delivery, and prevent or treat complications.

1. General Management

Initial Stabilization

Airway, Breathing, Circulation (ABC): Assess maternal vitals; administer oxygen (10 L/min via mask) if hypoxic.

IV Access: Two large-bore cannulae; infuse Ringer's lactate (1–2 L) to correct dehydration or shock.

Blood Transfusion: Cross-match 2–4 units of packed red cells for anemia (Hb <7 g/dL) or anticipated hemorrhage.

Antibiotics: Broad-spectrum (e.g., ampicillin 2 g IV + gentamicin 5 mg/kg IV) for prolonged rupture (>18 hours), fever, or suspected chorioamnionitis.

Analgesia: Parenteral opioids (e.g., pethidine 50–100 mg IM) or epidural if cesarean not imminent.

Catheterization: Insert Foley catheter to empty bladder (distended bladder may obstruct descent) and monitor urine output.

Fetal Monitoring: Continuous CTG or intermittent auscultation every 15 minutes. Non-reassuring FHR (e.g., bradycardia <110 bpm) indicates urgent delivery.

Maternal Support: Reassure patient and family; explain need for intervention (e.g., cesarean). Involve birth companion to reduce anxiety.

2. Specific Management by Cause

Cephalopelvic Disproportion (CPD)

Cesarean Section- Indication: Absolute CPD (e.g., obstetric conjugate <10 cm), failed trial of labor, or fetal distress.Preferred for macrosomia (EFW >4,500 g), severe holding (+3), or Bandl's ring. Technique: Lower segment cesarean section (LSCS) under spinal/general anesthesia. Risks: Infection, hemorrhage, prolonged recovery.

Trial of Labor (rare): For relative CPD with vertex presentation, favorable position (OA), and borderline pelvis. Monitor with partogram; proceed to cesarean if no progress after 2–4 hours in active phase.

Malpresentation/Malposition

Brow or Mento-Posterior Face: Cesarean section, as vaginal delivery is rarely feasible. Breech: Attempt external cephalic version (ECV) antenatally (36–37 weeks) if feasible; otherwise, cesarean. Vaginal breech delivery by skilled providers in select cases (e.g., frank breech, EFW <3,500 g).

Shoulder Presentation/Transverse Lie: Cesarean section; avoid internal podalic version due to rupture risk.

Occiput Posterior (OP) or Transverse (OT): Manual Rotation: Rotate to OA under anesthesia if station ≥0 and cervix fully dilated.

Assisted Vaginal Delivery: Forceps or vacuum for OP at +2 station, no CPD and skilled operator. Cesarean: If rotation fails or distress occurs.

Soft Tissue Obstruction

Fibroids/Cysts: Cesarean section; excise tumor if feasible.

Cervical Stenosis: Gentle dilatation under anesthesia or cesarean.

Vaginal Septa: Incise septum under local anesthesia if minor; cesarean for major obstructions.

Inefficient Contractions (Secondary to Obstruction)

Avoid Oxytocin: Contraindicated in obstruction, as it increases rupture risk.

Tocolytics: Administer terbutaline (0.25 mg IV) or nitroglycerin (50–100 mcg IV) to relax uterus if hypertonic or Bandl's ring present, facilitating cesarean.

Fetal Anomalies (e.g., Hydrocephalus)

Cephalocentesis: Drain cerebrospinal fluid under ultrasound guidance in non-viable fetuses to allow vaginal delivery (ethical considerations apply).

Cesarean: For viable fetuses or if cephalocentesis contraindicated.

3. Management of Complications

Uterine Rupture: Emergency Laparotomy: Repair uterus (if feasible) or hysterectomy; stabilize with IV fluids, blood transfusion, and antibiotics. Maternal Mortality: 5–10% without rapid surgery.

Fetal Distress: Intrauterine Resuscitation: Left lateral position, oxygen, IV fluids, stop oxytocin (if used).

Expedited Delivery: Cesarean (first stage or high station) or assisted vaginal delivery (second stage, station ≥+2).

Infection: Broad-spectrum antibiotics (e.g., ceftriaxone 1 g IV + metronidazole 500 mg IV).Monitor for sepsis (lactate >2 mmol/L, organ dysfunction); escalate to ICU if needed.

Postpartum Hemorrhage (PPH)

Uterotonics: Oxytocin 10 IU IM, misoprostol 600 mcg oral, or ergometrine 0.2 mg IM.

Uterine massage, bimanual compression, or balloon tamponade.

Surgical options: Uterine artery ligation, B-Lynch suture, or hysterectomy.

Obstetric Fistulae

Postpartum catheter for 14–21 days to promote spontaneous closure (small fistulae).

Surgical repair (fistulotomy) after 3–6 months by specialists.

Neonatal Asphyxia

Resuscitate per Helping Babies Breathe (HBB) or AAP guidelines: PPV, oxygen, chest compressions if heart rate <60 bpm.

Transfer to neonatal intensive care unit (NICU) for hypoxic-ischemic encephalopathy (HIE) management.

4. Postpartum Care

Maternal: Vitals, uterine tone, bleeding, and perineal condition every 15 minutes for 2 hours, then hourly. Neonatal: Apgar scores (1, 5, 10 minutes), temperature, feeding, and signs of sepsis or HIE.

Management

Maternal

Repair perineal tears/episiotomy under local anesthesia.

Continue antibiotics for 5–7 days if infection present.

Administer uterotonics (oxytocin 10 IU IV infusion) for PPH prevention.

Monitor urine output (indwelling catheter for 24–48 hours post-cesarean or fistula risk).

Neonatal

Initiate breastfeeding within 1 hour (if stable).

Administer vitamin K (1 mg IM), hepatitis B vaccine, and eye prophylaxis (erythromycin ointment).

Monitor for jaundice, seizures, or respiratory distress.

Prevention

Antenatal Care

Routine ultrasound to assess fetal size, presentation, and anomalies (e.g., hydrocephalus).

Clinical pelvimetry to identify contracted pelvis (e.g., diagonal conjugate <11.5 cm).

Manage diabetes to reduce macrosomia risk.

Perform ECV for breech at 36–37 weeks to achieve vertex presentation.

Education

Counsel on labor signs, hospital delivery, and risks of obstruction.

Train traditional birth attendants to refer prolonged labor cases early.

Promote birth preparedness via ASHA workers (India's NHM).

Nutrition

Address childhood malnutrition to prevent pelvic deformities (e.g., rickets).

Ensure adequate maternal weight gain to support pelvic development.

Conclusion

Obstructed labor is a critical obstetric emergency characterized by mechanical impedance to vaginal delivery, often due to cephalopelvic disproportion, malpresentation, or pelvic abnormalities. It leads to severe maternal complications (e.g., uterine rupture, fistulae) and fetal morbidity (e.g., asphyxia, stillbirth). Diagnosis relies on partogram monitoring, clinical examinations (abdominal, vaginal), and ultrasound to confirm obstruction and its cause. Management involves urgent cesarean section for most cases, with assisted delivery or manual rotation in select scenarios, supported by stabilization measures (fluids, antibiotics).

References

Dutta, D.C. (2020). Textbook of Obstetrics.

Cunningham, F.G., et al. (2022). Williams Obstetrics.

World Health Organization. (2018). WHO Recommendations: Intrapartum Care for a Positive Childbirth Experience.

World Health Organization. (2006). Managing Complications in Pregnancy and Childbirth.

American College of Obstetricians and Gynecologists. (2020). ACOG Practice Bulletin No. 49: Dystocia and Augmentation of Labor.

7.3 Occipito Posterior Position

(*Wazyeeya qazaliya khalfiya*)

Introduction

The occipito-posterior (OP) position is a common fetal malposition during labor, where the fetal occiput is oriented toward the posterior quadrant of the maternal pelvis, either as right occipito-posterior (ROP) or left occipito-posterior (LOP). While many fetus in the OP position rotate spontaneously to the optimal occipito-anterior (OA) position, persistent OP can lead to prolonged labor, increased maternal and fetal complications, and a higher likelihood of operative delivery. The OP position is significant in obstetrics due to its association with labor dystocia, perineal trauma and neonatal morbidity.

Definition

The occipito-posterior position is a vertex presentation in which the fetal head enters the pelvic inlet with the occiput aligned with the maternal posterior pelvis (sacrum), rather than the anterior pelvis (pubic symphysis). It is classified as:

Right Occipito-Posterior (ROP): Fetal occiput faces the maternal right posterior quadrant (most common, ~60–70% of OP cases).

Left Occipito-Posterior (LOP): Fetal occiput faces the maternal left posterior quadrant.

Direct Occipito-Posterior (DOP): Occiput directly aligns with the maternal sacrum (rare).

The OP position contrasts with the occipito-anterior (OA) position, where the occiput faces the maternal anterior pelvis, presenting the smallest fetal head diameter (suboccipitobregmatic, 9.5 cm) for delivery. In OP, the fetal head is often deflexed, presenting a larger diameter (occipitofrontal, 11.5 cm), which can impede labor progress.

Risk Factors: Higher incidence in primigravidas, epidural analgesia, anthropoid/android pelvis, and preterm labor.

Causes and Predisposing Factors

The OP position results from a combination of fetal, maternal and labor-related factors that prevent or delay rotation to OA.

1. Fetal Factors

Head Deflexion: The fetal head is partially extended (deflexed), presenting the occipitofrontal diameter (11.5 cm) instead of the suboccipitobregmatic (9.5 cm). Deflexion reduces engagement and alignment with the pelvic inlet.

Fetal Size: Macrosomia (EFW >4,000 g) increases the likelihood of OP due to limited pelvic space for rotation.

Fetal Anomalies: Rare anomalies (e.g., neck masses) may restrict head flexion.

2. Maternal Factors

Pelvic Shape:

Anthropoid Pelvis: Long anteroposterior diameter favors OP entry, as the occiput aligns with the sacrum.

Android Pelvis: Narrow transverse diameter and convergent sidewalls hinder rotation to OA.

Platypelloid Pelvis: Flattened inlet may trap the head in OP.

Contracted Pelvis: Reduced diameters (e.g., interspinous <9.5 cm) increase CPD risk, perpetuating OP.

Soft Tissue Resistance: Rigid pelvic floor or perineum (e.g., in primigravidas) impedes rotation.

Maternal Posture: Prolonged supine position or sedentary lifestyle antenatally may encourage posterior occiput alignment.

3. Labor-Related Factors

Epidural Analgesia: Relaxes pelvic floor muscles, reducing resistance needed for rotation, increasing persistent OP (2–3-fold risk).

Premature Rupture of Membranes (PROM): Early loss of amniotic fluid reduces cushioning, fixing the head in OP.

Inefficient Contractions: Weak or incoordinate uterine action (e.g., in primigravidas) delays descent and rotation.

Maternal Obesity: BMI >30 kg/m^2 increases OP risk due to altered pelvic dynamics and macrosomia.

Diagnosis

Accurate diagnosis of the OP position is essential for anticipating labor challenges and planning management. It relies on clinical examination, supplemented by imaging when needed.

1. History

Symptoms: Persistent back pain (back labor) due to occipital pressure on the maternal sacrum. Prolonged labor or slow progress reported by the patient. Urge to push before full dilatation (second stage) due to posterior head pressure on the rectum.

Risk Factors

Primigravidity, epidural use, or history of OP in prior deliveries. Antenatal ultrasound suggesting posterior occiput.

2. Physical Examination

Abdominal Examination: Leopold's Maneuvers

Fetal back felt in the maternal flank or laterally (less distinct than OA).

Limbs palpated anteriorly across the maternal abdomen (fetal abdomen faces forward).

Head often deflexed, with a higher fundal height than OA.

Engagement: Delayed or absent due to larger presenting diameter.

Contractions: Assess frequency, duration, and intensity (adequate contractions with no progress suggest OP or CPD).

Vaginal Examination (sterile, minimize to reduce infection):

Cervical Status

Dilatation: Slow progress (<1 cm/hour in active phase) suggests OP-related dystocia.

Effacement: May be incomplete due to uneven head pressure.

Position: Posterior cervix indicates poor application of the presenting part.

Presenting Part

Sutures and Fontanelles: Anterior fontanelle (bregma, diamond-shaped) felt centrally or anteriorly due to deflexion. Posterior fontanelle (lambda, Y-shaped) felt posteriorly or not palpable. Sagittal suture runs anteroposteriorly, with lambda toward the sacrum.

Position: Confirm ROP (occiput to maternal right posterior), LOP, or DOP.

Station: Often high (–1 to 0) due to delayed descent.

Moulding: Moderate to severe (+2 to +3) indicates prolonged pressure or CPD.

Caput Succedaneum: Swelling over the vertex, obscuring sutures in prolonged labor.

Pelvimetry

Assess diagonal conjugate (>11.5 cm), ischial spines (interspinous >9.5 cm), and pubic arch (>80°) to rule out CPD. Note pelvic shape (android/anthropoid predisposes to OP).

Amniotic Fluid: Meconium-staining suggests fetal distress in prolonged OP labor.

Fetal Heart Rate (FHR)

Auscultate every 15 minutes in active phase (normal: 110–160 bpm).

Abnormal: Bradycardia (<110 bpm), tachycardia (>160 bpm), or decelerations indicate distress, common in prolonged OP.

3. Partogram: WHO-recommended tool to monitor labor progress

Cervical Dilatation: Slow (<1 cm/hour from 4 cm) or arrested, crossing alert/action lines.

Fetal Descent: Delayed or stalled (station 0 or above).

Contractions: Adequate (3–5/10 minutes, 40–60 seconds) but ineffective, suggesting malposition. FHR: Non-reassuring patterns trigger intervention.

4. Ultrasound

Intrapartum Ultrasound

Confirms OP position (occiput at 6–9 o'clock for ROP, 3–6 o'clock for LOP).

Assesses head flexion (deflexed in OP), station, and angle of progression.

Rules out macrosomia (EFW >4,000 g) or anomalies.

Antenatal Ultrasound

Identifies persistent OP at 36–37 weeks, guiding delivery planning.

Mechanism of Labor in Occipito-Posterior Position

The mechanism of labor in OP differs from OA due to the larger presenting diameter and need for rotation. Approximately 80–90% of OP fetuses rotate to OA, but persistent OP alters the cardinal movements.

1. Normal Rotation to Occipito-Anterior (Long Rotation, 80–90%)

Engagement: Fetal head enters the pelvic inlet in ROP or LOP, with the occipitofrontal diameter (11.5 cm) aligned transversely or obliquely. Deflexed attitude delays engagement compared to OA.

Descent: Driven by uterine contractions and maternal pushing. Descent is slower due to larger diameter and poor head application to the cervix.

Flexion: As the head meets pelvic floor resistance (levator ani), it flexes, reducing the presenting diameter to suboccipitobregmatic (9.5 cm).

Internal Rotation: Head rotates 135° (ROP: counterclockwise; LOP: clockwise) to OA, aligning the occiput with the maternal pubic symphysis. Facilitated by pelvic floor muscles and a gynecoid pelvis.

Extension: Head extends under the symphysis pubis, delivering the occiput, forehead, and face.

Restitution and External Rotation: Head restitutes 45° to align with shoulders, then rotates further as shoulders align anteroposteriorly.

Expulsion: Shoulders and body deliver as in OA.

2. Persistent Occipito-Posterior (Short Rotation or No Rotation, 10–20%)

Engagement and Descent: Head remains deflexed, presenting occipitofrontal (11.5 cm) or rarely frontomental (13.5 cm) diameter. Descent is slow or arrested due to CPD or pelvic shape (android/anthropoid).

Internal Rotation (Partial or None): Head rotates 45° to direct OP (DOP) or fails to rotate, remaining ROP/LOP. Arrest at midpelvis (deep transverse arrest in OT) or outlet occurs.

Extension: In DOP, the head delivers face-to-pubes, with the occiput pivoting over the perineum and the forehead under the sacrum. Requires significant perineal stretching, increasing tear risk.

Expulsion: Shoulders follow, often with difficulty due to misalignment.

Outcomes: Prolonged second stage, higher operative delivery rate (forceps, vacuum, cesarean).

Complications of Occipito-Posterior Position

The OP position, particularly when persistent, increases maternal and fetal risks due to prolonged labor and mechanical challenges.

1. Maternal Complications

Prolonged Labor

First stage: Slow dilatation (<1 cm/hour) due to poor head application.

Second stage: >2 hours (primigravida) or >1 hour (multigravida) without epidural.

Perineal Trauma: Third/fourth-degree tears from face-to-pubes delivery or operative intervention.

Postpartum Hemorrhage (PPH): Uterine atony from prolonged labor or trauma.

Infection: Chorioamnionitis or endometritis from prolonged rupture of membranes (>18 hours) or frequent vaginal examinations.

Maternal Exhaustion: Dehydration, ketoacidosis, or psychological trauma from back pain and prolonged effort.

Operative Delivery: Increased cesarean (15–30%) or assisted vaginal delivery (10–20%) rates. Risks: Infection, hemorrhage, or anesthesia complications.

2. Fetal Complications

Birth Asphyxia: Prolonged labor or cord compression reduces placental perfusion. Incidence: 5–10%; risk of hypoxic-ischemic encephalopathy (HIE).

Neonatal Trauma: Facial bruising, cephalhematoma, or subgaleal hemorrhage from operative delivery or molding.

Neonatal Sepsis: From prolonged rupture or maternal infection.

Meconium Aspiration Syndrome: Meconium-stained fluid from distress in prolonged labor.

Long-Term: Rare neurodevelopmental delays from severe asphyxia.

Management of Occipito-Posterior Position

Management aims to facilitate rotation to OA, promote vaginal delivery, and prevent complications.

1. Antenatal Management

Screening: Ultrasound at 36–37 weeks to identify persistent OP. Assess fetal size (EFW), pelvic shape, and risk factors (e.g., diabetes, obesity).

Counseling: Educate on OP risks (prolonged labor, operative delivery) and benefits of hospital delivery. Promote active maternal postures (e.g., walking, pelvic tilts) to encourage OA rotation.

Prevention: Manage gestational diabetes to reduce macrosomia. Encourage upright or forward-leaning positions antenatally to align fetal occiput anteriorly.

2. Intrapartum Management

Management is tailored to labor stage, cervical dilatation, station and maternal/fetal condition.

First Stage

Expectant Management

Indication: Early labor (<4 cm), no distress, and adequate contractions.

Rationale: 80–90% of OP fetuses rotate to OA spontaneously.

Monitor with partogram (alert line: 1 cm/hour from 4 cm).

Supportive Care: Positioning

Encourage upright (standing, squatting) or lateral positions to promote rotation.

Hands-and-knees or forward-leaning positions align the fetal occiput anteriorly.

Avoid prolonged supine position (reduces pelvic outlet).

Hydration: IV fluids (Ringer's lactate, 125 mL/hour) to prevent exhaustion.

Pharmacological: Epidural (monitor for prolonged second stage), nitrous oxide, or pethidine (50–100 mg IM).

Amniotomy

Perform if cervix ≥4 cm, head engaged, and contractions inadequate.

Oxytocin Augmentation

Indication: Hypotonic contractions (<3/10 minutes) with slow dilatation (<1 cm/hour).

Monitoring

Part gram: Track dilatation, descent, contractions, and FHR.

FHR: Auscultate every 15–30 minutes (active phase); continuous CTG if high-risk.

Vaginal Examination: Every 2–4 hours to assess dilatation, station, and position.

Maternal Vitals: Every 4 hours (pulse, BP, temperature).

Second Stage

Expectant Management; Indication: Full dilatation, station ≥+1, and progress (descent) with pushing. Allow 1–2 hours (primigravida) or 30–60 minutes (multigravida) for spontaneous rotation or delivery.

Manual Rotation: Indication: Persistent OP at +1 or lower, no CPD, and skilled operator.

Technique: Under epidural or pudendal block, rotate head 135° (ROP: counterclockwise; LOP: clockwise) to OA. Use fingers to grasp occiput or apply pressure on parietal bones. Confirm rotation with ultrasound or vaginal examination.

Risks: Cord prolapse, fetal trauma (rare).

Assisted Vaginal Delivery: Indication: Persistent OP or OP rotated to OA, station ≥+2, full dilatation, no CPD, and prolonged second stage (>2 hours primigravida, >1 hour multigravida).

Techniques

Vacuum Extraction: Apply cup over flexing point (midline, 3 cm anterior to posterior fontanelle). Traction with contractions, avoiding excessive force. Preferred for OP due to lower maternal trauma.

Forceps Delivery:Use rotational forceps (e.g., Kielland's) to rotate OP to OA, then deliver. Higher risk of maternal tears (third/fourth-degree).

Cesarean Section: Indications-

Failed manual rotation or assisted delivery.

Arrest of descent (no progress after 1–2 hours of pushing).

Fetal distress (e.g., bradycardia, late decelerations).

Suspected CPD (e.g., excessive molding, interspinous <9.5 cm).

Persistent DOP with face-to-pubes delivery unfeasible.

Technique: Lower segment cesarean section (LSCS) under spinal/general anesthesia.

Monitoring: FHR every 5 minutes in second stage. Assess maternal effort and perineal condition during pushing. Watch for signs of obstruction (e.g., Bandl's ring, severe molding).

Third Stage: Active Management

Administer oxytocin 10 IU IM/IV within 1 minute of delivery to prevent PPH (increased risk in OP). Controlled cord traction (Brandt-Andrews maneuver) after placental separation signs. Uterine massage post-delivery.

Inspection: Examine placenta for completeness. Assess perineum for tears (third/fourth-degree common in OP).

Management: Repair tears under local anesthesia or in theater if severe. Monitor for PPH (uterine atony, trauma).

3. Postpartum Management

Monitoring: Maternal: Vitals, uterine tone, bleeding and perineal pain every 15 minutes for 2 hours. Neonatal: Apgar scores (1, 5, 10 minutes), temperature, feeding and signs of trauma or asphyxia.

Management

Maternal: Analgesics (paracetamol, ibuprofen) for perineal pain. Continue antibiotics if infection suspected (e.g., prolonged rupture). Catheterize if urinary retention (common post-epidural or tears).

Neonatal: Initiate breastfeeding within 1 hour. Administer vitamin K (1 mg IM), hepatitis B vaccine, and eye prophylaxis. Monitor for jaundice, seizures, or respiratory distress.

Counselling

Discuss cause, recurrence risk (10–15% in future pregnancies), and delivery options (e.g., trial of labor vs. cesarean).

Address psychological trauma from prolonged labor or operative delivery.

Educate on danger signs (fever, bleeding, neonatal lethargy).

Follow-Up: Postpartum visits at 1–2 weeks, 6 weeks to assess recovery and neonatal health.

7.4 Deep Transverse Arrest

(*Twaq-quf-e-mustariz ameeq*)

Introduction

Deep transverse arrest (DTA) is a serious complication of labor characterized by the failure of the fetal head to rotate and descend beyond the midpelvis, with the head arrested in the transverse position (occipito-transverse, OT) at or below the level of the ischial spines. It is a form of labor dystocia typically associated with malposition (e.g., persistent occipito-posterior or occipito-transverse), cephalopelvic disproportion (CPD), or inadequate uterine contractions.

Definition

Deep transverse arrest occurs when the fetal head, in a vertex presentation, is arrested in the midpelvis with the sagittal suture aligned in the transverse diameter of the maternal pelvis (occipito-transverse position), typically at a station of 0 to +2 relative to the ischial spines. The head fails to rotate to the occipito-anterior (OA) position or descend further, despite adequate uterine contractions. DTA is distinct from:

Occipito-Posterior (OP) Arrest: Where the occiput remains posterior, potentially delivering face-to-pubes.

High Transverse Arrest: Arrest above the ischial spines, often due to inlet CPD.

Obstructed Labor: Broader term encompassing DTA, OP arrest or other mechanical obstructions.

Incidence

1–3% of vertex deliveries, higher in primigravidas (2–5%).

Association with Malposition: Occurs in 10–20% of persistent occipito-transverse (OT) or occipito-posterior (OP) positions that fail to rotate.

Geographical Variation: More common in low- and middle-income countries (LMICs) due to higher rates of contracted pelvis, malnutrition, and delayed access to CEmOC.

Causes and Predisposing Factors

DTA results from a complex interplay of abnormalities in the three Ps of labor: Passenger (fetus), passage (maternal pelvis) and powers (uterine contractions), often compounded by maternal psychological factors (psyche).

1. Passenger (Fetus)

Malposition

Occipito-Transverse (OT): Persistent right occipito-transverse (ROT) or left occipito-transverse (LOT) position, failing to rotate 90° to OA.

Occipito-Posterior (OP): Partial rotation from OP (ROP or LOP) to OT, but arrest in midpelvis.

Deflexed head attitude presents a larger diameter (occipitofrontal, 11.5 cm vs. suboccipitobregmatic, 9.5 cm), impeding rotation.

Fetal Size

Macrosomia: Estimated fetal weight (EFW) >4,000 g increases biparietal diameter (BPD, ~9.5 cm), contributing to CPD. Common in gestational diabetes or post-term pregnancy (>41 weeks).

Lack of holding: Failure of cranial sutures to overlap reduces head adaptability to the pelvis.

Fetal Anomalies (rare): Hydrocephalus or neck masses prevent flexion or rotation.

2. Passage (Maternal Pelvis and Soft Tissues)

Cephalopelvic Disproportion (CPD)

Relative CPD: Borderline mismatch between fetal head and midpelvis, exacerbated by OT position or deflexion.

Absolute CPD: Severe mismatch (e.g., interspinous diameter <9 cm vs. BPD 9.5 cm).

Midpelvis Contraction

Interspinous diameter <9.5 cm (normal: 10–10.5 cm) or prominent ischial spines.

Convergent sidewalls or shallow sacral curve (android pelvis) trap the head.

Pelvic Shape

Android Pelvis: Narrow transverse diameter and straight sidewalls hinder rotation.

Anthropoid Pelvis: Long anteroposterior but narrow transverse diameter favors OT arrest.

Soft Tissue Resistance

Rigid pelvic floor (e.g., in primigravidas) or levator ani dysfunction prevents rotation.

Cervical edema or scarring (e.g., post-conization) impedes dilatation.

Pelvic Deformities

Congenital: Kyphoscoliosis, asymmetrical pelvis (e.g., Naegele's pelvis).

Acquired: Rickets, osteomalacia, or pelvic fractures.

3. Powers (Uterine Contractions)

Inefficient Contractions

Hypotonic contractions (weak, <3/10 minutes, or short, <40 seconds) fail to drive rotation or descent. Causes: Uterine overdistension (twins, polyhydramnios), maternal exhaustion, or grand multiparity.

Incoordinate Contractions

Irregular or asynchronous contractions reduce rotational force .Common in primigravidas or with epidural analgesia (reduces oxytocin).

Secondary Inertia: Contractions weaken after prolonged effort due to myometrial fatigue or obstruction.

4. Iatrogenic Factors

Epidural Analgesia: Relaxes pelvic floor, reducing resistance needed for rotation (2–3-fold risk of OT arrest).

Premature Amniotomy: Early rupture of membranes (ROM) fixes the head in OT, limiting rotation.

Oxytocin Misuse: Excessive augmentation without addressing CPD increases arrest risk.

Diagnosis

Accurate diagnosis of DTA is critical for timely intervention. It relies on clinical examination, partogram monitoring, and imaging when available.

1. History

Prolonged labor with slow or arrested progress despite strong contractions.

Severe back pain (back labor) if associated with OP origin.

Urge to push before full dilatation (second stage) due to head pressure on the rectum.

Maternal exhaustion, dehydration, or fever (suggests complications).

Primigravidity, short stature (<150 cm), obesity (BMI >30 kg/m^2), or diabetes (macrosomia).

Antenatal ultrasound showing OT or OP position.

History of pelvic trauma or contracted pelvis.

2. Physical Examination

Check for vitals, dehydration or exhaustion.

Abdominal Examination

Leopold's Maneuvers

Confirm vertex presentation and longitudinal lie.

Fetal back lateral (ROT or LOT), limbs anteriorly palpable.

Head deflexed, often not engaged or high (station –1 to 0).

Contractions: Palpate frequency (3–5/10 minutes), duration (40–60 seconds), and ntensity (adequate but ineffective).

Bandl's Ring: Pathological retraction ring (oblique ridge between upper and lower uterus) suggests impending obstruction (emergency).

Vaginal Examination (sterile, minimize to reduce infection)

Cervical Status

Dilatation: Full (10 cm) or near-full, but arrested.

Effacement: Complete, but cervix may be edematous.

Position: Anterior, indicating head pressure.

Presenting Part

Sutures and Fontanelles

Sagittal suture in transverse diameter (perpendicular to anteroposterior axis).

Anterior fontanelle (bregma) and posterior fontanelle (lambda) equidistant from pelvis, confirming OT.

ROT: Lambda to maternal right; LOT: Lambda to maternal left.

Station: 0 to +2 (at or below ischial spines), indicating midpelvis arrest.

Holding: Moderate to severe (+2 to +3), suggesting CPD or prolonged pressure.

Caput Succedaneum: Large, boggy swelling over vertex obscures sutures.

Pelvimetry

Interspinous diameter (<9.5 cm) or prominent spines suggest midpelvis contraction.

Sidewall convergence or shallow sacrum (android pelvis) impedes rotation.

Pubic arch angle (<80°) may contribute to arrest.

Amniotic Fluid: Meconium-stained (thick, green) indicates fetal distress; foul odor suggests chorioamnionitis.

Fetal Heart Rate (FHR)

Auscultate every 15 minutes in active phase, every 5 minutes in second stage (normal: 110–160 bpm). Abnormal: Bradycardia (<110 bpm), tachycardia (>160 bpm), or late/variable decelerations indicate distress.

3. Partogram: WHO-recommended tool to monitor labor progress:

Cervical Dilatation: Arrested or slow (<1 cm/hour) in active phase, crossing action line.

Fetal Descent: Stalled at station 0 to +2, confirming midpelvis arrest.

Contractions: Adequate (3–5/10 minutes, 40–60 seconds) but ineffective, suggesting mechanical issue.

FHR: Non-reassuring patterns trigger urgent intervention.

Maternal Vitals: Fever or tachycardia indicates infection or exhaustion.

4. Ultrasound

Intrapartum Ultrasound

Confirms OT position (sagittal suture transverse, occiput at 3 or 9 o'clock).

Assesses head flexion (deflexed in DTA), station, and angle of progression (<120° suggests arrest).

Rules out macrosomia (EFW >4,000 g) or anomalies (e.g., hydrocephalus).

Antenatal Ultrasound: Identifies OT or OP at 36–37 weeks, guiding delivery planning.

Mechanism of Deep Transverse Arrest

DTA occurs when the normal cardinal movements of labore are disrupted, preventing rotation and descent in the midpelvis.

Engagement: Head enters in OT (ROT or LOT) or rotates partially from OP, with occipitofrontal diameter (11.5 cm) due to deflexion.

Descent: Head reaches midpelvis (station 0 to +2), but stalls due to:

Failure of Rotation: Inadequate pelvic floor resistance, narrow midpelvis or deflexed attitude prevents 90° rotation to OA.

CPD: Interspinous diameter <9.5 cm or android pelvis traps the head transversely.

Arrest: Sagittal suture remains transverse, with no further descent or rotation.

Outcomes: Prolonged second stage or obstructed labor if untreated. Increased molding (+2 to +3) and caput from prolonged pressure.

Complications of Deep Transverse Arrest

DTA is a high-risk condition associated with significant maternal and fetal complications, particularly if intervention is delayed.

1. Maternal Complications

Prolonged Labor

Second stage >2 hours (primigravida) or >1 hour (multigravida) without epidural.

Increases exhaustion and dehydration.

Uterine Rupture

Incidence: 0.5–1%, higher in multiparous women or with oxytocin misuse.

Signs: Sudden pain, FHR abnormalities, vaginal bleeding, or shock.

Obstetric Fistulae

Vesicovaginal or rectovaginal fistulae from prolonged head pressure on pelvic tissues.

Incidence: 1–2% in LMICs with delayed CEmOC.

Postpartum Hemorrhage (PPH)

Uterine atony from prolonged labor or operative trauma. Incidence: 10–15%.

Infection: Chorioamnionitis or endometritis from prolonged rupture of membranes (>18 hours) or frequent vaginal examinations. Sepsis risk: 20–40% mortality if untreated.

Perineal Trauma: Third/fourth-degree tears from operative delivery (forceps/vacuum). Incidence: 5–10%.

Maternal Exhaustion: Dehydration, ketoacidosis, or psychological trauma.

Operative Risks: Cesarean or assisted delivery increases infection, hemorrhage or anesthesia complications.

2. Fetal Complications

Birth Asphyxia: Prolonged midpelvis compression or cord prolapse reduces placental perfusion.

Incidence: 5–10%; risk of hypoxic-ischemic encephalopathy (HIE).

Cephalhematoma, subgaleal hemorrhage, or facial bruising from operative delivery or molding. Incidence: 3–5%.

Neonatal Sepsis: From maternal infection or prolonged rupture. Incidence: 2–5%.

Meconium Aspiration Syndrome: Thick meconium from distress in prolonged labor. Incidence 1–3%.

Stillbirth or Neonatal Death: Incidence: 5–10% in untreated DTA, highest with rupture or severe asphyxia.

Long-Term: Cerebral palsy or developmental delays from HIE.

Management

Management aims to relieve the arrest, facilitate vaginal delivery if feasible, and prevent complications. It requires rapid decision-making, skilled intervention, and access to surgical facilities.

1. General Management

Initial Stabilization

Airway, Breathing, Circulation (ABC): Assess maternal vitals; administer oxygen (10 L/min via mask) if hypoxic.

IV Access: Two large-bore cannulae; infuse Ringer's lactate (1–2 L) for dehydration or shock.

Blood Transfusion: Cross-match 2–4 units of packed red cells for anemia (Hb <7 g/dL) or anticipated hemorrhage.

Antibiotics: Broad-spectrum (e.g., ampicillin 2 g IV + gentamicin 5 mg/kg IV) for prolonged rupture (>18 hours), fever, or chorioamnionitis.

Analgesia: Epidural or pudendal block for rotation/delivery; parenteral opioids (pethidine 50–100 mg IM) if cesarean not imminent.

Catheterization: Foley catheter to empty bladder (distended bladder impedes descent) and monitor urine output.

Fetal Monitoring

Continuous CTG or intermittent auscultation every 5 minutes in second stage.

Non-reassuring FHR (e.g., bradycardia <110 bpm) indicates urgent delivery.

Maternal Support

Reassure patient and family; explain need for intervention (e.g., rotation, cesarean).

Involve birth companion to reduce anxiety.

2. Specific Management

Management depends on station, cervical dilatation, maternal/fetal condition, and provider expertise.

First Stage (Rare, as DTA Typically Occurs in Second Stage)

Expectant Management

If DTA diagnosed early (cervix <10 cm, station 0), allow 1–2 hours for spontaneous rotation with adequate contractions.

Monitor with partogram; proceed to cesarean if no progress or distress.

Oxytocin Augmentation (Cautious)

Indication: Hypotonic contractions (<3/10 minutes) with no CPD.

Protocol: Start at 2–4 mU/min IV, increase by 1–2 mU/min every 15–30 minutes (max 20 mU/min).

Risks: Hyperstimulation, rupture (contraindicated if CPD suspected).

Cesarean Section

Indication: Arrested dilatation, fetal distress, or suspected CPD (e.g., interspinous <9 cm).

Second Stage (Primary Setting for DTA)

Manual Rotation

Indication: Full dilatation, station ≥+1, ROT/LOT, no CPD, and skilled operator.

Technique

Under epidural or pudendal block, rotate head 90° (ROT: counterclockwise; LOT: clockwise) to OA. Grasp occiput with fingers or apply pressure on parietal bones. Confirm rotation with ultrasound or vaginal examination. Success Rate: 60–80%; allows vaginal delivery or assisted delivery.

Risks: Cord prolapse, fetal trauma (rare).

Follow-Up: If successful, encourage pushing or proceed to assisted delivery.

Assisted Vaginal Delivery

Indication: DTA at +2 or lower, full dilatation, no CPD, and prolonged second stage (>2 hours primigravida, >1 hour multigravida).

Techniques

Vacuum Extraction: Apply cup over flexing point (midline, 3 cm anterior to posterior fontanelle). Traction with contractions, rotating to OA if needed. Preferred due to lower maternal trauma.

Forceps Delivery: Use rotational forceps (e.g., Kielland's) to rotate OT to OA, then deliver. Higher risk of third/fourth-degree tears.

Risks: Neonatal trauma (cephalhematoma, facial marks), maternal tears, or hemorrhage.

Cesarean Section

Third Stage

Active Management

Oxytocin 10 IU IM/IV within 1 minute of delivery to prevent PPH (increased risk in DTA).

Controlled cord traction (Brandt-Andrews maneuver) after placental separation.

Uterine massage post-delivery.

Inspection

Examine placenta for completeness. Assess perineum for tears (third/fourth-degree common in operative delivery).

Management

Repair tears under local anesthesia or in theater if severe. Monitor for PPH (atony, trauma).

3. Management of Complications

Uterine Rupture: Emergency laparotomy; repair uterus or hysterectomy. Stabilize with IV fluids, blood transfusion, and antibiotics.

Fetal Distress: Intrauterine resuscitation: Left lateral position, oxygen, IV fluids.

Expedited delivery: Cesarean (first stage or high station) or assisted delivery (second stage, station ≥+2).

Infection: Broad-spectrum antibiotics (e.g., ceftriaxone 1 g IV + metronidazole 500 mg IV). Monitor for sepsis (lactate >2 mmol/L); escalate to ICU if needed.

PPH: Uterotonics: Oxytocin, misoprostol (600 mcg oral), or ergometrine (0.2 mg IM).

Uterine massage, bimanual compression, or balloon tamponade.

Surgical options: Uterine artery ligation, B-Lynch suture, or hysterectomy.

Fistulae: Postpartum catheter for 14–21 days (small fistulae). Surgical repair after 3–6 months by specialists.

Neonatal Asphyxia: Resuscitate per Helping Babies Breathe (HBB): PPV, oxygen, chest compressions if heart rate <60 bpm. Transfer to NICU for HIE management.

4. Postpartum Care

Monitoring: Maternal: Vitals, uterine tone, bleeding, and perineal pain every 15 minutes for 2 hours.

Neonatal: Apgar s cores (1, 5, 10 minutes), temperature, feeding, and signs of trauma or asphyxia.

Management:

Maternal

Analgesics (paraceta mol, ibuprofen) for perineal pain.

Continue antibiotics for 5–7 days if infection present.

Catheterize if urinary retention (post-epidural or tears).

Neonatal

Initiate breastfeeding within 1 hour (if stable).

Administer vitamin K (1 mg IM), hepatitis B vaccine, and eye prophylaxis.

Monitor for jaundice, seizures, or respiratory distress.

Prevention

Antenatal Care

Ultrasound at 36–37 weeks to identify OT/OP or macrosomia.

Clinical pelvimetry (diagonal conjugate >11.5 cm, interspinous >9.5 cm).

Manage diabetes to reduce macrosomia.

Maternal Positioning: Encourage hands-and-knees, pelvic tilts, or forward-leaning exercises in late pregnancy to promote OA.

Nutrition: Address childhood malnutrition to prevent pelvic deformities (e.g., rickets). Ensure adequate maternal weight gain.

Conclusion

Deep transverse arrest is a critical labor complication where the fetal head arrests in the midpelvis in the occipito-transverse position, often due to CPD, malposition, or inefficient contractions. It leads to prolonged labor, maternal complications (e.g., fistulae, rupture) and fetal risks (e.g., asphyxia, trauma). Diagnosis relies on partogram monitoring, vaginal examination (sagittal suture transverse, station 0 to +2), and ultrasound. Management includes manual rotation, assisted vaginal delivery (vacuum, forceps), or cesarean section, with stabilization measures (fluids, antibiotics).

References

Dutta, D.C. (2020). Textbook of Obstetrics.

Cunningham, F.G., et al. (2022). Williams Obstetrics.

World Health Organization. (2018). WHO Recommendations: Intrapartum Care for a Positive Childbirth Experience.

American College of Obstetricians and Gynecologists. (2020). ACOG Practice Bulletin No. 49: Dystocia and Malposition.

7.5 Breech Presentation

(*Maji-e-maqadee*)

Introduction

Breech presentation is a fetal malpresentation in which the buttocks or lower limbs present at the maternal pelvic inlet, rather than the head (vertex). Breech presentation poses challenges in labor management, as vaginal delivery requires specific skills and conditions to minimize complications such as cord prolapse, head entrapment, or birth asphyxia. The management of breech presentation has evolved with evidence from trials like the Term Breech Trial (2000), favoring planned cesarean section in many cases, though vaginal breech delivery remains an option with skilled providers and strict criteria.

Definition

Breech presentation is defined as a longitudinal fetal lie where the buttocks, feet, or both are the presenting parts at the maternal pelvic inlet. The fetal head is positioned at the uterine fundus, and the fetus is oriented with the pelvis or lower limbs entering the birth canal first during labor. Breech presentation is classified into three main types based on fetal attitude and leg position:

1. Frank Breech (50–70%): Hips flexed, knees extended, with buttocks as the presenting part (feet near the head).
2. Complete Breech (5–10%): Hips and knees flexed, with buttocks and feet presenting together.
3. Incomplete Breech (10–30%): One or both hips extended, with one or both feet or knees presenting (e.g., footling or knee presentation).

Incidence

Overall: 3–4% of singleton pregnancies at term (≥37 weeks).

Gestational Age

Early pregnancy (28 weeks): 20–25%, as fetuses frequently change position.

Term (37–40 weeks): 3–4%, as most fetuses spontaneously turn to vertex.

Recurrence: 9–10% risk in subsequent pregnancies.

Geographical Variation: Higher in low- and middle-income countries (LMICs) due to preterm births, congenital anomalies, or limited antenatal ultrasound.

Causes and Predisposing Factors

Breech presentation results from factors that prevent the fetus from assuming a vertex presentation or restrict spontaneous version to cephalic. These include fetal, maternal and placental/uterine factors.

1. Fetal Factors

Preterm Gestation: Higher incidence in preterm fetuses (<37 weeks) due to increased intrauterine space and incomplete fetal turning.

Fetal Anomalies: Congenital anomalies (e.g., hydrocephalus, anencephaly, meningomyelocele) alter fetal shape or mobility, preventing version.

Multiple Gestation: Twins or higher-order multiples increase breech risk due to crowding (e.g., second twin often breech).

Fetal Mobility: Neuromuscular disorders (e.g., spina bifida) reduce fetal movement, favoring breech.

2. Maternal Factors

Uterine Abnormalities: Bicornuate, septate or unicornuate uterus restricts fetal movement. Uterine fibroids (especially lower segment) block head descent.

Pelvic Shape: Contracted pelvis (e.g., interspinous diameter <9.5 cm) or android pelvis limits space for version. Pelvic tumors (e.g., ovarian cysts) obstruct head entry.

Maternal Posture: Prolonged sitting or sedentary lifestyle may favor breech positioning.

Parity: Higher in primigravidas due to tighter uterine tone, limiting fetal turning.

3. Placental and Uterine Factors

Placenta Previa: Placenta in the lower uterine segment prevents head engagement.

Polyhydramnios: Excessive amniotic fluid (AFI >25 cm) allows excessive fetal movement, delaying version.

Oligohydramnios: Reduced amniotic fluid (AFI <5 cm) restricts fetal movement, trapping the fetus in breech.

Cord Abnormalities: Short umbilical cord or nuchal cord may limit fetal turning.

4. Other Factors

Previous Breech Delivery: Increases recurrence risk (9–10%).

Maternal Obesity: BMI >30 kg/m^2 alters uterine dynamics.

Diagnosis

1. History

Symptom: Maternal sensation of fetal head under ribs (hard, ballotable mass). Kicking felt in the lower abdomen (footling breech). Reduced fetal movements in cases of oligohydramnios or anomalies.

Risk Factors: Preterm gestation, primigravidity, previous breech or uterine anomalies. Antenatal records indicating breech on prior ultrasound.

2. Physical Examination

Abdominal Examination: Leopold's Maneuvers

First Maneuver: Hard, round, ballotable head at the fundus.

Second Maneuver: Soft, irregular buttocks in the lower uterus; back may be lateral.

Third Maneuver: Buttocks or feet (soft, non-ballotable) at the pelvic inlet.

Fourth Maneuver: Head not engaged; fingers meet resistance at fundus.

Fundal Height: May be higher than expected due to longitudinal lie and head position.

Fetal Heart Rate (FHR): Heard higher on the abdomen (near umbilicus) than in vertex.

Vaginal Examination (sterile, during labor or if ROM)

Presenting Part

Frank Breech: Smooth, soft buttocks with sacrum palpable; no feet felt.

Complete Breech: Buttocks with feet or knees palpable; sacrum and ischial tuberosities form a triangle.

Incomplete Breech: Foot or knee presenting (e.g., single/double footling).

Cervical Status: Assess dilatation, effacement, and position (often posterior in early labor).

Station: High (–2 to 0) in early labor; lower (+1 to +2) in second stage.

Membranes: Note if intact or ruptured (increased cord prolapse risk with ROM).

Pelvimetry: Measure diagonal conjugate (>11.5 cm), interspinous diameter (>9.5 cm), and pubic arch (>80°) to rule out CPD.

Amniotic Fluid: Meconium-stained fluid suggests distress, common in breech labor.

FHR: Auscultate every 15 minutes in active phase (normal: 110–160 bpm). Abnormal: Bradycardia or decelerations indicate distress or cord prolapse.

3. Ultrasound

Antenatal Ultrasound (routine at 36–37 weeks)

Confirms breech type (frank, complete, incomplete).

Assesses fetal lie (longitudinal), presentation, and attitude (hip/knee flexion).

Measures estimated fetal weight (EFW, ideally 2,500–3,800 g for vaginal delivery).

Evaluates head flexion (hyperextended head increases entrapment risk).

Checks placental location (rule out previa), amniotic fluid index (AFI), and anomalies.

Intrapartum Ultrasound

Verifies presentation and position during labor, especially if vaginal delivery planned.

Assesses station and cord position (to exclude prolapse).

Complications of Breech Presentation

Breech presentation increases risks for both mother and fetus, particularly with vaginal delivery, due to mechanical challenges and potential for obstructed labor.

1. Maternal Complications

Prolonged Labor

First stage: Slow dilatation due to uneven pressure from buttocks.

Second stage: Delayed descent of aftercoming head.

Perineal Trauma: Third/fourth-degree tears from rapid head delivery or operative maneuvers.

Postpartum Hemorrhage (PPH): Uterine atony from prolonged labor or trauma.

Infection: Chorioamnionitis or endometritis from prolonged rupture of membranes (>18 hours) or frequent examinations.

Operative Delivery: Cesarean section (70–85% of term breeches) or assisted vaginal delivery increases risks of infection, hemorrhage, or anesthesia complications.

Uterine Rupture (rare): Risk with injudicious oxytocin or obstructed labor.

Maternal Exhaustion: Prolonged labor or back pain from sacral pressure.

2. Fetal Complications

Birth Asphyxia: Cord compression or prolapse during delivery reduces oxygenation. Head entrapment in incompletely dilated cervix or pelvis.

Birth Trauma: Fractures (clavicle, humerus, femur) from traction maneuvers. Brachial plexus injury (Erb's palsy) or spinal cord injury from hyperextended head. Intracranial hemorrhage from rapid head compression.

Cord Prolapse: Higher risk in incomplete breech (footling, 5–10%) due to poor fit of presenting part. Incidence: 1–2% in frank breech, 5–10% in footling.

Neonatal Sepsis: From prolonged rupture or maternal infection.

Perinatal Mortality: Higher in vaginal breech (1–3%) vs. cesarean (<1%), per Term Breech Trial.

Long-Term: Neurodevelopmental delays or cerebral palsy from asphyxia or trauma (rare).

Management of Breech Presentation

Management aims to optimize maternal and fetal outcomes through early diagnosis, version attempts, and delivery planning. Options include external cephalic version (ECV), vaginal breech delivery, or cesarean section and patient factors.

1. Antenatal Management

Diagnosis and Counseling

Confirm breech at 36–37 weeks via ultrasound.

Discuss risks/benefits of ECV, vaginal delivery, and cesarean section.

Address recurrence risk (9–10%) and anomaly screening.

External Cephalic Version (ECV)

Indication: Singleton breech at 36–37 weeks, no contraindications.

Technique: Perform in hospital with ultrasound, CTG, and cesarean backup. Administer tocolytic (e.g., terbutaline 0.25 mg SC) to relax uterus. Operator lifts buttocks from pelvis and rotates fetus to cephalic (forward/backward somersault).

Success Rate: 50–60% (higher in multiparas, frank breech, or adequate fluid).

Contraindications

Absolute: Placenta previa, previous cesarean, severe fetal anomalies.

Relative: Oligohydramnios (AFI <5 cm), fetal growth restriction (FGR), or hyperextended head.

Risks: Placental abruption, cord compression, or fetal distress (1–2%); emergency cesarean if persistent FHR abnormalities.

2. Delivery Planning

Delivery mode depends on breech type, maternal/fetal factors, provider expertise, and patient preference.

Vaginal Breech Delivery

Indication (ACOG, WHO criteria)

Frank or complete breech (not footling due to cord prolapse risk).

EFW 2,500–3,800 g (avoid macrosomia >4,000 g).

Adequate pelvis (diagonal conjugate >11.5 cm, interspinous >9.5 cm).

Flexed fetal head (no hyperextension on ultrasound).

No fetal/maternal contraindications (e.g., FGR, previa).

Skilled provider and CEmOC access.

Informed maternal consent.

Contraindications

Incomplete breech (footling/knee).

CPD (e.g., interspinous <9 cm).

Fetal anomalies (e.g., hydrocephalus).

Fetal distress or non-reassuring FHR.

Lack of skilled provider or surgical backup.

Technique (Assisted Breech Delivery)

Preparation: Perform in operating theater with cesarean capability.

Ensure IV access, cross-matched blood, and anesthesia team.

Empty maternal bladder; avoid epidural (impairs pushing).

First Stage: Monitor with partogram (dilatation ≥1 cm/hour, active phase).

Avoid premature pushing or amniotomy (cord prolapse risk).

Continuous CTG or auscultation every 15 minutes.

Second Stage: Allow spontaneous descent to umbilicus with maternal pushing.

Pinard's Maneuver: Flex knees to deliver legs (if not spontaneous).

Løvset Maneuver: Rotate trunk to deliver shoulders (scapulae visible).

Mauriceau-Smellie-Veit or Burns-Marshall: Deliver aftercoming head by flexing neck (MSV: fingers on maxilla; BM: feet lifted upward).

Avoid traction on head to prevent spinal injury.

Third Stage: Active management with oxytocin 10 IU IM to prevent PPH.

Risks: Head entrapment (1–2%), cord prolapse, or asphyxia. Higher perinatal morbidity (3–5%) vs. cesarean (<1%).

Monitoring: FHR every 5 minutes in second stage. Assess descent, station, and head flexion during delivery.

Cesarean Section

Indication (preferred, per Term Breech Trial):

Term breech with any contraindication to vaginal delivery.

Failed ECV or patient preference for cesarean.

Preterm breech (<37 weeks, higher head entrapment risk).

Footling breech, hyperextended head, or EFW >3,800 g.

Lack of skilled provider or CEmOC.

Technique: Lower segment cesarean section (LSCS) under spinal/general anesthesia. Ensure fetal head extraction (may require vertical incision if preterm or impacted).

Benefits: Reduces perinatal mortality (0.5% vs. 2–3% vaginal) and morbidity (1% vs. 5%). Avoids head entrapment or cord prolapse.

Risks: Maternal: Infection, hemorrhage, longer recovery.

Neonatal: Respiratory distress (preterm), transient tachypnea.

Future pregnancies: Increased placenta previa/accreta risk.

Timing: Planned at 39 weeks to avoid labor onset. Emergency if labor, distress, or cord prolapse.

Preterm Breech

Management: Cesarean preferred (<37 weeks) due to higher head entrapment risk (immature pelvis, larger head-to-body ratio). Administer antenatal corticosteroids (betamethasone 12 mg IM, 2 doses 24 hours apart) for lung maturity (<34 weeks). Vaginal delivery considered only if imminent, frank breech, and skilled provider.

Risks: Higher perinatal mortality (5–10%) due to prematurity and trauma.

3. Intrapartum Management

Spontaneous Labor

Assess breech type, station, and FHR on admission.

If vaginal delivery planned, follow strict criteria and monitor with partogram.

Prepare for emergency cesarean if progress stalls or distress occurs.

Cord Prolapse

Signs: Sudden FHR abnormalities (bradycardia, variable decelerations) post-ROM.

Management: Elevate presenting part (vaginal hand or knee-chest position). Administer oxygen, IV fluids, and tocolytics (terbutaline 0.25 mg IV). Immediate cesarean section.

Head Entrapment

Signs: Failure of head delivery after body, with cervix or pelvis constricting.

Management

Duhrssen's Incisions: Cervical incisions at 2, 6, and 10 o'clock (rare, high bleeding risk).

Zavanelli Maneuver: Replace fetus into uterus, proceed to cesarean (last resort).

Symphysiotomy: Widen pelvis.

Prevention: Confirm full dilatation and adequate pelvis before vaginal delivery.

4. Postpartum Management

Monitoring: Maternal: Vitals, uterine tone, bleeding, and perineal condition every 15 minutes for 2 hours. Neonatal: Apgar scores (1, 5, 10 minutes), temperature, feeding, and signs of trauma or asphyxia.

Management:

Maternal: Repair perineal tears under local anesthesia or in theatre if severe. Continue antibiotics if infection suspected (e.g., prolonged ROM). Monitor for PPH (oxytocin 10 IU IV infusion).

Neonatal: Initiate breastfeeding within 1 hour (if stable). Administer vitamin K (1 mg IM), hepatitis B vaccine, and eye prophylaxis. Monitor for respiratory distress, jaundice, or neurological signs (e.g., seizures). Orthopedic evaluation for hip dysplasia (increased in breech, 5–10%).

Prevention

Antenatal Care: Routine ultrasound at 36 weeks to detect breech and offer ECV.

Screen for anomalies, placenta previa, or abnormal fluid (poly-/oligohydramnios).

Assess pelvic adequacy (clinical pelvimetry).

Maternal Health: Manage diabetes to reduce macrosomia.

Correct uterine anomalies or fibroids preconceptionally if feasible.

Conclusion

Breech presentation, where the buttocks or feet present first, occurs in 3–4% of term pregnancies and poses significant risks of perinatal morbidity, cord prolapse, and operative delivery. Diagnosis involves clinical examination (Leopold's maneuvers, vaginal exam) and ultrasound to confirm type (frank, complete, incomplete) and assess suitability for vaginal delivery. Management includes ECV at 36–37 weeks, vaginal breech delivery with strict criteria and skilled providers, or cesarean section (preferred for most term breeches). Complications such as head entrapment or asphyxia necessitate rapid intervention.

References

Dutta, D.C. (2020). Textbook of Obstetrics.

Cunningham, F.G., et al. (2022). Williams Obstetrics.

World Health Organization. (2018). WHO Recommendations: Intrapartum Care for a Positive Childbirth Experience.

American College of Obstetricians and Gynecologists. (2020). *ACOG Practice Bulletin No. 161: External Cephalic Version.

Hannah, M.E., et al. (2000). Planned Caesarean Section versus Planned Vaginal Birth for Breech Presentation at Term: A Randomised Multicentre Trial (Term Breech Trial).

7.6 Face Presentation

(***Maji-e-wajhee***)

Introduction

Face presentation is a rare fetal malpresentation in which the fetal head is hyperextended, presenting the face (chin or mentum) as the leading part at the maternal pelvic inlet, rather than the vertex. It is a significant obstetric condition due to its association with prolonged labor, increased risk of operative delivery, and potential maternal and fetal complications

Definition

Face presentation is a longitudinal cephalic presentation where the fetal head is fully extended, with the face (from forehead to chin) as the presenting part. The presenting diameter is the submentobregmatic (9.5 cm), compared to the suboccipitobregmatic (9.5 cm) in vertex presentation. The position is defined by the fetal chin (mentum) relative to the maternal pelvis

Mento-Anterior (MA): Chin faces the maternal pubic symphysis (e.g., right mento-anterior, RMA; left mento-anterior, LMA).

Mento-Posterior (MP): Chin faces the maternal sacrum (e.g., right mento-posterior, RMP; left mento-posterior, LMP).

Mento-Transverse (MT): Chin aligns with the maternal transverse diameter (rare, transitional).

Mento-anterior positions may permit vaginal delivery, while mento-posterior positions typically result in arrest, necessitating operative intervention.

Incidence

Overall: 0.1–0.2% of singleton deliveries (1 in 500–1,000 births).

Gestational Age: More common in preterm (<37 weeks) due to smaller fetal size and increased intrauterine space.

Parity: Slightly higher in multiparas due to lax uterine tone.

Recurrence: Low, unless caused by persistent maternal or fetal factors (e.g., pelvic contracture, anencephaly).

Causes and Predisposing Factors

Face presentation results from factors that promote hyperextension of the fetal head or prevent flexion, involving the fetus, maternal pelvis, or uterine environment.

1. Fetal Factors

Fetal Anomalies

Anencephaly: Absence of cranial vault leads to hyperextension (10–20% of face presentations).

Neck Masses: Goiter, cystic hygroma, or teratomas force head extension.

Neuromuscular Disorders: Reduced tone (e.g., fetal akinesia) prevents head flexion.

Fetal Size

Preterm Fetus: Smaller size allows hyperextension in spacious uterus.

Macrosomia: Large shoulders or abdomen tilt the head backward.

Multiple Gestation: Crowding (e.g., second twin) promotes atypical head positions.

Cord Abnormalities: Nuchal cord or short cord restricts head flexion.

2. Maternal Factors

Pelvic Abnormalities

Contracted Pelvis: Inlet contraction (obstetric conjugate <10 cm) or android pelvis favors hyperextension as the head aligns with a narrower diameter.

Pelvic Tumors: Fibroids or ovarian cysts displace the head upward.

Uterine Factors

Polyhydramnios: Excessive fluid (AFI >25 cm) allows head hyperextension.

Uterine Anomalies: Bicornuate or septate uterus restricts head flexion.

High Parity: Lax uterine tone in grand multiparas (>5 deliveries) permits atypical positions.

Maternal Posture: Prolonged supine position may encourage posterior head tilt.

3. Other Factors

Placenta Previa: Low-lying placenta displaces the head upward.

Premature Rupture of Membranes (PROM): Early ROM fixes the head in extension.

Iatrogenic: Limited antenatal screening in LMICs misses face presentation early.

Diagnosis

Accurate diagnosis is critical for delivery planning and anticipating complications. It relies on clinical examination and ultrasound confirmation.

1. History

Symptoms: Maternal sensation of irregular fetal movements or discomfort from head under ribs. Prolonged labor or back pain (mento-posterior positions).

Risk Factors: Preterm gestation, multiparity, previous malpresentation, or known fetal anomalies. Antenatal ultrasound indicating face presentation or hyperextended head.

2. Physical Examination

Abdominal Examination: Leopold's Maneuvers

First Maneuver: Breech (soft, irregular) at the fundus.

Second Maneuver: Fetal back lateral or anterior; limbs on opposite side.

Third Maneuver: Hard, smooth head (hyperextended) at the pelvic inlet, often not engaged.

Fourth Maneuver: Fingers meet resistance at chin or forehead, not occiput.

Fundal Height: Normal or slightly increased due to head extension.

FHR: Heard near maternal umbilicus, similar to vertex.

Vaginal Examination (sterile, during labor or if ROM)

Presenting Part: Palpate facial features: Chin (mentum), mouth, nose or orbital ridges.

Mento-Anterior: Chin toward pubis, mouth accessible, nose posterior.

Mento-Posterior: Chin toward sacrum, forehead anterior, mouth less palpable.

Mento-Transverse: Chin lateral, transitional position.

Edema (caput succedaneum) over face may obscure features in prolonged labor.

Cervical Status

Dilatation: Slow progress (<1 cm/hour) in mento-posterior.

Effacement: Incomplete if head poorly applied.

Position: Posterior, indicating uneven pressure.

Station: High (–2 to 0) in early labor; lower (+1 to +2) in second stage.

Molding: Over forehead or chin, increasing submentobregmatic diameter.

Pelvimetry

Diagonal conjugate (<11.5 cm) or interspinous (<9.5 cm) suggests CPD.

Pubic arch (<80°) or android pelvis impedes delivery.

Amniotic Fluid: Meconium-stained fluid indicates distress; foul odor suggests infection.

FHR: Bradycardia, tachycardia, or decelerations suggest distress.

3. Ultrasound

Antenatal Ultrasound (36–37 weeks)

Confirms face presentation (hyperextended head, chin leading).

Identifies position (mento-anterior, posterior, transverse).

Assesses estimated fetal weight (EFW, ideally 2,500–3,800 g for vaginal delivery).

Evaluates anomalies (e.g., anencephaly), placental location, and amniotic fluid index (AFI).

Intrapartum Ultrasound

Verifies position and station during labor.

Rules out cord prolapse or head entrapment risk.

4. Other Imaging (rare)

X-ray: Historical use to confirm hyperextension or pelvic adequacy; replaced by ultrasound.

MRI: For complex anomalies or pelvic assessment in high-resource settings.

Mechanism of Labor in Face Presentation

The mechanism of labor in face presentation differs from vertex due to head hyperextension and the submentobregmatic diameter (9.5 cm). Outcomes vary by position (mento-anterior vs. mento-posterior).

1. Mento-Anterior (MA) Position (60–70% of Face Presentations)

Engagement: Head enters pelvic inlet in RMA or LMA, with submentobregmatic diameter aligned transversely or obliquely. Engagement may be delayed due to deflexion.

Descent: By uterine contractions and maternal pushing. Chin leads, with face applying to cervix.

Internal Rotation: Chin rotates 90° from transverse/oblique to anterior (pubic symphysis), aligning submentobregmatic diameter anteroposteriorly. Facilitated by pelvic floor (levator ani) and gynecoid pelvis.

Extension: Chin delivers under symphysis pubis, followed by nose, forehead, and occiput. Head flexes post-delivery to align with body.

Restitution and External Rotation: Head restitutes 45° to align with shoulders, then rotates as shoulders align anteroposteriorly.

Expulsion: Shoulders and body deliver as in vertex.

Outcome: Vaginal delivery possible in 80–90% of MA cases with adequate pelvis and no CPD.

2. Mento-Posterior (MP) Position (20–30%)

Engagement and Descent: Head enters in RMP or LMP, with chin toward sacrum. Descent is slow due to larger presenting diameter (mento-occipital, ~13 cm in deflexion) and poor cervical application.

Internal Rotation: Rotation to mento-anterior fails due to sacrum resistance and deflexed attitude. Arrest occurs in midpelvis or outlet, as chin cannot pivot under sacrum.

Outcome: Persistent MP is incompatible with vaginal delivery in most cases (90–95%). Cesarean section required unless spontaneous rotation to MA occurs (rare, <5%).

3. Mento-Transverse (MT) Position (rare)

Transitional: Head arrests transversely, often progressing to MA or MP.

Outcome: Depends on rotation; cesarean if arrested.

Complications of Face Presentation

Face presentation increases maternal and fetal risks due to prolonged labor and operative interventions.

1. Maternal Complications

Prolonged Labor

Obstructed Labor

Uterine Rupture (rare)

Perineal Trauma

Postpartum Hemorrhage (PPH)

Infection

Operative Delivery

Maternal Exhaustion

2. Fetal Complications

Birth Asphyxia: Cord compression or prolonged labor reduces oxygenation.

Facial Trauma: Edema, bruising, or lacerations over face (chin, lips, eyes) from pressure.

Neonatal Sepsis: From prolonged rupture or maternal infection.

Intracranial Hemorrhage: From rapid compression during delivery or operative trauma.

Perinatal Mortality: Higher in vaginal delivery (1–2%) vs. cesarean (<1%), especially with anomalies or MP.

Long-Term: Neurodevelopmental delays from asphyxia (rare).

Management of Face Presentation

Management aims to optimize outcomes through early diagnosis, labor monitoring and delivery planning. Vaginal delivery is feasible in mento-anterior positions with strict criteria, while mento-posterior positions typically require cesarean section.

1. Antenatal Management

Diagnosis: Ultrasound at 36–37 weeks to confirm face presentation, position (MA/MP), and anomalies. Assess EFW, pelvic adequacy and fluid (AFI).

External Cephalic Version (ECV): Rarely attempted due to hyperextension and anomaly risk. Considered if no contraindications (e.g., normal fetus, adequate fluid).

2. Intrapartum Management

Management depends on position, labor progress and maternal/fetal condition.

First Stage

Diagnosis: Confirm face presentation and position via vaginal examination and ultrasound.

Assess cervical dilatation, station and pelvimetry.

Expectant Management

Indication: Mento-anterior, early labor (<4 cm), no distress.

Monitor with partogram (dilatation ≥1 cm/hour in active phase). Allow spontaneous progress if MA and adequate pelvis.

Supportive Care: Positioning: Upright or lateral positions promote descent in MA.

Hydration: IV fluids (Ringer's lactate, 125 mL/hour) to prevent exhaustion.

Amniotomy (Cautious)

Perform only if head engaged, cervix ≥4 cm, and MA position.

Risks: Cord prolapse, meconium aspiration (monitor FHR post-ARM).

Oxytocin Augmentation (Rare)

Indication: Hypotonic contractions in MA with no CPD.

Protocol: Start at 2–4 mU/min IV, increase by 1–2 mU/min every 15–30 minutes (max 20 mU/min).

Contraindications: MP, CPD, or fetal distress.

Monitoring

Partogram: Track dilatation, descent, contractions, and FHR.

FHR: Auscultate every 15–30 minutes (active phase); continuous CTG if high-risk.

Vaginal examination every 2–4 hours. Maternal vitals every 4 hours.

Second Stage

Mento-Anterior (MA):

Vaginal Delivery

Indication: Full dilatation, station ≥+2, adequate pelvis, no distress.

Technique: Allow spontaneous descent with maternal pushing. Maintain head extension (avoid flexion attempts, risks cervical spine injury). Deliver chin under symphysis pubis, followed by nose, forehead, and occiput. Episiotomy may be needed to reduce perineal trauma.

Success Rate: 80–90% in MA with skilled provider.

Risks: Facial edema, perineal tears, or asphyxia.

Assisted Vaginal Delivery

Indication: Prolonged second stage (>2 hours primigravida, >1 hour multigravida) or maternal exhaustion.

Technique: Vacuum extraction (apply cup over chin, avoid eyes/mouth). Forceps (e.g., Simpson's) to guide chin delivery (rare, high trauma risk).

Risks: Facial trauma, lacerations, or hemorrhage.

Mento-Posterior (MP)

Expectant Management: Allow 1–2 hours for spontaneous rotation to MA (rare, <5%). Monitor FHR and descent closely.

Manual Rotation (Rare): Attempt to rotate chin to MA under anesthesia if station ≥+1 and no CPD.

Success rate: <20%; high risk of cord prolapse or trauma.

Cesarean Section: Indication

Persistent MP with no rotation.

Arrest of descent or dilatation.

Fetal distress (e.g., bradycardia, late decelerations).

CPD (e.g., interspinous <9.5 cm).

Technique: Lower segment cesarean section (LSCS) under spinal/general anesthesia.

Risks: Infection, hemorrhage, prolonged recovery.

Monitoring: FHR every 5 minutes in second stage. Assess descent, position, and maternal effort. Watch for obstruction (e.g., severe molding, cervical edema).

Third Stage

Active Management: Oxytocin 10 IU IM/IV within 1 minute of delivery to prevent PPH. Controlled cord traction (Brandt-Andrews) after placental separation. Uterine massage post-delivery.

Inspection: Examine placenta for completeness. Assess perineum for tears (third/fourth-degree in MA).

Management: Repair tears under local anesthesia or in theater if severe. Monitor for PPH (atony, trauma).

3. Management of Complications

Obstructed Labor: Cesarean for persistent MP, CPD or Bandl's ring. Tocolytics (e.g., nitroglycerin 50–100 mcg IV) if hypertonic contractions.

Fetal Distress: Intrauterine resuscitation: Left lateral position, oxygen, IV fluids. Expedited delivery: Cesarean (first stage) or assisted delivery (second stage, MA).

Infection: Broad-spectrum antibiotics (e.g., ceftriaxone 1 g IV + metronidazole 500 mg IV). Monitor for sepsis (lactate >2 mmol/L).

PPH: Uterotonics: Oxytocin, misoprostol (600 mcg oral), or ergometrine (0.2 mg IM).

Uterine massage, bimanual compression, or balloon tamponade.

Surgical options: Uterine artery ligation, hysterectomy.

Facial Trauma: Pediatric evaluation for bruising, lacerations or airway obstruction. Monitor for feeding difficulties or infection.

4. Postpartum Management

Monitoring-Maternal: Vitals, uterine tone, bleeding, and perineal pain every 15 minutes for 2 hours. Neonatal: Apgar scores (1, 5, 10 minutes), temperature, feeding, and signs of trauma or asphyxia.

Management

Maternal: Analgesics (paracetamol, ibuprofen) for perineal pain. Continue antibiotics for 5–7 days, if infection present. Catheterize if urinary retention (post-epidural or tears).

Neonatal: Initiate breastfeeding within 1 hour (if stable). Administer vitamin K (1 mg IM), hepatitis B vaccine and eye prophylaxis. Monitor for facial edema, respiratory distress or neurological signs.

Counseling: Discuss cause (e.g., anomaly, pelvis), recurrence risk (low) and future delivery options. Address psychological trauma from prolonged labor or caesarean. Educate on danger signs (fever, bleeding, neonatal lethargy).

Follow-Up: Maternal: Postpartum visits at 1–2 weeks, 6 weeks. Neonatal: Pediatric follow-up for anomalies, growth, or trauma sequelae.

Prevention

Antenatal Care: Routine ultrasound at 36 weeks to detect face presentation and anomalies. Assess pelvic adequacy (clinical pelvimetry). Screen for polyhydramnios or placenta previa.

Maternal Health: Correct uterine anomalies or fibroids preconceptionally. Promote active postures (e.g., walking) to encourage vertex presentation.

Conclusion

Face presentation, a rare cephalic malpresentation, occurs when the fetal head is hyperextended, presenting the face (chin) first, with an incidence of 0.1–0.2%. It is associated with anomalies (e.g., anencephaly), contracted pelvis, or polyhydramnios. Diagnosis involves abdominal/vaginal examination and ultrasound to confirm position (mento-anterior, posterior) and assess suitability for vaginal delivery. Mento-anterior positions may allow vaginal delivery with skilled providers, while mento-posterior positions typically require cesarean due to arrest. Complications include prolonged labor, facial trauma and asphyxia.

References

Dutta, D.C. (2020). Textbook of Obstetrics.

Cunningham, F.G., et al. (2022). Williams Obstetrics.

World Health Organization. (2018). WHO Recommendations: Intrapartum Care for a Positive Childbirth Experience.

American College of Obstetricians and Gynecologists. (2020). ACOG Practice Bulletin No. 49: Dystocia and Malposition.

7.7 Brow Presentation

(*Maji-e-jabhee*)

Definition

Brow presentation is a type of malpresentation in which the fetal head is partially extended, with the forehead as the presenting part, resulting in the largest diameter of the fetal head (occipitomental diameter, approximately 13–14 cm) entering the maternal pelvis. It is an unstable and rare presentation, occurring in approximately 0.02–0.1% of all deliveries.

Etiology

Brow presentation is often associated with factors that prevent full flexion or promote extension of the fetal head:

Maternal factors: Cephalopelvic disproportion, Contracted pelvis, Uterine anomalies (e.g., fibroids, bicornuate uterus), Placenta previa.

Fetal factors: Macrosomia, Polyhydramnios, Fetal anomalies (e.g., neck tumors, anencephaly), Prematurity.

Other factors: Multiple gestation, Abnormal uterine contractions, Deflexed head due to cord around the neck or other mechanical factors.

Mechanism of Presentation

In brow presentation, the fetal head is midway between full flexion (vertex presentation) and full extension (face presentation). The presenting part is the area between the anterior fontanelle (bregma) and the orbital ridges.

The fetal head engages in the pelvis with the occipitomental diameter, which is significantly larger than the suboccipitobregmatic diameter (9.5 cm) seen in vertex presentation, making vaginal delivery difficult or impossible in most cases.

The attitude of the fetal head is one of partial extension, and the presentation is typically unstable, often transitioning to either a vertex or face presentation during labor.

Diagnosis

Clinical Examination

1. Vaginal examination: The presenting part feels high, with palpable landmarks including the anterior fontanelle, frontal sutures and orbital ridges. The absence of the sagittal suture in the midline differentiates it from vertex presentation.

2. Abdominal examination (Leopold's maneuvers): The head may feel high and not well-engaged. The fetal heart tones are typically heard higher than in vertex presentations.

Ultrasound: The gold standard for confirming brow presentation. It visualizes the partially extended head, with the forehead as the presenting part and the occipitomental diameter aligned with the pelvic inlet.

X-ray (rarely used): May confirm the extended head position but is largely replaced by ultrasound.

Types of Brow Presentation

Transient: The brow presentation may convert to a vertex or face presentation as labor progresses, especially in early labor or with a small fetus.

Persistent: The brow presentation remains fixed, often due to cephalopelvic disproportion or other obstructing factors, leading to obstructed labor.

Positions

Brow presentation is described based on the position of the fetal forehead relative to the maternal pelvis:

Left mento-anterior (LMA)

Right mento-anterior (RMA)

Left mento-posterior (LMP)

Right mento-posterior (RMP)

Mento-transverse positions (left or right)

Management

The management of brow presentation depends on the stage of labor, maternal and fetal condition, and the likelihood of vaginal delivery.

1. Antenatal Diagnosis

If diagnosed antenatally via ultrasound, assess for underlying causes (e.g., fetal anomalies, pelvic abnormalities). Counsel the patient about the potential need for cesarean delivery, especially if the presentation persists or if associated risk factors (e.g., macrosomia) are present.

2. During Labor

Early labor: Monitor closely with continuous fetal heart rate monitoring and regular vaginal examinations. If the brow presentation is transient, it may convert to a vertex or face presentation with adequate contractions and time. Avoid artificial rupture of membranes (ARM) as it may commit the fetus to an unfavorable position.

Persistent brow presentation: Vaginal delivery is rarely possible due to the large presenting diameter (occipitomental, 13–14 cm) compared to the pelvic inlet (average 11–12 cm). Attempted vaginal delivery carries risks of prolonged labor, obstructed labor, uterine rupture, and fetal distress.

Cesarean section is the preferred mode of delivery in most cases of persistent brow presentation, especially in primigravidas or when cephalopelvic disproportion is suspected.

Trial of labor: May be considered in multiparous women with a proven pelvis, a small fetus, and favorable mento-anterior position, under close supervision. Requires adequate labor progress, absence of fetal distress, and availability of immediate cesarean section facilities.

External cephalic version (ECV): Rarely attempted in brow presentation due to the risk of cord prolapse or fetal distress. If attempted, it should be done early in labor with tocolytics and ultrasound guidance.

3. Contraindications to Vaginal Delivery

Persistent brow presentation in active labor, Cephalopelvic disproportion, Fetal distress, Macrosomia, Maternal or fetal compromise.

Complications

Maternal: Prolonged or obstructed labor, Uterine rupture, Postpartum hemorrhage, Perineal trauma (if vaginal delivery is attempted), Increased risk of infection due to prolonged labor.

Fetal: Fetal distress due to cord compression or prolonged labor, Birth trauma (e.g., facial bruising, skull fractures), Hypoxia or asphyxia, Intracranial hemorrhage (rare, but possible with traumatic delivery).

Prognosis

With timely cesarean delivery, maternal and fetal outcomes are generally excellent.

Vaginal delivery, if successful, may occur in rare cases (e.g., small fetus, multiparous mother, mento-anterior position) but carries significant risks. Persistent brow presentation without intervention is associated with high perinatal morbidity and mortality.

Prevention

Routine antenatal ultrasound to identify malpresentations early.

Address modifiable risk factors (e.g., maternal obesity, polyhydramnios).

Careful labor management to avoid premature ARM or oxytocin augmentation in suspected malpresentations.

Key Points

Brow presentation is a rare and unstable malpresentation that often requires cesarean delivery.

Diagnosis is confirmed by ultrasound, with vaginal examination identifying key landmarks (anterior fontanelle, orbital ridges).

Persistent brow presentation is incompatible with vaginal delivery in most cases due to the large occipitomental diameter.

Management prioritizes fetal and maternal safety, with cesarean section being the standard of care for persistent cases.

7.8 Transverse Lie

(*Vijah mustariza*)

Definition

Transverse lie is a malpresentation in which the long axis of the fetus is perpendicular to the long axis of the maternal spine, with the fetal shoulder, back or abdomen presenting at the pelvic inlet. It occurs in approximately 0.3–0.5% of term pregnancies and is incompatible with vaginal delivery without intervention due to the inability of the fetus to engage in the pelvis.

Etiology

Transverse lie results from factors that prevent the fetus from assuming a longitudinal lie (vertex or breech presentation). Common causes include:

Maternal factors

Multiparity (lax uterine and abdominal muscles)

Contracted pelvis or cephalopelvic disproportion

Uterine anomalies (e.g., bicornuate uterus, fibroids)

Placenta previa

Pelvic tumors

Fetal factors

Prematurity (more common due to increased fetal mobility)

Polyhydramnios (excess amniotic fluid allows excessive fetal movement)

Multiple gestation (e.g., twins, where one fetus may lie transversely)

Fetal anomalies (e.g., hydrocephalus, abdominal distension)

Macrosomia

Other factors

Short umbilical cord or cord entanglement

Abnormal uterine contractions or poor uterine tone

Mechanism of Presentation

In transverse lie, the fetus lies horizontally across the uterus, with the head on one side of the maternal pelvis and the lower limbs on the opposite side.

The presenting part is typically the shoulder (acromion process), but the back, abdomen, or ribs may also present.

The lie is described as dorso-anterior (fetal back facing the maternal anterior) or

dorso-posterior (fetal back facing the maternal posterior), with variations such as right or left acromion presentation.

The transverse lie is inherently unstable in labor, as the fetus cannot engage in the pelvis, leading to obstructed labor if uncorrected.

Diagnosis

Clinical Examination

Abdominal examination (Leopold's maneuvers)

The fetal head is palpable in one flank, and the breech is felt on the opposite side.

The uterus appears wider than usual, and the fundus is lower than expected for gestational age.

Fetal heart tones are typically heard in the mid-abdomen rather than lower in the pelvis.

Vaginal examination

In early labor, the cervix may be high and difficult to reach. The presenting part (shoulder, arm, or ribs) may be felt, or no presenting part is palpable if the fetus is high. A prolapsed arm or cord may be detected in advanced labor.

Ultrasound: The definitive diagnostic tool, confirming the transverse lie, fetal position, and associated conditions (e.g., placenta previa, polyhydramnios, fetal anomalies).

X-ray (rarely used): May confirm fetal lie but is largely replaced by ultrasound.

Types of Transverse Lie

Unstable/Transient: Common in preterm pregnancies, where the fetus may spontaneously convert to a longitudinal lie as gestation progresses or early in labor.

Persistent: Fixed transverse lie, often associated with underlying maternal or fetal factors, persisting into labor and requiring intervention.

Positions

The position is described based on the presenting part (usually the shoulder) and its orientation:

Right acromion anterior (RAA): Right shoulder presenting, fetal back anterior.

Left acromion anterior (LAA): Left shoulder presenting, fetal back anterior.

Right acromion posterior (RAP): Right shoulder presenting, fetal back posterior.

Left acromion posterior (LAP): Left shoulder presenting, fetal back posterior.

Dorso-superior or dorso-inferior positions may also occur, depending on whether the fetal back is directed upward or downward.

Management

The management of transverse lie depends on gestational age, labor status, and associated maternal and fetal conditions.

1. Antenatal Diagnosis

Before 36 weeks

Observation is appropriate, as many fetuses spontaneously convert to a longitudinal lie as term approaches. Ultrasound to identify underlying causes (e.g., placenta previa, uterine anomalies). Consider external cephalic version (ECV) at 36–37 weeks if the lie remains transverse, provided there are no contraindications.

ECV

Performed under ultrasound guidance with tocolytics (e.g., terbutaline) to relax the uterus.

Success rate is approximately 50–70%, higher in multiparous women.

Contraindications include placenta previa, fetal distress, multiple gestation, or

urine anomalies.

Risks include placental abruption, cord prolapse, or fetal distress, necessitating immediate access to cesarean facilities.

2. During Labor

Early labor: Confirm diagnosis with ultrasound. Attempt ECV if not previously performed and conditions are favorable (e.g., adequate amniotic fluid, no fetal distress). Avoid artificial rupture of membranes (ARM), as it increases the risk of cord prolapse or arm prolapse.

Persistent transverse lie: Vaginal delivery is not possible without correction to a longitudinal lie.

Cesarean section is the standard of care for persistent transverse lie in labor, especially in primigravidas, term pregnancies, or cases with associated risk factors (e.g., placenta previa, fetal distress).

A low transverse incision is usually sufficient, but a vertical (classical) incision may be required for preterm fetuses, multiple gestations, or difficult fetal extraction.

Internal podalic version (rare):

Considered only in exceptional circumstances (e.g., second twin in a multiple gestation, experienced obstetrician, no cesarean facilities). Involves manually rotating the fetus to a breech position under anesthesia, followed by breech extraction. High risk of uterine rupture, cord prolapse, and fetal trauma; rarely performed in modern practice.

Contraindications to Vaginal Delivery

Persistent transverse lie in active labor

Cord prolapse or arm prolapse

Fetal distress

Placenta previa

Cephalopelvic disproportion

Maternal or fetal compromise

Complications

Maternal

Obstructed labor

Uterine rupture (especially if labor is prolonged or oxytocin is used)

Postpartum hemorrhage

Infection due to prolonged labor or ruptured membranes

Trauma to the birth canal (if vaginal delivery is attempted)

Fetal

Cord prolapse (high risk, especially after membrane rupture)

Fetal distress due to cord compression or prolonged labor

Birth trauma (e.g., brachial plexus injury, fractures) if vaginal delivery is attempted

Perinatal asphyxia or death if delivery is delayed

Prognosis

With timely cesarean delivery, maternal and fetal outcomes are excellent.

Without intervention, persistent transverse lie in labor is associated with high risks of maternal and fetal morbidity and mortality.

Successful ECV can allow vaginal delivery, but careful monitoring is required.

Prevention

Routine antenatal ultrasound to detect transverse lie early.

Address modifiable risk factors (e.g., polyhydramnios, maternal obesity).

Antenatal ECV at 36–37 weeks to correct the lie in appropriate candidates.

Careful labor management, avoiding premature ARM or oxytocin in suspected malpresentations.

Key Points

Transverse lie is a rare malpresentation that precludes vaginal delivery without correction to a longitudinal lie.

Diagnosis is confirmed by ultrasound, with abdominal and vaginal examinations providing initial clues.

Cesarean section is the preferred management for persistent transverse lie in labor.

ECV may be attempted antenatally or in early labor to avoid cesarean delivery, but it carries risks and requires expertise.

Transverse lie is associated with significant maternal and fetal complications, particularly cord prolapse and obstructed labor.

Early recognition and appropriate intervention are critical for optimizing outcomes.

7.9 Compound Presentation

(*Maji-e-murakkab*)

Definition

Compound presentation is a rare malpresentation in which two or more parts of the fetus present simultaneously at the pelvic inlet, typically involving a fetal extremity (most commonly an arm or hand) alongside the presenting part (usually the vertex). It occurs in approximately 0.04–0.1% of deliveries and is associated with increased risks of labor complications.

Etiology

Compound presentation results from conditions that prevent the fetus from assuming a fully flexed vertex presentation or allow excessive mobility of fetal parts. Contributing factors include:

Maternal factors

Multiparity (lax uterine and abdominal muscles)

Premature rupture of membranes (PROM)

Polyhydramnios (increased amniotic fluid allowing fetal mobility)

Contracted pelvis or cephalopelvic disproportion

Uterine anomalies (e.g., bicornuate uterus, fibroids)

Fetal factors

Prematurity (smaller fetal size allows greater mobility)

Multiple gestation (e.g., twins, where crowding may lead to abnormal positioning)

Fetal anomalies (e.g., anencephaly, hydrocephalus)

Small-for-gestational-age fetus

Other factors

Cord entanglement or short umbilical cord

Abnormal fetal lie or attitude (e.g., deflexed head)

Inadequate uterine contractions

Mechanism of Presentation

In compound presentation, the most common scenario is a hand or arm prolapsing alongside the vertex (head), but other combinations, such as a foot or shoulder with the vertex, may occur. The presenting parts (e.g., vertex and hand) enter the pelvic inlet together, potentially obstructing descent or complicating engagement.

The presentation is often unstable and may resolve spontaneously if the prolapsed extremity retracts or the fetus adjusts to a vertex presentation during labor. Persistent compound presentation can lead to obstructed labor due to the increased diameter of the presenting parts or mechanical interference.

Diagnosis

Clinical Examination: Abdominal examination (Leopold's maneuvers)

May reveal an irregular fetal outline or difficulty palpating the presenting part clearly.

The fetal head may not be well-engaged, and fetal heart tones may be higher than expected.

Vaginal examination

The hallmark is palpation of a fetal extremity (e.g., hand, arm, or foot) alongside the presenting part (usually the vertex).

The prolapsed extremity may be felt as a soft, irregular structure next to the head or breech.

Care must be taken to differentiate a prolapsed hand from a cord prolapse, which is a medical emergency.

Ultrasound: The definitive diagnostic tool, confirming the presence of a fetal extremity alongside the presenting part and assessing fetal lie, position, and associated anomalies (e.g., polyhydramnios, cord position).

Types of Compound Presentation

Vertex-hand/arm: The most common type, where a hand or arm presents alongside the fetal head.

Vertex-foot: Rare, where a foot prolapses alongside the vertex.

Breech-hand/arm: Seen in breech presentations with a prolapsed upper extremity.

Other combinations: Less common, such as shoulder and arm or multiple extremities in multiple gestations.

Positions

Described based on the presenting part and the side of the prolapsed extremity (e.g., left hand with vertex, right foot with breech).

The position of the vertex (e.g., occiput anterior, occiput posterior) may also influence management and outcomes.

Management

The management of compound presentation depends on the stage of labor, the specific presenting parts, and maternal and fetal conditions.

1. Antenatal Diagnosis

If detected antenatally via ultrasound, assess for underlying causes (e.g., polyhydramnios, fetal anomalies).

Counsel the patient about potential labor complications and the possible need for cesarean delivery.

In preterm pregnancies, compound presentation may resolve spontaneously as the fetus grows and assumes a longitudinal lie.

2. During Labor

Early labor: Monitor closely with continuous fetal heart rate monitoring and regular vaginal examinations. In many cases, the prolapsed extremity may retract spontaneously as labor progresses, allowing the vertex to engage and proceed to vaginal delivery. Avoid artificial rupture of membranes (ARM) to prevent cord prolapse or further descent of the extremity.

Gentle repositioning of the prolapsed extremity may be attempted by an experienced clinician during vaginal examination to encourage spontaneous resolution, but this should be done cautiously to avoid fetal distress or cord compression.

Persistent compound presentation

If the prolapsed extremity does not retract and obstructs labor, vaginal delivery may be impossible.

Cesarean section is indicated in cases of:

Persistent compound presentation with failure to progress.

Fetal distress (e.g., abnormal fetal heart rate patterns).

Cord prolapse (a common complication).

Cephalopelvic disproportion or macrosomia.

Prolapsed arm with risk of trauma or shoulder dystocia-like complications.

A low transverse incision is usually sufficient, but a classical incision may be needed in rare cases (e.g., preterm fetus, multiple gestation).

Trial of labor: May be considered in multiparous women with a small fetus, adequate pelvis, and no signs of obstruction or fetal distress. Requires close monitoring, experienced obstetric staff, and immediate access to cesarean facilities.

Internal podalic version or manipulative delivery: Extremely rare in modern practice due to high risks of fetal and maternal trauma.May be considered in exceptional cases (e.g., second twin in a multiple gestation) by a skilled obstetrician with no cesarean facilities available.

Complications

Maternal: Prolonged or obstructed labor, Uterine rupture (rare, but possible with forceful contractions or oxytocin use), Postpartum hemorrhage, Perineal or cervical trauma if vaginal delivery is attempted, Increased risk of infection due to prolonged labor or ruptured membranes.

Fetal: Cord prolapse (high risk, especially after membrane rupture), Fetal distress due to cord compression or prolonged labor, Birth trauma (e.g., brachial plexus injury, fractures of the prolapsed extremity), Hypoxia or asphyxia if delivery is delayed, Perinatal mortality (rare with timely intervention).

Prognosis

With timely recognition and management, maternal and fetal outcomes are generally favorable.

Spontaneous resolution occurs in many cases, particularly in multiparous women or preterm pregnancies, allowing vaginal delivery.

Persistent compound presentation or associated complications (e.g., cord prolapse) significantly increases risks, necessitating cesarean delivery.

Early cesarean section in cases of persistent presentation or fetal distress minimizes adverse outcomes.

Prevention

Routine antenatal ultrasound to identify malpresentations or risk factors (e.g., polyhydramnios, multiple gestation). Address modifiable risk factors (e.g., maternal obesity, polyhydramnios management).

Avoid premature ARM or oxytocin augmentation in suspected malpresentations.

Careful labor monitoring to detect compound presentation early and intervene appropriately.

Key Points

Compound presentation is a rare malpresentation involving two or more fetal parts (typically a hand/arm with the vertex) presenting simultaneously.

Diagnosis is confirmed by vaginal examination and ultrasound, with the prolapsed extremity palpable alongside the presenting part.

Many cases resolve spontaneously, but persistent presentation often requires cesarean delivery due to risks of obstruction or cord prolapse.

Management prioritizes fetal and maternal safety, with close monitoring and readiness for surgical intervention.

Complications include cord prolapse, fetal distress, and birth trauma, emphasizing the need for prompt recognition and intervention.

7.10 Shoulder Presentation and Dystocia

(*Maji-e-ktafi aur Usr-al-Wilada*)

Definition

Shoulder presentation is a type of malpresentation in which the fetus lies transversely across the maternal pelvis, with the shoulder (typically the acromion process) as the presenting part. This is a subset of transverse lie, occurring in approximately 0.2–0.3% of term deliveries. Shoulder dystocia, more broadly, is an obstetric emergency characterized by the inability to deliver the fetal shoulders after the head has been delivered, typically in vertex presentations, but it can also complicate shoulder presentations if labor is mismanaged.

Shoulder Presentation

Etiology

Shoulder presentation arises from conditions that prevent the fetus from assuming a longitudinal lie (vertex or breech). Common causes include:

Maternal factors

Multiparity (lax uterine and abdominal muscles)

Contracted pelvis or cephalopelvic disproportion

Uterine anomalies (e.g., bicornuate uterus, fibroids)

Placenta previa

Pelvic tumors

Fetal factors

Prematurity (increased fetal mobility in preterm gestations)

Polyhydramnios (excess amniotic fluid allows excessive movement)

Multiple gestation (e.g., twins, where one fetus may lie transversely)

Fetal anomalies (e.g., hydrocephalus, anencephaly, abdominal distension)

Macrosomia

Other factors

Short umbilical cord or cord entanglement

Abnormal uterine contractions or poor uterine tone

Mechanism of Presentation

In shoulder presentation, the fetus lies horizontally, with the head in one maternal flank and the breech in the other, and the shoulder (acromion) or upper arm presents at the pelvic inlet.

The long axis of the fetus is perpendicular to the maternal spine, making engagement in the pelvis impossible without correction to a longitudinal lie.

Positions include:

Right acromion anterior (RAA): Right shoulder presenting, fetal back anterior.

Left acromion anterior (LAA): Left shoulder presenting, fetal back anterior.

Right acromion posterior (RAP): Right shoulder presenting, fetal back posterior.

Left acromion posterior (LAP): Left shoulder presenting, fetal back posterior.

Dorso-superior or dorso-inferior: Fetal back directed upward or downward.

If labor progresses, the shoulder may become impacted in the pelvis, leading to neglected transverse lie, a dangerous condition associated with obstructed labor and severe complications.

Diagnosis

Clinical Examination: Abdominal examination (Leopold's maneuvers)

The uterus appears wider than usual, with a lower fundal height than expected.

The fetal head is palpable in one flank, and the breech is felt on the opposite side.

Fetal heart tones are typically heard in the mid-abdomen, not low in the pelvis.

Vaginal examination

The presenting part is the shoulder, arm, or ribs, often high and non-engaged.

A prolapsed arm or cord may be palpated, especially after membrane rupture.

No presenting part may be felt if the fetus is high in the uterus.

Ultrasound: The gold standard, confirming transverse lie, shoulder presentation, and associated conditions (e.g., placenta previa, polyhydramnios, fetal anomalies).

X-ray (rarely used): May confirm the transverse lie but is largely replaced by ultrasound.

Management

The management of shoulder presentation depends on gestational age, labor status, and maternal/fetal conditions.

1. Antenatal Diagnosis

Before 36 weeks: Observation is reasonable, as many fetuses spontaneously convert to a longitudinal lie as term approaches. Ultrasound to identify underlying causes (e.g., uterine anomalies, placenta previa). Plan for external cephalic version (ECV) at 36–37 weeks if the lie remains transverse, provided no contraindications exist.

ECV (External Cephalic Version)

Performed under ultrasound guidance with tocolytics (e.g., terbutaline) to relax the uterus.

Success rate: 50–70%, higher in multiparous women.

Contraindications: Placenta previa, fetal distress, multiple gestation, uterine anomalies.

Risks: Placental abruption, cord prolapse, fetal distress; requires immediate access to cesarean facilities.

2. During Labor

Early labor: Confirm diagnosis with ultrasound. Attempt ECV if not previously performed, provided labor is not advanced, membranes are intact, and conditions are favorable. Avoid artificial rupture of membranes (ARM) to prevent cord prolapse or arm prolapse. Monitor closely with continuous fetal heart rate monitoring.

Persistent shoulder presentation: Vaginal delivery is not possible without correction to a longitudinal lie. Cesarean section is the standard of care for persistent shoulder presentation in labor, particularly in: Primigravidas

Term pregnancies

Cases with risk factors (e.g., placenta previa, fetal distress)

A low transverse incision is typically sufficient, but a classical (vertical) incision may be needed for preterm fetuses, multiple gestations, or difficult extractions.

Internal podalic version (rare): Considered only in exceptional cases (e.g., second twin in multiple gestation, no cesarean facilities, experienced obstetrician). Involves manually rotating the fetus to a breech position under anesthesia, followed by breech extraction.

High risk of uterine rupture, cord prolapse, and fetal trauma; rarely performed in modern practice.

3. Contraindications to Vaginal Delivery

Persistent shoulder presentation in active labor, Cord prolapse or arm prolapse, Fetal distress, Placenta previa, Cephalopelvic disproportion, Maternal or fetal compromise.

Complications

Maternal: Obstructed labor, Uterine rupture (especially in neglected cases or with oxytocin use) Postpartum hemorrhage, Infection due to prolonged labor or ruptured membranes, Trauma to the birth canal if vaginal delivery is attempted

Fetal: Cord prolapse (high risk after membrane rupture), Fetal distress due to cord compression or prolonged labor, Birth trauma (e.g., brachial plexus injury, fractures), Perinatal asphyxia or death if delivery is delayed.

Prognosis

Timely cesarean delivery ensures excellent maternal and fetal outcomes. Neglected shoulder presentation (e.g., prolonged labor without intervention) is associated with high risks of maternal and fetal morbidity/mortality. Successful ECV may allow vaginal delivery, but close monitoring is essential.

Prevention

Routine antenatal ultrasound to detect transverse lie early. Address modifiable risk factors (e.g., polyhydramnios, maternal obesity). Perform ECV at 36–37 weeks in appropriate candidates. Avoid premature ARM or oxytocin in suspected malpresentations.

Shoulder dystocia

Definition: Shoulder dystocia is an obstetric emergency occurring when the fetal shoulders fail to deliver spontaneously after delivery of the head, typically due to impaction of the anterior shoulder against the maternal pubic symphysis or the posterior shoulder against the sacral promontory.

Incidence: 0.2–3% of vaginal deliveries in vertex presentations; rare in shoulder presentations unless labor is mismanaged.

Risk Factors

Maternal

Diabetes mellitus (gestational or pre-existing)

Obesity

Previous history of shoulder dystocia

Contracted pelvis

Fetal

Macrosomia (birth weight >4,000 g)

Post-term pregnancy

Labor-related

Prolonged second stage of labor

Operative vaginal delivery (forceps or vacuum)

Precipitous labor

Inappropriate management of shoulder presentation (e.g., failure to recognize transverse lie)

Mechanism

In vertex presentations, the anterior shoulder becomes impacted behind the pubic symphysis, preventing delivery.

In shoulder presentations, dystocia may occur if the shoulder is forcibly engaged in the pelvis (e.g., during neglected labor or failed version), leading to impaction or entrapment.

The bisacromial diameter (distance between the shoulders) is too wide to pass through the pelvic inlet or outlet without rotation.

Diagnosis

Clinical Features

Difficulty delivering the shoulders after the head is delivered in vertex presentation (classic "turtle sign": head retracts against the perineum).

In shoulder presentation, failure of the shoulder to engage or progress in labor, often with a prolapsed arm or cord.

Prolonged second stage or lack of descent despite adequate contractions.

Ultrasound: Not typically used in active labor but may identify risk factors (e.g., macrosomia) antenatally.

Vaginal examination: Confirms impaction of the shoulder or presence of a prolapsed extremity.

Management

Shoulder dystocia requires rapid, systematic intervention to prevent fetal hypoxia and maternal trauma. The ALSO (Advanced Life Support in Obstetrics) mnemonic HELPERR guides management:

1. H – Help:

Call for assistance (obstetrician, neonatologist, anesthesiologist, additional staff).

Ensure availability of cesarean facilities.

2. E – Evaluate for Episiotomy:

Consider episiotomy to facilitate maneuvers, though it does not directly resolve shoulder impaction.

Rarely needed with modern techniques but may aid access for posterior arm delivery.

3. L – Legs (McRoberts Maneuver):

Hyperflex the maternal hips (knees to chest) to flatten the sacrum and increase pelvic outlet diameter. First-line maneuver; effective in 40–60% of cases.

4. P – Pressure (Suprapubic):

Apply suprapubic pressure (not fundal pressure) to dislodge the anterior shoulder from the pubic symphysis. Performed by an assistant, using a rocking motion or continuous pressure.

5. E – Enter (Rotational Maneuvers):

Rubin II: Rotate the anterior shoulder to the oblique diameter by applying pressure behind the anterior shoulder.

Woods screw: Rotate the posterior shoulder to dislodge the anterior shoulder.

Reverse Woods screw: Rotate the fetus in the opposite direction.

6. R – Remove the Posterior Arm:

Deliver the posterior arm by sweeping it across the fetal chest, reducing the bisacromial diameter.

Requires skill to avoid fracture of the humerus or brachial plexus injury.

7. R – Roll (All-Fours Position):

Turn the mother onto her hands and knees (Gaskin maneuver) to dislodge the shoulder using gravity and pelvic repositioning.

Effective in some cases, particularly in multiparous women.

Advanced Maneuvers (if HELPERR fails):

Zavanelli maneuver: Push the fetal head back into the uterus and perform an emergency cesarean section (rare, high risk).

Deliberate clavicle fracture: Intentionally fracture the fetal clavicle to reduce shoulder width (rare, used as a last resort).

Symphysiotomy: Surgical division of the pubic symphysis (extremely rare, high maternal morbidity).

Management in Shoulder Presentation

If shoulder presentation is mistaken for a vertex presentation and labor progresses, shoulder dystocia may occur due to impaction of the shoulder in the pelvis. Immediate recognition of the transverse lie and cesarean delivery is critical to avoid dystocia-related complications.

Attempted vaginal delivery or version in shoulder presentation significantly increases the risk of dystocia and should be avoided.

Complications

Maternal

Postpartum hemorrhage (most common)

Perineal tears (third- or fourth-degree)

Uterine rupture (especially in neglected shoulder presentation)

Pelvic floor injury

Psychological trauma

Fetal

Brachial plexus injury (e.g., Erb's palsy, 5–15% of cases)

Clavicle or humerus fracture

Hypoxic-ischemic encephalopathy due to prolonged delivery time

Perinatal asphyxia or death (rare with prompt intervention)

Cord prolapse (in shoulder presentation)

Prognosis

Prompt recognition and management of shoulder dystocia (within 5–7 minutes) minimize adverse outcomes. In shoulder presentation, cesarean delivery prevents dystocia and ensures favorable maternal and fetal outcomes. Delayed intervention increases risks of permanent fetal injury (e.g., brachial plexus damage) or mortality.

Prevention

Antenatal: Identify risk factors (e.g., macrosomia, diabetes) via ultrasound and clinical assessment.

Consider elective cesarean for estimated fetal weight >4,500 g in non-diabetic mothers or >4,000 g in diabetic mothers.

Perform ECV for transverse lie/shoulder presentation at 36–37 weeks.

Intrapartum: Avoid operative vaginal delivery in high-risk cases (e.g., prolonged second stage, suspected macrosomia).

Ensure experienced staff and emergency protocols are in place for high-risk deliveries.

Early recognition of shoulder presentation via ultrasound or examination to avoid labor mismanagement.

Key Points

Shoulder presentation is a transverse lie with the shoulder as the presenting part, precluding vaginal delivery without correction.

Diagnosis relies on abdominal/vaginal examination and ultrasound, with cesarean section as the standard management for persistent cases.

Shoulder dystocia is an emergency primarily associated with vertex presentations but can occur in shoulder presentations if mismanaged.

The HELPERR mnemonic guides shoulder dystocia management, prioritizing rapid, systematic maneuvers to deliver the fetus.

Complications include maternal hemorrhage, fetal brachial plexus injury, and hypoxia, emphasizing the need for timely intervention.

Prevention involves antenatal risk assessment, early detection of malpresentations, and preparedness for emergency delivery.

7.11 Cord Presentation and Cord Prolapse

(*Maji-e-surri aur tadalliy-e-habl-us-surrah*)

Definition

Cord Presentation: A condition in which the umbilical cord lies below or alongside the presenting part of the fetus (e.g., vertex, breech, or shoulder) with intact membranes. The cord is positioned between the presenting part and the cervix but has not yet prolapsed into the vagina.

Cord Prolapse: An obstetric emergency where the umbilical cord descends through the cervix into the vagina or beyond, either before or alongside the presenting part, after the membranes have ruptured. This can lead to cord compression, compromising fetal oxygenation and requiring urgent intervention.

Incidence

Cord presentation: Exact incidence is difficult to quantify as it is often asymptomatic and detected only by ultrasound or during labor.

Cord prolapse: Occurs in approximately 0.1–0.6% of all deliveries, with higher rates in malpresentations (e.g., breech, transverse lie, shoulder presentation).

Etiology

Both cord presentation and prolapse are associated with conditions that allow excessive mobility of the fetus or cord, or prevent proper engagement of the presenting part. Risk factors include:

Maternal factors

Multiparity (lax uterine and abdominal muscles)

Cephalopelvic disproportion or contracted pelvis

Uterine anomalies (e.g., bicornuate uterus, fibroids)

Placenta previa (low-lying placenta increases cord malposition risk)

Premature rupture of membranes (PROM)

Fetal factors

Malpresentations (e.g., breech, transverse lie, shoulder presentation, compound presentation)

Prematurity (smaller fetus, more amniotic fluid)

Polyhydramnios (excess amniotic fluid allows cord mobility)

Multiple gestation (e.g., twins, where one fetus may have an abnormal lie)

Fetal anomalies (e.g., anencephaly, hydrocephalus)

Other factors

Long umbilical cord

Cord entanglement or abnormal cord insertion (e.g., velamentous insertion)

Artificial rupture of membranes (ARM) in the presence of a high or poorly applied presenting part

Obstetric interventions (e.g., amniotomy, external cephalic version, or internal podalic version)

Mechanism

Cord Presentation

The umbilical cord lies below or beside the presenting part but is protected by intact amniotic membranes. It is often transient and may resolve spontaneously, if the fetus repositions or the presenting part engages. Risk of progression to cord prolapse increases if membranes rupture spontaneously or artificially.

Cord Prolapse

Occurs when the membranes rupture, and the cord slips through the cervix into the vagina or external genitalia, either overtly (visible or palpable in the vagina) or occultly (compressed beside the presenting part without descending into the vagina).

Cord compression occurs due to pressure from the presenting part or uterine contractions, leading to reduced blood flow and fetal hypoxia.

The risk is highest in malpresentations (e.g., transverse lie: 10–20% risk; breech: 5–10% risk) compared to vertex presentations (<1% risk).

Types of Cord Prolapse

Overt cord prolapse: The cord is palpable or visible in the vagina or beyond, below the presenting part.

Occult cord prolapse: The cord is compressed alongside the presenting part but not visible or palpable in the vagina.

Funic presentation: Synonymous with cord presentation, where the cord is below the presenting part with intact membranes.

Diagnosis

Cord Presentation

Antenatal: Often asymptomatic and detected incidentally on routine ultrasound.

Ultrasound: Identifies the cord below or beside the presenting part, often using color Doppler to visualize cord position and blood flow. Clinical suspicion arises in high-risk cases (e.g., malpresentation, polyhydramnios).

Intrapartum: Vaginal examination: May detect the cord as a soft, pulsatile structure below the presenting part, with intact membranes.

Ultrasound: Confirms diagnosis if suspected during labor.

Fetal heart rate abnormalities (e.g., variable decelerations) may suggest cord compression, even with intact membranes.

Cord Prolapse

Clinical Features

Sudden fetal distress: Variable or prolonged decelerations, bradycardia, or loss of variability on fetal heart rate monitoring, especially after membrane rupture.

Vaginal examination: Overt prolapse is diagnosed by palpating or visualizing the cord in the vagina or beyond. Occult prolapse may be suspected if fetal distress occurs without visible cord.

Cord prolapse is often precipitated by ARM or spontaneous rupture of membranes in the presence of a high or malpresented fetus.

Ultrasound: May confirm cord position in occult cases but is rarely feasible in an emergency due to time constraints.

Management

Cord Presentation

1. Antenatal: If detected on ultrasound, assess for underlying causes (e.g., malpresentation, placenta previa, polyhydramnios). Monitor closely with serial ultrasounds to assess fetal lie and cord position.

Consider external cephalic version (ECV) at 36–37 weeks for malpresentations (e.g., transverse lie, breech) to reduce the risk of cord prolapse during labor. Counsel the patient about the risk of progression to cord prolapse and the potential need for cesarean delivery. Avoid ARM in outpatient settings if cord presentation is suspected.

2. Intrapartum

Early labor: Confirm diagnosis with ultrasound if suspected. Avoid ARM until the presenting part is well-applied to the cervix to prevent prolapse. Monitor fetal heart rate continuously to detect early signs of cord compression.

If the fetus is in a longitudinal lie (e.g., vertex, breech) and the presenting part engages, vaginal delivery may be possible with close monitoring.

Persistent cord presentation: In cases of persistent malpresentation (e.g., transverse lie), plan for elective cesarean section to avoid prolapse risk. If labor begins with cord presentation and the fetus remains non-engaged, proceed to cesarean delivery.

Cord Prolapse

Cord prolapse is an obstetric emergency requiring immediate action to prevent fetal hypoxia and death.

1. Immediate Actions

Call for help

Relieve cord compression

Manual elevation: If the cord is prolapsed, gently elevate the presenting part (e.g., head or shoulder) by placing a hand in the vagina to lift it off the cord, reducing compression.

Positioning: Place the mother in a knee-chest position (face down, knees to chest) or Trendelenburg position (head down, pelvis elevated) to use gravity to reduce cord compression.

Tocolysis: Administer a tocolytic (e.g., terbutaline 0.25 mg IV) to reduce uterine contractions and improve fetal oxygenation.

Bladder filling: In some cases, filling the bladder with 500–700 mL of saline via a Foley catheter can elevate the presenting part and relieve cord compression temporarily.

Avoid cord manipulation: Do not attempt to replace the prolapsed cord, as this may cause vasospasm or further compromise blood flow.

Oxygen administration: Provide supplemental oxygen to the mother to optimize fetal oxygenation.

2. Delivery: Emergency cesarean section

The preferred management for overt or occult cord prolapse in most cases, especially if the fetus is viable and labor is not imminent.

Performed urgently to minimize fetal hypoxia (target delivery within 10–20 minutes of diagnosis).

General or regional anesthesia is used, depending on urgency and maternal condition.

Manual elevation of the presenting part is maintained during transport to the operating room and until the fetus is delivered.

Vaginal delivery: Considered only if delivery is imminent (e.g., fully dilated cervix, vertex presentation, head at +2 station or lower) and can be achieved rapidly (e.g., via spontaneous pushing or operative vaginal delivery with forceps/vacuum).

Rarely feasible in malpresentations like transverse lie or shoulder presentation.

3. Contraindications to Vaginal Delivery

Non-viable fetus (e.g., pre-viable gestation or confirmed fetal demise)

Persistent cord compression with fetal distress

Malpresentation (e.g., transverse lie, shoulder presentation)

Cervix not fully dilated or presenting part not engaged

Complications

Maternal

Postpartum hemorrhage

Uterine rupture (rare, associated with prolonged labor or aggressive interventions)

Infection (prolonged labor or ruptured membranes)

Psychological trauma from emergency delivery

Fetal

Hypoxic-ischemic encephalopathy

Perinatal asphyxia

Neurological sequelae (e.g., cerebral palsy)

Fetal death (5–10% mortality rate in overt prolapse without rapid intervention)

Cord trauma or vasospasm (rare, from excessive manipulation)

Prognosis

Cord Presentation: Good prognosis if detected early and managed with cesarean delivery or spontaneous resolution before membrane rupture. Risk of progression to prolapse necessitates vigilant monitoring.

Cord Prolapse: Prognosis depends on the speed of intervention:

Delivery via cesarean section results in favorable outcomes in most cases.

Delayed intervention increases risks of fetal hypoxia, neurological injury, or death.

Perinatal mortality is significantly reduced with modern obstetric practices and access to emergency cesarean facilities.

Prevention

Antenatal

Routine ultrasound to identify malpresentations, polyhydramnios, or cord presentation.

Perform ECV at 36–37 weeks for breech or transverse lie to reduce prolapse risk. Counsel high-risk patients (e.g., those with polyhydramnios or multiple gestation) about signs of PROM and the need for immediate medical attention.

Intrapartum

Avoid ARM in cases of high, non-engaged, or malpresented fetuses.

Confirm fetal presentation and engagement via ultrasound or vaginal examination before ARM.

Use continuous fetal heart rate monitoring in high-risk cases to detect early signs of cord compression.

Plan elective cesarean section for persistent malpresentations (e.g., transverse lie, shoulder presentation) to avoid labor-related prolapse.

Key Points

Cord presentation involves the umbilical cord lying below or beside the presenting part with intact membranes, while cord prolapse is an emergency where the cord descends into the vagina after membrane rupture.

Both conditions are associated with malpresentations, prematurity, and polyhydramnios, with prolapse carrying a high risk of fetal hypoxia due to cord compression.

Diagnosis relies on ultrasound (antenatal) and vaginal examination (intrapartum), with fetal distress often indicating prolapse.

Management of cord presentation involves avoiding ARM and planning cesarean delivery for persistent cases; cord prolapse requires immediate relief of cord compression and urgent cesarean section in most cases.

Complications include fetal hypoxia, neurological injury, and maternal trauma, emphasizing the need for rapid intervention. Prevention includes early detection of risk factors, careful labor management and avoiding premature ARM in high-risk cases.

Long Answer Questions (LAQs)

Define prolonged labor and describe its causes.

Explain the maternal complications of prolonged labor.

Describe fetal complications associated with prolonged labor.

Discuss diagnosis and monitoring of prolonged labor.

Explain management of prolonged labor in primigravida and multigravida.

Short Answer Questions (SAQs)

Define prolonged labor.

Mention causes of prolonged labor.

List maternal complications of prolonged labor.

List fetal complications of prolonged labor.

What is the role of partograph in prolonged labor?

Multiple Choice Questions (1 Mark Each)

1. Prolonged labor is defined as labor lasting more than:

A. 12 hours B. 18 hours

C. 24 hours D. 36 hours

Answer: C

2. Most common cause of prolonged labor is:
A. Fetal distress   B. Inefficient uterine contractions
C. Placenta previa   D. Cord prolapse
Answer: B
3. Which of the following is a maternal complication of prolonged labor?
A. Birth asphyxia   B. Meconium aspiration
C. Uterine exhaustion   D. Caput succedaneum
Answer: C
4. Fetal complication commonly seen in prolonged labor is:
A. Shoulder dystocia   B. Birth asphyxia
C. Cephalhematoma   D. Congenital anomaly
Answer: B
5. Partograph is mainly used to:
A. Diagnose pregnancy   B. Detect fetal anomalies
C. Monitor progress of labor   D. Assess placental position
Answer: C
6. Prolonged labor increases the risk of:
A. Post-term pregnancy   B. Pre-eclampsia
C. Postpartum hemorrhage   D. Ectopic pregnancy
Answer: C
7. In prolonged labor, dehydration occurs due to:
A. Blood loss   B. Fever
C. Long duration without oral intake   D. Infection
Answer: C
8. Which factor does NOT contribute to prolonged labor?
A. Cephalopelvic disproportion   B. Malpresentation
C. Polyhydramnios   D. Poor uterine contractions
Answer: C
9. First sign of maternal exhaustion in prolonged labor is:
A. Hypotension   B. Tachycardia
C. Bradycardia   D. Cyanosis
Answer: B
10. Best prevention of prolonged labor is:
A. Early induction   B. Antibiotics
C. Proper monitoring of labor   D. Elective cesarean
Answer: C

08

Medical & Gynecological Disorders in Pregnancy

(Dauran-e-haml lahq hone wale Mualajati aur Niswani Amrad)

8.1 *Qay'al Haml aur Qay'al haml Mufriat* (Emesis & Hyperemesis Gravidarum)
8.2 *Faqr-al-Dam* (Anemia)
8.3 Dhayabitus Harr aur Dhayabitus Harr Hamli (Diabetes Mellitus & GDM)
8.4 *Kahla-i-Ghudda Darqiyay* (Thyroid Dysfunction)
8.5 *Tamniy -i-rahayee iswi* (Rh Isoimmunization)
8.6 *Mi'di Mi'wi Amrad* (Gastrointestinal Disorders)
8.7 *Kabisi, marari aur banqarasi Amrad* (Hepatic, Biliary & Pancreatic Disorder)
8.8 *Qalbi 'Uruqi amrad* (Cardiovascular Disorders)
8.9 *Amrad-i-Kulya wa Majra-i-Bawl* (Renal & Urinary Tract Disorders)
8.10 *Daurane Haml fairoosu, jarasimi, tufeli aur awali ibteka wa ta'diya* (Viral, Bacterial, Parasitic & Protozoal Infestation & Infection in pregnancy)
8.11 *Daurane Haml lahaq hone wale niswani Amrad* (Gynecological disorders in pregnancy)

Learning Objective (At the end of the session, the students should be able to)

Identify Emesis & Hyperemesis Gravidarum & explore etiopathology, diagnosis, complications & management of Emesis Gravidarum

Identify Anemia in pregnancy & Describe its classification, etiopathology, diagnosis, management & Complications

Describe the classification, screening & complications of Diabetes Mellitus & Gestational DM.

Discuss the diagnosis & complications of Hyper & Hypothyroidism in pregnancy

Describe the etiopathology, diagnosis & complications of Gastrointestinal Disorders with Hepatic, Biliary & Pancreatic Disorders in pregnancy

Explain pathophysiology, diagnosis, complications & prevention of Rh Isoimmunization

Explain the types, effects & diagnosis of Cardiovascular Disorders in pregnancy

Elaborate causes, diagnosis & complications of Renal & Urinary Tract Disorders in pregnancy

Discuss Viral, Bacterial, Parasitic & Protozoal Infestations & Infections in pregnancy and its classification, diagnosis & complications

Describe etiology, diagnosis, management & complications of Gynecological disorders in pregnancy

8.1 Emesis & Hyperemesis Gravidarum

(*Qay'al Haml aur Qay'al haml Mufriat*)

Definition

Emesis (Nausea and Vomiting of Pregnancy, NVP): A common condition characterized by nausea, with or without vomiting, during pregnancy, typically occurring in the first trimester. It affects approximately 50–80% of pregnant women and is usually mild and self-limiting.

Hyperemesis Gravidarum (HG): A severe form of NVP, characterized by persistent, excessive vomiting leading to dehydration, weight loss (>5% of pre-pregnancy weight), electrolyte imbalances, and potential complications. It occurs in 0.3–2% of pregnancies and may require hospitalization.

Etiology

The exact cause of NVP and HG is multifactorial and not fully understood, but several factors are implicated:

Hormonal Changes

Elevated levels of human chorionic gonadotropin (hCG), particularly in the first trimester, correlate with the onset of symptoms. Higher hCG levels (e.g., in multiple gestations or molar pregnancies) are associated with increased severity. Estrogen and progesterone surges may contribute by altering gastrointestinal motility and gastric emptying. Other hormones, such as thyroid-stimulating hormone (TSH) analogs and cortisol, may play a role.

Gastrointestinal Factors

Delayed gastric emptying due to progesterone-mediated smooth muscle relaxation. Increased sensitivity to gastric irritants or altered gastric pH. Possible role of Helicobacter pylori infection, with some studies showing an association with HG.

Genetic and Environmental Factors

Genetic predisposition: Family history or previous HG increases risk.

Environmental triggers: Stress, dietary factors (e.g., high-fat meals) or odors may exacerbate symptoms.

Maternal Factors

Multiparity or nulliparity

Multiple gestations (e.g., twins, triplets)

Molar pregnancy or gestational trophoblastic disease

Pre-existing gastrointestinal disorders (e.g., reflux, irritable bowel syndrome)

Psychological factors (e.g., stress, anxiety) may exacerbate symptoms, though not primary causes.

Other Factors

Younger maternal age

Obesity

History of motion sickness or migraines

Previous history of HG in prior pregnancies

Female fetus (slightly higher risk)

History of eating disorders

Hyperthyroidism or transient gestational thyrotoxicosis (often associated with high hCG levels)

Pathophysiology

Nausea and Vomiting of Pregnancy (NVP)

Likely results from the interaction of hormonal changes (hCG, estrogen, progesterone) with the chemoreceptor trigger zone in the brainstem and altered gastrointestinal motility.

Increased vagal stimulation and heightened olfactory sensitivity may contribute.

Usually peaks at 8–12 weeks gestation, resolving by 16–20 weeks in most cases.

Hyperemesis Gravidarum

Severe, persistent vomiting leads to dehydration, starvation ketosis, and metabolic disturbances. Electrolyte imbalances: Hypokalemia, hyponatremia, and metabolic alkalosis (from loss of gastric acid) or acidosis (from ketosis).

Nutritional deficiencies: Depletion of thiamine (vitamin B1), leading to risks of Wernicke's encephalopathy if untreated.

Hepatic and renal effects: Elevated liver enzymes (transaminases) and mild hyperbilirubinemia in severe cases; acute kidney injury may occur due to dehydration.

Thyroid dysfunction: Transient gestational thyrotoxicosis due to hCG's thyroid-stimulating effects, with suppressed TSH and elevated free T4 in some cases.

Clinical Features

Nausea and Vomiting of Pregnancy (NVP)

Symptoms typically begin at 5–6 weeks gestation, peak at 8–12 weeks, and resolve by 16–20 weeks.

Mild to moderate nausea, often worse in the morning ("morning sickness") but can occur throughout the day.

Occasional vomiting, usually not severe enough to cause dehydration or weight loss.

No significant impact on maternal weight, hydration, or nutrition in most cases.

Normal physical examination findings, with stable vital signs and no evidence of dehydration.

Hyperemesis Gravidarum

Severe, persistent vomiting (multiple episodes daily), leading to inability to retain food or fluids.

Dehydration: Dry mucous membranes, reduced skin turgor, tachycardia, hypotension, and oliguria.

Weight loss: >5% of pre-pregnancy body weight.

Ketosis: Ketonuria or ketonemia due to starvation and fat metabolism.

Electrolyte disturbances: Hypokalemia, hyponatremia, or metabolic alkalosis/acidosis.

Other symptoms

Fatigue, weakness, or dizziness

Epigastric pain or hematemesis (from esophageal irritation or Mallory-Weiss tears)

Jaundice (rare, in severe cases with liver involvement)

Neurological symptoms (e.g., confusion, ataxia) if thiamine deficiency progresses to Wernicke's encephalopathy.

Physical examination

Signs of dehydration (e.g., sunken eyes, dry tongue, orthostatic hypotension)

Weight loss

Possible jaundice or neurological signs in severe cases

Diagnosis

Nausea and Vomiting of Pregnancy: Diagnosis is clinical, based on

History of nausea and/or vomiting in early pregnancy.

Absence of other causes (e.g., gastroenteritis, appendicitis, cholecystitis).

Normal physical examination and laboratory findings.

Pregnancy-Unique Quantification of Emesis (PUQE) score: A validated tool to assess severity (mild: ≤6; moderate: 7–12; severe: ≥13).

Investigations (if needed)

Urine dipstick to rule out ketonuria.

Basic blood work (e.g., electrolytes, renal function) if symptoms are prolonged or severe.

Hyperemesis Gravidarum: Diagnosis is based on

Persistent vomiting with inability to tolerate oral intake.

Weight loss >5% of pre-pregnancy weight.

Evidence of dehydration (e.g., elevated hematocrit, reduced urine output).

Ketonuria or ketonemia on urine dipstick or serum testing.

Laboratory Investigations

Electrolytes: Check for hypokalemia, hyponatremia, or metabolic alkalosis/acidosis.

Renal function: Elevated blood urea nitrogen (BUN) or creatinine in dehydration.

Liver function tests: Mild elevation of transaminases (AST/ALT) or bilirubin in severe cases.

Thyroid function tests: Suppressed TSH and elevated free T4 (transient thyrotoxicosis, seen in 50–60% of HG cases).

Urinalysis: Ketonuria, possible proteinuria in severe dehydration.

Complete blood count (CBC): Hemoconcentration (elevated hematocrit) due to dehydration.

Serum thiamine levels (if Wernicke's encephalopathy is suspected).

Ultrasound: To rule out multiple gestation, molar pregnancy, or other causes of elevated hCG.

Differential Diagnosis

Gastrointestinal: Appendicitis, cholecystitis, pancreatitis, gastroenteritis, peptic ulcer disease, H. pylori infection.

Metabolic: Diabetic ketoacidosis, Addison's disease, hyperthyroidism.

Neurological: Migraine, intracranial pathology (e.g., mass, raised intracranial pressure).

Other: Pyelonephritis, drug side effects, eating disorders.

Management

Nausea and Vomiting of Pregnancy

Management focuses on symptom relief and lifestyle modifications, with pharmacotherapy for persistent cases.

1. Non-Pharmacological

Dietary modifications

Small, frequent, bland meals (e.g., dry toast, crackers).

Avoid spicy, fatty, or odorous foods.

Stay hydrated with clear fluids (e.g., water, electrolyte drinks).

Lifestyle changes

Rest and stress reduction.

Avoid triggers (e.g., strong smells, motion).

2. Pharmacological (if non-pharmacological measures fail):

Pyridoxine (Vitamin B6): 10–25 mg orally 2–3 times daily (first-line, safe in pregnancy).

Doxylamine: 12.5–25 mg at bedtime, often combined with pyridoxine.

Antihistamines: Dimenhydrinate (50–100 mg every 4–6 hours) or diphenhydramine (25–50 mg every 6 hours).

Metoclopramide: 5–10 mg every 6–8 hours (prokinetic, improves gastric emptying).

Ondansetron: 4–8 mg every 8 hours (second-line, effective for nausea but monitor for QT prolongation).

3. Monitoring

Regular follow-up to assess symptom resolution.

Escalate to HG management if symptoms worsen, weight loss occurs, or ketonuria develops.

Hyperemesis Gravidarum

Management requires aggressive treatment of dehydration, electrolyte imbalances, and nutritional deficiencies, often necessitating hospitalization.

1. Hospitalization Indications

Persistent vomiting with inability to tolerate oral intake.

Weight loss >5% of pre-pregnancy weight.

Dehydration (e.g., ketonuria, abnormal electrolytes, oliguria).

Failure of outpatient management.

2. Initial Management

Intravenous (IV) fluids

Normal saline or Ringer's lactate (1–2 L initially, then maintenance fluids).

Add dextrose (e.g., D5NS) once ketosis resolves to prevent hypoglycemia.

Correct electrolytes (e.g., potassium, magnesium) based on lab results.

Thiamine supplementation

Administer 100 mg IV thiamine daily for 2–3 days before dextrose-containing fluids to prevent Wernicke's encephalopathy.

Antiemetics (escalate as needed)

First-line: Pyridoxine (10–25 mg IV/oral) + doxylamine (12.5–25 mg).

Second-line: Metoclopramide (5–10 mg IV/oral every 6–8 hours) or ondansetron (4–8 mg IV/oral every 8 hours).

Third-line: Promethazine (12.5–25 mg IV/IM/oral every 4–6 hours) or prochlorperazine (5–10 mg IV/IM).

Refractory cases: Corticosteroids (e.g., methylprednisolone 16 mg IV/oral every 8 hours for 3 days, then taper) may be considered after 10 weeks gestation.

3. Nutritional Support

Enteral feeding: If oral intake remains inadequate, consider nasogastric or nasojejunal feeding.

Parenteral nutrition: Reserved for severe, refractory cases unable to tolerate enteral feeding (risks include infection, thrombosis).

4. Treat Underlying Conditions

Test for H. pylori (stool antigen or serology) and treat if positive (e.g., amoxicillin, clarithromycin, proton pump inhibitor).

Manage transient thyrotoxicosis symptomatically (antithyroid drugs rarely needed).

5. Monitoring

Daily assessment of hydration, weight and urine output.

Regular labs (electrolytes, renal function, liver function, ketonuria).

Fetal monitoring via ultrasound to assess growth and amniotic fluid.

6. Psychosocial Support

Address psychological distress (e.g., anxiety, depression) with counseling or support groups.

HG can significantly impact quality of life, requiring empathetic care.

Refractory Cases

Consider multidisciplinary consultation (obstetrics, gastroenterology, nutrition).

Rarely, termination of pregnancy may be discussed in extreme cases unresponsive to treatment, with severe maternal morbidity.

Complications

Nausea and Vomiting of Pregnancy

Usually self-limiting with minimal complications.

Rare: Prolonged symptoms leading to dehydration, weight loss, or progression to HG.

Hyperemesis Gravidarum

Maternal: Dehydration and acute kidney injury. Electrolyte imbalances (e.g., hypokalemia, hyponatremia) leading to cardiac arrhythmias or seizures. Wernicke's encephalopathy (thiamine deficiency, presenting as confusion, ataxia, nystagmus). Mallory-Weiss tears or esophageal rupture from forceful vomiting. Nutritional deficiencies (e.g., vitamin deficiencies, anemia). Psychological impact (e.g., depression, anxiety).

Fetal

Intrauterine growth restriction (IUGR) in severe, prolonged cases. Preterm birth (if maternal condition worsens).No direct evidence of increased congenital anomalies, but severe malnutrition may affect fetal development.

Pregnancy Outcomes

Increased risk of preterm delivery and low birth weight in severe HG. No significant increase in perinatal mortality with proper management.

Prognosis

NVP: Typically resolves by 16–20 weeks gestation, with excellent maternal and fetal outcomes. Recurrence is common in subsequent pregnancies but usually mild.

HG: With timely treatment, most women recover fully, with symptoms resolving by mid-pregnancy. Recurrence risk in future pregnancies is high (15–80%). Severe cases may lead to prolonged hospitalization or rare complications like Wernicke's encephalopathy.

Prevention

Antenatal

Early identification of risk factors (e.g., history of HG, multiple gestation).

Preconception counseling for women with prior HG to discuss prophylactic measures (e.g., early pyridoxine, dietary planning).

Lifestyle

Encourage small, frequent meals and hydration before pregnancy symptoms begin.

Avoid known triggers (e.g., strong odors, high-fat foods).

Prophylactic Treatment

In women with a history of HG, consider starting pyridoxine ± doxylamine at the onset of pregnancy or before symptoms develop.

Early intervention for NVP to prevent progression to HG.

Key Points

NVP is common, affecting 50–80% of pregnancies, and is usually mild, resolving by 16–20 weeks.

HG is a severe form of NVP, characterized by persistent vomiting, weight loss (>5%), dehydration, and ketosis, requiring aggressive management.

Hormonal changes (hCG, estrogen, progesterone) and gastrointestinal factors play a key role in etiology.

Diagnosis is clinical for NVP; HG requires laboratory confirmation of dehydration, ketosis, and electrolyte imbalances.

Management of NVP includes dietary/lifestyle changes and antiemetics (e.g., pyridoxine, doxylamine); HG requires IV fluids, thiamine, antiemetics, and possibly nutritional support.

Complications of HG include Wernicke's encephalopathy, electrolyte disturbances, and IUGR; timely intervention improves outcomes.

Prevention involves early recognition of risk factors, trigger avoidance, and prophylactic treatment in high-risk cases.

8.2 Anemia

(*Faqr-al-Dam*)

Definition

Anemia in pregnancy is defined as a hemoglobin (Hb) concentration below the normal range for gestational age, typically <11 g/dL in the first and third trimesters or <10.5 g/dL in the second trimester, according to the World Health Organization (WHO). It is a common complication of pregnancy, affecting 20–40% of pregnant women globally, with higher prevalence in low-resource settings.

Etiology

Anemia in pregnancy results from physiological changes, increased nutritional demands, or pathological conditions. The major causes include:

1. Physiological Anemia

Plasma volume expansion: During pregnancy, plasma volume increases by 30–50% (1–2 L), peaking at 28–34 weeks, while red blood cell (RBC) mass increases by only 15–30%. This disproportionate expansion causes hemodilution, lowering Hb concentration.

Typically mild and not associated with adverse outcomes if nutritional needs are met.

2. Nutritional Deficiencies

Iron deficiency anemia (IDA): The most common cause (50–75% of cases).

Increased iron demand (1,000–1,200 mg total in pregnancy) for fetal growth, placental development, and maternal RBC expansion.

Inadequate dietary intake, poor absorption (e.g., due to phytates, tea, or calcium), or pre-existing iron deficiency.

Folate deficiency: Common in populations with poor dietary folate intake or malabsorption.

Increased folate requirements (400–600 μg/day) for DNA synthesis and fetal development.

Leads to megaloblastic anemia.

Vitamin B12 deficiency: Rare, seen in vegans, malabsorption syndromes (e.g., pernicious anemia), or gastric disorders.

Causes megaloblastic anemia and potential neurological complications.

Other deficiencies: Vitamin A, zinc, or copper deficiencies (less common).

3. Hemoglobinopathies

Sickle cell disease: Autosomal recessive disorder causing hemolytic anemia, vaso-occlusive crises, and increased infection risk.

Thalassemias: Inherited disorders of hemoglobin synthesis (α- or β-thalassemia), leading to microcytic anemia.

Other hemoglobin variants: HbC, HbE, or other rare variants.

4. Chronic Diseases

Chronic infections (e.g., malaria, HIV, tuberculosis).

Chronic renal disease, autoimmune disorders, or malignancies.

Inflammatory states causing anemia of chronic disease (impaired iron utilization).

5. Hemorrhagic Causes

Acute blood loss: Ectopic pregnancy, miscarriage, placenta previa, placental abruption, or postpartum hemorrhage.

Chronic blood loss: Gastrointestinal bleeding (e.g., hookworm, peptic ulcer), menorrhagia pre-pregnancy.

6. Other Causes

Aplastic anemia: Rare, due to bone marrow suppression (e.g., drugs, viral infections).

Hemolytic anemias: Autoimmune, drug-induced, or hereditary (e.g., G6PD deficiency, hereditary spherocytosis).

Maternal infections: Malaria, hookworm, or schistosomiasis, particularly in endemic areas.

Risk Factors

Low socioeconomic status or poor access to nutrition.

Multiparity or short interpregnancy intervals.

Pre-pregnancy anemia or malnutrition.

Multiple gestation (increased iron and folate demands).

Chronic medical conditions or infections.

Vegetarian/vegan diet (risk of B12 or iron deficiency).

Adolescent pregnancy (increased nutritional needs).

Residence in malaria-endemic areas.

Pathophysiology

1. Physiological Anemia: Hemodilution due to greater plasma volume expansion compared to RBC mass. Compensatory mechanisms include increased cardiac output and oxygen delivery to tissues.

2. Iron Deficiency Anemia: Depletion of iron stores leads to reduced hemoglobin synthesis, resulting in microcytic, hypochromic RBCs.

Stages: Depleted iron stores (low ferritin) → reduced iron supply (low transferrin saturation) → anemia (low Hb, low MCV).

3. Megaloblastic Anemia: Folate or B12 deficiency impairs DNA synthesis, leading to ineffective erythropoiesis, large RBCs (high MCV), and megaloblastic changes in bone marrow.

4. Hemoglobinopathies

   a. Sickle cell disease: Abnormal HbS causes RBC sickling, hemolysis, and vaso-occlusion.
   b. Thalassemias: Reduced globin chain production leads to microcytic anemia and ineffective erythropoiesis.

5. Hemolytic Anemia: Increased RBC destruction (e.g., autoimmune, malaria, or hereditary causes) reduces Hb levels and increases reticulocytes.

6. Anemia of Chronic Disease: Inflammatory cytokines (e.g., IL-6) increase hepcidin, reducing iron availability for erythropoiesis despite adequate stores.

Clinical Features

Symptoms (depend on severity and type)

Mild anemia (Hb 10–11 g/dL): Often asymptomatic, detected on routine screening.

Moderate anemia (Hb 7–9.9 g/dL)

Fatigue, weakness or lethargy, dyspnea on exertion, palpitations or tachycardia.

Pallor (skin, conjunctiva, mucous membranes).

Severe anemia (Hb <7 g/dL)

Severe fatigue, dizziness, or syncope.

Shortness of breath at rest.

Chest pain or angina (rare).

Signs of high-output cardiac failure (e.g., edema, bounding pulses).

Specific to underlying cause

Iron deficiency: Koilonychia, angular cheilitis, pica (craving non-food substances, e.g., ice, clay).

Folate/B12 deficiency: Glossitis, neuropathy (B12), or jaundice (hemolysis in severe cases).

Sickle cell disease: Pain crises, jaundice, splenomegaly (in children), or leg ulcers.

Thalassemia: Hepatosplenomegaly, skeletal changes (in severe cases).

Signs

Pallor (conjunctiva, tongue, nail beds, palms).

Tachycardia or bounding pulse.

Systolic flow murmur (due to increased cardiac output).

Signs of heart failure in severe cases (e.g., edema, hepatomegaly, crackles).

Specific findings based on etiology (e.g., jaundice in hemolytic anemia, splenomegaly in hemoglobinopathies).

Diagnosis

Screening-Routine complete blood count (CBC) at the first prenatal visit and again at 24–28 weeks gestation.

WHO criteria for anemia in pregnancy

First trimester: Hb <11 g/dL.

Second trimester: Hb <10.5 g/dL.

Third trimester: Hb <11 g/dL.

Severe anemia: Hb <7 g/dL.

Laboratory Investigations

1) Complete Blood Count (CBC)

Hb and hematocrit: Low in anemia.

Mean corpuscular volume (MCV)

Microcytic (<80 fL): Iron deficiency, thalassemia.

Normocytic (80–100 fL): Acute blood loss, chronic disease, early IDA.

Macrocytic (>100 fL): Folate or B12 deficiency.

Mean corpuscular hemoglobin (MCH) and MCH concentration (MCHC): Low in IDA, normal/high in spherocytosis.

Red cell distribution width (RDW): High in IDA, normal in thalassemia.

2) Peripheral Smear

Microcytic, hypochromic RBCs in IDA or thalassemia.

Macrocytic RBCs with hypersegmented neutrophils in folate/B12 deficiency.

Sickle cells or target cells in hemoglobinopathies.

Spherocytes in hereditary spherocytosis or autoimmune haemolysis.

3) Iron Studies

Serum ferritin Low (<15 μg/L) in IDA; normal/high in anaemia of chronic disease.

Serum iron and total iron-binding capacity (TIBC): Low iron, high TIBC in IDA; low iron, low TIBC in chronic disease.

Transferrin saturation: Low in IDA.

4. Folate and B12 Levels

Serum folate: Low in folate deficiency.

Serum B12: Low in B12 deficiency.

Homocysteine and methylmalonic acid: Elevated in B12 deficiency; homocysteine elevated in folate deficiency.

5. Reticulocyte Count

Low in IDA, folate/B12 deficiency, or aplastic anemia.

High in hemolytic anemia or acute blood loss.

6. Additional Tests (based on suspected etiology)

Hemoglobin electrophoresis: For sickle cell disease or thalassemia.

Direct Coombs test: For autoimmune hemolytic anemia.

Malaria smear or rapid diagnostic test: In endemic areas.

Stool for occult blood or parasites (e.g., hookworm).

Bone marrow biopsy: Rarely needed for aplastic anemia or malignancy.

Differential Diagnosis

Physiological anemia (hemodilution).

Nutritional anemias (iron, folate, B12 deficiency).

Hemoglobinopathies (sickle cell, thalassemia).

Hemolytic anemias (autoimmune, G6PD deficiency, malaria).

Anemia of chronic disease (infections, inflammation).

Acute or chronic blood loss.

Management

Management depends on the severity, etiology, and gestational age. The goals are to correct anemia, prevent complications, and optimize maternal and fetal outcomes.

1. Physiological Anemia

No specific treatment required if Hb is within normal limits for pregnancy and no symptoms.

Ensure adequate nutrition and routine iron/folate supplementation.

2. Iron Deficiency Anemia

Prevention: WHO recommends universal supplementation: 30–60 mg elemental iron and 400 μg folic acid daily for all pregnant women.

Dietary counselling: Increase intake of iron-rich foods (e.g., red meat, lentils, spinach) and vitamin C to enhance absorption.

Treatment

Oral iron: First-line (e.g., ferrous sulfate 200 mg 1–2 times daily, providing 60–120 mg elemental iron). Take with vitamin C (e.g., orange juice) to improve absorption.

Side effects: Nausea, constipation, dark stools; consider alternative formulations (e.g., ferrous gluconate) if poorly tolerated.

Expected response: Hb rise of 0.3–1 g/dL per week after 2–3 weeks.

Parenteral iron

Indicated for severe anemia (Hb <7 g/dL) near term, poor oral tolerance, malabsorption, or non-compliance.

Options: Iron sucrose, ferric carboxymaltose, or low-molecular-weight iron dextran.

Administered IV in divided doses or as a single infusion; monitor for anaphylaxis or infusion reactions.

Blood transfusion

Reserved for severe anemia (Hb <6 g/dL) with symptoms of heart failure, impending delivery, or acute blood loss. Transfuse packed RBCs slowly with diuretic cover (e.g., furosemide) to prevent volume overload.

Monitoring: Repeat CBC after 4–6 weeks of treatment; aim for Hb >11 g/dL by delivery.

3. Folate Deficiency Anemia

Supplementation: Folic acid 1–5 mg daily orally (higher doses for confirmed deficiency).

Dietary counselling: Increase intake of leafy greens, citrus fruits, and fortified cereals.

Prevention: Routine folate supplementation (400 µg/day) starting preconception or early pregnancy to prevent neural tube defects and anemia.

4. Vitamin B12 Deficiency

Treatment: Intramuscular (IM) cyanocobalamin or hydroxocobalamin (1 mg weekly for 4–6 weeks, then maintenance).

Dietary counselling: Increase intake of animal products (e.g., meat, eggs, dairy) or fortified foods for vegetarians.

Investigate cause: Test for pernicious anemia (anti-intrinsic factor antibodies) or malabsorption.

5. Hemoglobinopathies

Sickle cell disease

Multidisciplinary care (obstetrician, hematologist).

Folic acid 1 mg daily to support erythropoiesis.

Hydration and oxygenation to prevent crises.

Hydroxyurea avoided in pregnancy; manage crises with analgesics, hydration, and oxygen.

Transfusion for severe anemia or complications (e.g., acute chest syndrome).

Thalassemia

Folic acid supplementation.

Transfusion for severe anemia (e.g., Hb <7 g/dL).

Chelation therapy (e.g., deferoxamine) deferred until postpartum.

Genetic counseling for future pregnancies.

6. Hemolytic Anemia

Treat underlying cause (e.g., antimalarials for malaria, steroids for autoimmune hemolytic anemia).

Transfusion for severe anemia or fetal compromise.

Monitor for jaundice, hemoglobinuria, or renal dysfunction.

7. Anemia of Chronic Disease

Treat underlying condition (e.g., antibiotics for infections, antimalarials).

Iron supplementation if coexisting IDA; avoid if ferritin is normal/high.

Erythropoiesis-stimulating agents rarely used in pregnancy.

8. Severe Anemia

Cesarean section planning: Ensure blood is available for transfusion.

Intrapartum management: Avoid excessive blood loss, use oxytocin to prevent postpartum hemorrhage.

Postpartum: Continue iron/folate supplementation for 3–6 months to replenish stores.

Complications

Maternal

Fatigue, reduced quality of life.

Increased risk of preterm labor, preeclampsia, or postpartum hemorrhage.

Cardiac failure in severe anemia (Hb <6 g/dL).

Increased infection susceptibility.

Postpartum depression or prolonged recovery.

Fetal

Intrauterine growth restriction (IUGR).

Preterm birth.

Low birth weight.

Fetal distress or stillbirth (in severe, untreated anemia).

Neural tube defects (folate deficiency).

Neurodevelopmental delays (severe B12 deficiency or chronic hypoxia).

Pregnancy Outcomes

Increased risk of perinatal mortality in severe anemia.

Higher rates of cesarean delivery and maternal morbidity in anemic women.

Prognosis

Mild/moderate anemia: Excellent prognosis with timely treatment; most women achieve normal Hb by delivery.

Severe anemia: Good outcomes with aggressive management (e.g., transfusion, parenteral iron), but untreated cases carry high maternal and fetal risks.

Hemoglobinopathies: Outcomes depend on disease severity and complications; multidisciplinary care improves prognosis.

Prevention

Antenatal

Routine iron (30–60 mg/day) and folate (400 µg/day) supplementation for all pregnant women.

Dietary counseling to ensure adequate intake of iron, folate, and B12.

Screen for anemia at booking visit and 24–28 weeks.

Treat pre-pregnancy anemia before conception.

Public Health Measures

Food fortification (e.g., iron, folate in grains).

Control of infections (e.g., malaria, hookworm) in endemic areas.

Access to prenatal care and nutritional support in low-resource settings.

High-Risk Populations

Early screening and higher-dose supplementation for women with multiple gestations, short interpregnancy intervals, or hemoglobinopathies.

Prophylactic antimalarials or deworming in endemic areas.

Key Points

Anemia in pregnancy is common, primarily due to iron deficiency, with physiological hemodilution contributing to mild cases.

Defined by Hb <11 g/dL (first/third trimesters) or <10.5 g/dL (second trimester); severe anemia (Hb <7 g/dL) requires urgent treatment.

Iron deficiency is the most common cause, followed by folate/B12 deficiency and hemoglobinopathies.

Diagnosis involves CBC, peripheral smear, iron studies, and specific tests (e.g., hemoglobin electrophoresis) based on suspected etiology.

Management includes oral or parenteral iron for IDA, folate/B12 supplementation for megaloblastic anemia and transfusion for severe cases.

Complications include maternal cardiac failure, preterm birth, IUGR and perinatal mortality, emphasizing timely intervention.

Prevention relies on universal iron/folate supplementation, dietary counseling and early screening/treatment of risk factors.

8.3 Diabetes Mellitus and Gestational Diabetes Mellitus

(*Dhayabitus Har aur Dhayabitus Har Hamli*)

Definition

Diabetes Mellitus (DM): A chronic metabolic disorder characterized by hyperglycemia due to insulin deficiency (Type 1 DM), insulin resistance (Type 2 DM), or other causes (e.g., monogenic diabetes). In pregnancy, pre-existing DM (Type 1 or Type 2) is termed pregestational diabetes

Gestational Diabetes Mellitus (GDM): Glucose intolerance first diagnosed during pregnancy, typically in the second or third trimester, that does not meet criteria for overt diabetes. GDM affects approximately 2–10% of pregnancies worldwide, with higher prevalence in high-risk populations.

Etiology and Classification

Pregestational Diabetes Mellitus

Type 1 DM: Autoimmune destruction of pancreatic β-cells leading to absolute insulin deficiency. Usually diagnosed before pregnancy, but rare new diagnoses may occur.

Type 2 DM: Insulin resistance with relative insulin deficiency, often associated with obesity, metabolic syndrome, or genetic predisposition. Increasingly common in reproductive-age women.

Other Types: Monogenic diabetes (e.g., MODY), secondary diabetes (e.g., due to pancreatitis, cystic fibrosis), or drug-induced diabetes.

Gestational Diabetes Mellitus

Caused by pregnancy-induced insulin resistance, primarily due to placental hormones (e.g., human placental lactogen, cortisol, progesterone) that impair insulin action.

Risk factors include:

Maternal obesity (BMI ≥30 kg/m^2).

Advanced maternal age (>35 years).

Family history of Type 2 DM.

Previous GDM or macrosomic infant (>4,000 g).

Polycystic ovary syndrome (PCOS).

Ethnicity (e.g., South Asian, Hispanic, African, Indigenous populations).

Sedentary lifestyle or excessive gestational weight gain.

Multiple gestation

Pathophysiology

Pregestational DM

Type 1 DM: Absolute insulin deficiency leads to uncontrolled hyperglycemia, risk of ketoacidosis, and dependence on exogenous insulin.

Type 2 DM: Insulin resistance with progressive β-cell dysfunction causes hyperglycemia, often exacerbated by pregnancy's metabolic demands.

Pregnancy increases insulin requirements due to placental hormones, weight gain, and increased maternal metabolism, worsening glycemic control.

Gestational Diabetes Mellitus

Pregnancy induces insulin resistance, peaking in the second and third trimesters, to ensure adequate glucose supply to the fetus.

In GDM, maternal β-cells cannot compensate with increased insulin production, leading to hyperglycemia.

Maternal-fetal effects

Maternal hyperglycemia crosses the placenta, stimulating fetal hyperinsulinemia.

Fetal hyperinsulinemia promotes excessive growth (macrosomia), fat deposition, and metabolic stress.

Placental transfer of glucose but not insulin creates a unique fetal environment prone to complications.

Clinical Features

Pregestational DM

Symptoms: Often asymptomatic in well-controlled cases; poorly controlled DM may present with polyuria, polydipsia, weight loss, fatigue, or recurrent infections.

Pregnancy effects: Worsening glycemic control, increased insulin needs, and higher risk of complications (e.g., hypoglycemia, ketoacidosis).

Physical examination: May reveal signs of chronic DM (e.g., retinopathy, neuropathy) or obesity (Type 2 DM).

Gestational Diabetes Mellitus

Symptoms: Usually asymptomatic; detected through routine screening.

Rare symptoms: Polyuria, polydipsia, or fatigue in severe cases.

Physical examination: Typically normal; may show obesity or signs of insulin resistance (e.g., acanthosis nigricans).

Diagnosis

Pregestational DM

Diagnosed before pregnancy based on standard criteria (American Diabetes Association, ADA)

Fasting plasma glucose (FPG) ≥126 mg/dL (7.0 mmol/L).

2-hour plasma glucose ≥200 mg/dL (11.1 mmol/L) during 75 g oral glucose tolerance test (OGTT).

Random plasma glucose ≥200 mg/dL (11.1 mmol/L) with symptoms.

HbA1c ≥6.5%.

In pregnancy, confirm diagnosis and assess glycemic control with HbA1c and self-monitored blood glucose (SMBG).

Gestational Diabetes Mellitus

Screening

Universal or selective screening at 24–28 weeks gestation.

High-risk women (e.g., obesity, prior GDM, family history) may be screened at the first prenatal visit to detect overt diabetes or early GDM.

Diagnostic Tests (based on guidelines, e.g., ADA, WHO)

One-step approach (International Association of Diabetes and Pregnancy Study Groups, IADPSG)

75 g OGTT at 24–28 weeks.

Diagnostic thresholds (one or more values met/exceeded)

Fasting: ≥92 mg/dL (5.1 mmol/L).

1-hour: ≥180 mg/dL (10.0 mmol/L).

2-hour: ≥153 mg/dL (8.5 mmol/L).

Two-step approach (Carpenter-Coustan or NIH criteria)

Step 1: 50 g glucose challenge test (GCT), non-fasting; if 1-hour glucose ≥130–140 mg/dL, proceed to step 2.

Step 2: 100 g OGTT, fasting; diagnostic if two or more values met/exceeded:

Fasting: ≥95 mg/dL (5.3 mmol/L).

1-hour: ≥180 mg/dL (10.0 mmol/L).

2-hour: ≥155 mg/dL (8.6 mmol/L).

3-hour: ≥140 mg/dL (7.8 mmol/L).

Early screening (first trimester)

HbA1c ≥6.5% or FPG ≥126 mg/dL indicates overt diabetes (not GDM).

HbA1c 5.7–6.4% or FPG 110–125 mg/dL may warrant early OGTT to diagnose GDM.

Differential Diagnosis

Overt diabetes (pre-existing Type 1 or Type 2 DM).

Monogenic diabetes (e.g., MODY).

Secondary causes (e.g., corticosteroid use, pancreatic disease).

Management

The goals of management are to achieve euglycemia, prevent maternal and fetal complications, and optimize pregnancy outcomes. Multidisciplinary care (obstetrician, endocrinologist, dietician) is essential.

Pregestational DM

1. Preconception Care

Optimize glycemic control before pregnancy (HbA1c <6.5%, ideally <6.0% if safe).

Switch to insulin if on oral agents (e.g., metformin safe, but others like sulfonylureas avoided).

Folic acid 5 mg daily to reduce neural tube defect risk.

Assess for complications (e.g., retinopathy, nephropathy, neuropathy) and treat as needed.

Counsel on risks of poor control (e.g., congenital anomalies, miscarriage).

2. Antenatal Management

Glycemic targets (ADA recommendations)

Fasting: <95 mg/dL (5.3 mmol/L).

1-hour postprandial: <140 mg/dL (7.8 mmol/L).

2-hour postprandial: <120 mg/dL (6.7 mmol/L).

HbA1c: <6–6.5% (avoid hypoglycemia).

Self-monitored blood glucose (SMBG): 4–6 times daily (fasting, pre/post-meals).

Insulin therapy

Basal-bolus regimen (e.g., long-acting insulin like glargine + rapid-acting insulin like aspart) or insulin pump.

Adjust doses frequently due to increasing insulin resistance.

Medical nutrition therapy (MNT)

Balanced diet (40–50% carbohydrates, 20–25% protein, 30–35% fat).

Small, frequent meals to avoid glucose spikes.

Fetal monitoring

Early ultrasound (10–12 weeks) to assess viability and anomalies.

Detailed anomaly scan at 18–20 weeks (e.g., cardiac defects, neural tube defects).

Fetal echocardiography for Type 1 DM or poorly controlled Type 2 DM.

Serial growth scans (every 4 weeks from 28 weeks) to detect macrosomia or IUGR.

Non-stress test (NST) or biophysical profile from 32 weeks if complications present.

Complication screening

Retinal exam each trimester (diabetic retinopathy may worsen).

Renal function (creatinine, urine albumin/creatinine ratio) for nephropathy.

Monitor for hypertension or preeclampsia (increased risk).

3. Intrapartum Management

Timing of delivery

Well-controlled DM: Deliver at 39–40 weeks.

Poorly controlled DM or complications: Consider delivery at 37–38 weeks.

Severe complications (e.g., IUGR, preeclampsia): May require earlier delivery.

Glycemic control

Maintain glucose 70–110 mg/dL (3.9–6.1 mmol/L) during labor.

Use IV insulin drip with dextrose infusion if needed.

Mode of delivery

Vaginal delivery preferred if no complications.

Cesarean section for macrosomia (>4,500 g), fetal distress, or maternal complications.

4. Postpartum Management

Reduce insulin doses (50–60% of pregnancy dose) due to decreased insulin resistance post-delivery.

Monitor for hypoglycemia, especially in breastfeeding mothers.

Resume pre-pregnancy medications (e.g., metformin for Type 2 DM) if safe.

Screen for postpartum thyroiditis in Type 1 DM.

Encourage contraception and preconception planning for future pregnancies.

Gestational Diabetes Mellitus

1. Initial Management

Medical nutrition therapy (MNT)

Individualized diet plan (similar to pregestational DM).

Carbohydrate counting (30–45 g/meal, 15–30 g/snack).

Avoid refined sugars and high-glycemic-index foods.

Physical activity: 30 minutes of moderate exercise (e.g., walking) most days, unless contraindicated.

SMBG: Fasting and 1- or 2-hour postprandial glucose 4 times daily.

Targets: Fasting <95 mg/dL, 1-hour postprandial <140 mg/dL, 2-hour <120 mg/dL.

2. Pharmacotherapy (if MNT fails to achieve targets after 1–2 weeks):

Insulin: Preferred if glucose levels remain elevated. Rapid-acting (e.g., aspart, lispro) for postprandial control; basal insulin (e.g., NPH, glargine) for fasting control. Safe in pregnancy, titrated based on SMBG.

Metformin: Alternative for mild GDM (crosses placenta, long-term fetal effects unclear).

Dose: 500–2,000 mg daily in divided doses.

Glyburide: Rarely used due to risk of fetal hypoglycemia and inconsistent efficacy.

Monitor closely; 15–20% of GDM patients require insulin.

3. Fetal Monitoring

Ultrasound at 28–32 weeks to assess fetal growth (macrosomia or IUGR).

NST or biophysical profile from 32–34 weeks if insulin-dependent or complications present.

No additional monitoring needed for well-controlled GDM on MNT alone.

4. Intrapartum Management

Timing of delivery

Well-controlled GDM on MNT: Deliver at 39–40 weeks.

Insulin-dependent or complications: Consider delivery at 37–39 weeks.

Macrosomia (>4,500 g): Discuss cesarean section to avoid shoulder dystocia.

Glycemic control

Maintain glucose 70–110 mg/dL during labor.

Insulin drip rarely needed unless glucose is uncontrolled.

Mode of delivery: Vaginal delivery preferred unless macrosomia or complications.

5. Postpartum Management

GDM resolves in most cases post-delivery, but 50–70% of women develop Type 2 DM within 5–10 years.

Screening: 75 g OGTT at 6–12 weeks postpartum to detect persistent diabetes or prediabetes.

Normal: FPG <100 mg/dL, 2-hour glucose <140 mg/dL.

Prediabetes: FPG 100–125 mg/dL or 2-hour glucose 140–199 mg/dL.

Diabetes: FPG ≥126 mg/dL or 2-hour glucose ≥200 mg/dL.

Discontinue insulin or metformin post-delivery unless overt diabetes is diagnosed.

Encourage weight loss, exercise, and healthy diet to reduce Type 2 DM risk.

Breastfeeding: Safe and encouraged; may improve insulin sensitivity.

Contraception and preconception counseling for future pregnancies.

Complications

Maternal: Pregestational DM

Worsening diabetic complications (retinopathy, nephropathy, neuropathy).

Diabetic ketoacidosis (DKA): More common in Type 1 DM, triggered by stress, infection, or poor control.

Hypoglycemia: Due to tight control or reduced oral intake.

Preeclampsia (2–4 times higher risk).

Cesarean delivery (increased risk due to macrosomia or complications).

Postpartum hemorrhage or infection.

GDM

Increased risk of preeclampsia.

Higher cesarean delivery rates.

Progression to Type 2 DM (50–70% lifetime risk).

Fetal/Neonatal

Congenital anomalies (pregestational DM, especially with poor preconception control):

Cardiac (e.g., ventricular septal defect, transposition of great arteries).

Neural tube defects (e.g., spina bifida, anencephaly).

Caudal regression syndrome (rare, specific to DM).

Macrosomia: Fetal weight >4,000–4,500 g due to hyperinsulinemia; increases risk of shoulder dystocia, birth trauma, and cesarean delivery.

Intrauterine growth restriction (IUGR): More common in pregestational DM with vascular complications (e.g., nephropathy, hypertension).

Preterm birth: Due to maternal complications or iatrogenic delivery.

Neonatal hypoglycemia: Caused by fetal hyperinsulinemia post-delivery.

Respiratory distress syndrome: Due to delayed lung maturation.

jaundice and polycythemia: From increased RBC turnover.

Stillbirth: Higher risk in poorly controlled DM or with vascular complications.

Long-term risks: Increased risk of obesity, Type 2 DM, and metabolic syndrome in offspring.

Prognosis

Pregestational DM: Good outcomes with tight glycemic control, preconception planning, and multidisciplinary care. Poor control increases maternal and fetal morbidity/mortality.

GDM: Excellent prognosis with early diagnosis and management. Recurrence risk in future pregnancies is 30–65%. Long-term maternal risk of Type 2 DM requires follow-up.

Prevention

Pregestational DM

Preconception counseling to achieve HbA1c <6.5% before pregnancy.

Optimize weight, diet, and exercise in Type 2 DM.

Screen and treat diabetic complications before conception.

GDM

Pre-pregnancy weight loss in obese women.

Healthy diet and regular exercise before and during pregnancy.

Early screening in high-risk women to detect overt diabetes or early GDM.

Public health measures: Education on nutrition, weight management, and diabetes risk.

Key Points

Pregestational DM (Type 1 or 2) requires preconception optimization and tight glycemic control (HbA1c <6.5%) to reduce congenital anomalies and complications.

GDM is glucose intolerance diagnosed in pregnancy, caused by insulin resistance, and screened at 24–28 weeks using OGTT.

Diagnosis of GDM uses one-step (IADPSG) or two-step (Carpenter-Coustan) criteria; early screening for high-risk women.

Management involves MNT, exercise, SMBG and insulin (or metformin) if needed; pregestational DM requires insulin therapy.

Complications include maternal preeclampsia, cesarean delivery, and fetal macrosomia, anomalies (pregestational DM), neonatal hypoglycemia and stillbirth.

Prevention includes preconception care, weight management, and early screening; postpartum OGTT is critical for GDM patients to detect Type 2 DM risk.

8.4 Thyroid Dysfunction

(*Kahla-i-Ghudda Darqiyay*)

Definition

Thyroid dysfunction in pregnancy encompasses disorders of thyroid hormone production or action, including hypothyroidism, hyperthyroidism and subclinical forms of these conditions. These disorders can significantly impact maternal and fetal health due to the critical role of thyroid hormones in metabolism, fetal neurodevelopment and pregnancy maintenance. Thyroid dysfunction is common, affecting 2–3% of pregnant women, with hypothyroidism being more prevalent than hyperthyroidism.

Physiology of Thyroid Function in Pregnancy

Maternal Changes

Increased thyroid hormone production: Pregnancy increases thyroid hormone demand by 20–50% due to higher maternal metabolism, placental growth and fetal needs.

Human chorionic gonadotropin (hCG): hCG, structurally similar to thyroid-stimulating hormone (TSH), stimulates the thyroid, causing transient hyperthyroidism in early pregnancy (peak at 8–12 weeks).

Increased thyroxine-binding globulin (TBG): Estrogen-induced TBG rise (2–3-fold) increases total T4 and T3 levels, but free T4 (fT4) and free T3 (fT3) remain stable in euthyroid women.

Iodine requirements: Rise to 250 μg/day due to increased renal clearance and fetal thyroid needs.

Fetal Thyroid Function

Fetal thyroid begins functioning at 10–12 weeks gestation; until then, the fetus relies on maternal T4, critical for neurodevelopment.

Placental deiodinase enzymes regulate thyroid hormone transfer, protecting the fetus from excess maternal hormone.

Etiology

1. Hypothyroidism

Overt Hypothyroidism: TSH above the trimester-specific upper limit (e.g., >2.5–4.0 mU/L in first trimester) with low fT4.

Primary causes: Autoimmune thyroiditis (Hashimoto's thyroiditis): Most common, associated with anti-thyroid peroxidase (TPO) antibodies.

Iodine deficiency: Common in iodine-deficient regions.

Previous thyroidectomy or radioactive iodine ablation.

Congenital hypothyroidism or pituitary/hypothalamic disorders (rare).

Secondary/tertiary hypothyroidism: Pituitary or hypothalamic dysfunction (e.g., Sheehan's syndrome post-delivery).

Subclinical Hypothyroidism: Elevated TSH with normal fT4; affects 2–5% of pregnancies. Often due to early Hashimoto's thyroiditis or iodine deficiency.

Risk factors

Personal or family history of thyroid disease.

Type 1 diabetes or other autoimmune disorders.

History of miscarriage, preterm birth, or infertility.

Residence in iodine-deficient areas.

2. Hyperthyroidism

Overt Hyperthyroidism: Suppressed TSH (<0.1 mU/L) with elevated fT4 or fT3.

Primary causes

Graves' disease: Most common (80–90% of cases), an autoimmune condition with TSH receptor antibodies (TRAb).

Toxic multinodular goiter or solitary toxic adenoma (rare in pregnancy).

Subacute thyroiditis or drug-induced (e.g., amiodarone).

Transient gestational thyrotoxicosis: hCG-mediated, usually in first trimester, often associated with hyperemesis gravidarum.

Subclinical Hyperthyroidism: Suppressed TSH with normal fT4 and fT3; often transient and hCG-related.

Risk factors

History of Graves' disease or thyroid nodules.

Multiple gestation or molar pregnancy (high hCG levels).

Hyperemesis gravidarum.

3. Other Thyroid Disorders

Isolated hypothyroxinemia: Normal TSH with low fT4; rare and controversial in terms of clinical significance.

Thyroid nodules or cancer: May be detected during pregnancy; usually managed postpartum unless aggressive.

Postpartum thyroiditis: Autoimmune inflammation post-delivery, presenting as transient hyperthyroidism followed by hypothyroidism (1–6 months postpartum).

Clinical Features

Hypothyroidism

Overt Hypothyroidism

Symptoms: Fatigue, weight gain, cold intolerance, constipation, dry skin, hair loss, muscle cramps, depression.

Signs: Bradycardia, goiter, delayed reflexes, edema, hoarse voice.

Pregnancy-specific: Increased risk of miscarriage, preeclampsia, preterm birth, or placental abruption.

Subclinical Hypothyroidism

Often asymptomatic or mild symptoms (e.g., fatigue, mild weight gain).

May be detected only through screening in high-risk women.

Hyperthyroidism

Overt Hyperthyroidism (e.g., Graves' disease):

Symptoms: Weight loss, heat intolerance, palpitations, anxiety, tremors, diarrhea, insomnia.

Signs: Tachycardia, goiter, exophthalmos (Graves'), lid lag, warm skin, thyroid bruit.

Pregnancy-specific: Increased risk of preeclampsia, preterm birth, heart failure, or thyroid storm.

Transient Gestational Thyrotoxicosis

Mild symptoms (nausea, vomiting) often linked to hyperemesis gravidarum.

No goiter or ophthalmopathy (unlike Graves' disease).

Subclinical Hyperthyroidism: Usually asymptomatic; detected on routine screening.

Postpartum Thyroiditis

Hyperthyroid phase (1–3 months postpartum): Palpitations, anxiety, fatigue.

Hypothyroid phase (3–6 months postpartum): Fatigue, depression, weight gain.

Up to 20% progress to permanent hypothyroidism.

Diagnosis

Screening: Universal vs. targeted screening

Universal screening for thyroid dysfunction in pregnancy is controversial; targeted screening is recommended for high-risk women (e.g., history of thyroid disease, Type 1 diabetes, autoimmune disorders, infertility, or miscarriage).

Screen at first prenatal visit with TSH and fT4.

Trimester-specific reference ranges (due to physiological changes)

First trimester: TSH 0.1–2.5 mU/L; fT4 varies by assay (typically 0.8–1.8 ng/dL).

Second trimester: TSH 0.2–3.0 mU/L.

Third trimester: TSH 0.3–3.0 mU/L.

If lab-specific ranges are unavailable, use non-pregnant ranges adjusted downward (TSH upper limit reduced by 0.5–1.0 mU/L).

Diagnostic Tests

1. Thyroid Function Tests

TSH: Primary screening test; elevated in hypothyroidism, suppressed in hyperthyroidism.

Free T4 (fT4): Confirms overt hypo/hyperthyroidism; normal in subclinical forms.

Free T3 (fT3): Measured if hyperthyroidism is suspected and fT4 is normal.

Total T4/T3: Less reliable due to TBG increase; adjust by 1.5x for pregnancy.

2. Antibody Testing

Anti-TPO antibodies: Positive in Hashimoto's thyroiditis; associated with increased miscarriage risk.

TSH receptor antibodies (TRAb): Positive in Graves' disease; assess for fetal/neonatal hyperthyroidism risk.

3. Ultrasound

Thyroid ultrasound for goiter, nodules, or suspected malignancy.

Fetal ultrasound to assess for signs of thyroid dysfunction (e.g., goiter, growth restriction).

4. Other Tests

Urinary iodine to assess deficiency (if suspected).

TRAb or thyroid-stimulating immunoglobulin (TSI) in hyperthyroidism to differentiate Graves' disease from transient thyrotoxicosis.

Radioactive iodine uptake contraindicated in pregnancy due to fetal risk.

Differential Diagnosis

Hypothyroidism: Iodine deficiency, Hashimoto's thyroiditis, post-thyroidectomy, pituitary dysfunction, drug-induced (e.g., amiodarone, lithium).

Hyperthyroidism: Graves' disease, transient gestational thyrotoxicosis, toxic adenoma, subacute thyroiditis, molar pregnancy or hyperemesis gravidarum.

Non-thyroid causes: Fatigue, depression or anemia mimicking hypothyroidism; anxiety or cardiac conditions mimicking hyperthyroidism.

Management

Hypothyroidism

1. Overt Hypothyroidism

Levothyroxine (LT4): Start at 1–2 μg/kg/day (typically 50–100 μg daily) or higher if severe (e.g., TSH >10 mU/L). Adjust dose every 4–6 weeks to maintain TSH within trimester-specific range. Increase dose by 20–30% in early pregnancy for women on pre-pregnancy LT4 due to increased demand.

Monitoring: Check TSH and fT4 every 4–6 weeks; aim for TSH 0.1–2.5 mU/L in first trimester, 0.2–3.0 mU/L later.

Preconception: Optimize LT4 to achieve TSH <2.5 mU/L before pregnancy to reduce miscarriage risk.

2. Subclinical Hypothyroidism

Treat if TSH >4 mU/L or TSH >2.5 mU/L with positive anti-TPO antibodies due to increased miscarriage and preterm birth risk. LT4 starting dose: 25–50 µg daily, titrated to maintain TSH <2.5–3.0 mU/L. Controversial if TSH 2.5–4.0 mU/L without antibodies; consider treatment in high-risk women (e.g., infertility history).

3. Iodine Supplementation

Ensure 250 µg/day iodine intake (via prenatal vitamins or diet) to prevent deficiency. Avoid excessive iodine (>500 µg/day), which can cause fetal goiter.

Hyperthyroidism

1. Overt Hyperthyroidism (eg. Graves' Disease)

Antithyroid drugs (ATDs)

Propylthiouracil (PTU): Preferred in first trimester (50–150 mg daily in divided doses) due to lower teratogenicity.

Methimazole (MMI): Preferred after first trimester (5–20 mg daily) due to lower hepatotoxicity risk. Titrate to maintain fT4 at upper-normal or slightly above-normal range to minimize fetal hypothyroidism.

Risks: PTU (hepatotoxicity), MMI (teratogenicity, e.g., aplasia cutis, choanal atresia in first trimester).

β-Blockers: Propranolol (10–40 mg every 6–8 hours) for symptom control (e.g., tachycardia, tremors) in early treatment; taper once ATDs take effect.

Surgery: Thyroidectomy (rare) in second trimester for severe cases unresponsive to ATDs or with drug intolerance.

Radioactive iodine: Contraindicated in pregnancy due to fetal thyroid destruction.

Monitoring: Check TSH, fT4, and fT3 every 2–4 weeks. Monitor TRAb in Graves' disease; high levels indicate risk of fetal/neonatal hyperthyroidism. Fetal ultrasound for goiter, growth restriction, or hydrops.

2. Transient Gestational Thyrotoxicosis: Usually self-limiting; no ATDs required unless severe symptoms. Supportive care: Hydration, antiemetics (for hyperemesis), and β-blockers (e.g., propranolol) for symptomatic relief. Monitor thyroid function to confirm resolution by 14–20 weeks.

3. Subclinical Hyperthyroidism: No treatment needed; usually transient and hCG-mediated. Monitor for progression to overt hyperthyroidism.

Postpartum Thyroiditis

Hyperthyroid phase: β-Blockers for symptoms; avoid ATDs unless persistent (distinguish from Graves' recurrence via TRAb or uptake scan postpartum).

Hypothyroid phase: LT4 (25–100 µg daily) if symptomatic or TSH >10 mU/L; taper after 6–12 months if transient.

Monitor annually for permanent hypothyroidism.

Intrapartum Management

Hypothyroidism: Continue LT4; no special considerations unless severe (e.g., myxedema coma, rare).

Hyperthyroidism: Monitor for thyroid storm (fever, tachycardia, altered mental status); treat with β-blockers, ATDs, and supportive care.

Delivery timing

Well-controlled thyroid disease: Deliver at 39–40 weeks.

Poorly controlled or complications (e.g., preeclampsia, fetal growth issues): Earlier delivery (37–38 weeks).

Postpartum Management

Hypothyroidism: Reduce LT4 dose by 20–30% post-delivery; check TSH/fT4 at 6 weeks postpartum.

Hyperthyroidism: Continue ATDs at lowest effective dose; MMI preferred if breastfeeding. Monitor for postpartum thyroiditis or Graves' flare.

Breastfeeding: PTU and low-dose MMI (<20 mg/day) are safe; monitor infant thyroid function if TRAb is high.

Complications

Maternal

Hypothyroidism

Preeclampsia, gestational hypertension.

Placental abruption, preterm birth.

Postpartum hemorrhage.

Increased cesarean delivery rates.

Myxedema coma (rare, life-threatening).

Hyperthyroidism

Preeclampsia, heart failure.

Thyroid storm (rare, triggered by infection, labor, or surgery).

Preterm labor, miscarriage.

Postpartum thyroiditis or Graves' flare.

Fetal/Neonatal

Hypothyroidism

Miscarriage, stillbirth.

Intrauterine growth restriction (IUGR).

Preterm birth.

Neurodevelopmental impairment (e.g., low IQ, cognitive delays) if untreated in early pregnancy.

Congenital hypothyroidism (rare, if maternal iodine deficiency or untreated severe disease).

Hyperthyroidism

Fetal hyperthyroidism (due to transplacental TRAb): Fetal tachycardia, goiter, hydrops, or growth restriction.

Neonatal thyrotoxicosis (5–10% of infants of mothers with Graves' disease).

Preterm birth, low birth weight.

Congenital anomalies (if exposed to high-dose MMI in first trimester).

Pregnancy Outcomes

Increased risk of adverse outcomes with poor control; well-managed thyroid dysfunction has near-normal outcomes.

Subclinical hypothyroidism may increase miscarriage and preterm birth risk, especially with anti-TPO antibodies.

Prognosis

Hypothyroidism: Excellent with LT4 treatment; untreated overt hypothyroidism significantly increases maternal and fetal risks.

Hyperthyroidism: Good outcomes with controlled Graves' disease or transient thyrotoxicosis; thyroid storm or fetal hyperthyroidism carries high morbidity.

Postpartum Thyroiditis: 80% resolve spontaneously; 20% develop permanent hypothyroidism requiring lifelong LT4.

Prevention

Preconception

Optimize thyroid function (TSH <2.5 mU/L) in women with known thyroid disease.

Screen high-risk women (e.g., Type 1 diabetes, autoimmune history) before pregnancy.

Ensure adequate iodine intake (150 μg/day pre-pregnancy, 250 μg/day in pregnancy).

Antenatal

Targeted screening at first prenatal visit for high-risk women.

Routine iodine supplementation via prenatal vitamins.

Avoid unnecessary ATD use or excessive iodine intake.

Education: Counsel women on risks of untreated thyroid disease and importance of adherence to therapy.

Key Points

Thyroid dysfunction in pregnancy includes hypothyroidism (often Hashimoto's) and hyperthyroidism (often Graves' or transient thyrotoxicosis), with subclinical forms common.

Pregnancy alters thyroid physiology (increased TBG, hCG stimulation, iodine needs), requiring trimester-specific TSH/fT4 ranges.

Diagnosis involves TSH, fT4, and antibody testing (anti-TPO, TRAb); ultrasound for structural abnormalities or fetal monitoring.

Hypothyroidism: Treat with levothyroxine to maintain TSH <2.5–3.0 mU/L; untreated cases risk miscarriage and neurodevelopmental issues.

Hyperthyroidism: Use PTU in first trimester, MMI later; monitor for fetal hyperthyroidism in Graves' disease.

Complications include preeclampsia, preterm birth, and fetal anomalies; well-managed cases have good outcomes.

Prevention includes preconception optimization, iodine supplementation, and targeted screening for high-risk women.

8.5 Rh Isoimmunization

(*Tamniy -i-rahayee iswi*)

Definition

Rh isoimmunization, also known as Rh alloimmunization or Rh incompatibility, is an immune-mediated condition in which a pregnant woman who is Rh-negative (lacking the RhD antigen on red blood cells) develops antibodies against the RhD antigen of an Rh-positive fetus. This can lead to hemolytic disease of the fetus and newborn (HDFN), causing fetal anemia, hydrops fetalis, or neonatal jaundice. Rh isoimmunization is a significant cause of perinatal morbidity and mortality if untreated, but preventive measures have significantly reduced its incidence.

Etiology

RhD Antigen: The RhD antigen is a protein on the surface of red blood cells (RBCs), present in approximately 85% of individuals (Rh-positive) and absent in 15% (Rh-negative).

Sensitization: Occurs when an Rh-negative mother is exposed to Rh-positive fetal RBCs, triggering her immune system to produce anti-D antibodies (IgG). Common sensitizing events include:

Fetomaternal hemorrhage (FMH) during pregnancy or delivery (e.g., miscarriage, ectopic pregnancy, abortion, placental abruption, trauma, amniocentesis, chorionic villus sampling, or vaginal/cesarean delivery).

Blood transfusion with Rh-positive blood.

External cephalic version or manual removal of placenta.

Risk Factors

Rh-negative mother carrying an Rh-positive fetus (determined by paternal Rh status).

Previous pregnancies or sensitizing events without Rh immunoglobulin (RhIg) prophylaxis.

Large-volume FMH (>30 mL) increases sensitization risk.

Inadequate or absent RhIg administration post-sensitizing event.

Pathophysiology

Primary Sensitization: Initial exposure to RhD-positive RBCs stimulates the maternal immune system to produce anti-D IgG antibodies, typically in low titers during the first affected pregnancy. This rarely causes significant fetal harm in the index pregnancy.

Secondary Immune Response: In subsequent pregnancies with an Rh-positive fetus, maternal anti-D IgG antibodies cross the placenta, bind to fetal Rh-positive RBCs, and cause hemolysis. This leads to:

Fetal anemia: Due to destruction of RBCs.

Extramedullary hematopoiesis: Liver and spleen compensate, leading to hepatosplenomegaly.

Hydrops fetalis: Severe anemia causes high-output cardiac failure, resulting in edema, ascites, pleural/pericardial effusions, and polyhydramnios.

Neonatal jaundice: Hemolysis increases bilirubin, which can lead to kernicterus if untreated.

Severity: Depends on maternal antibody titers, timing of sensitization, and fetal Rh status. Other Rh antigens (e.g., C, c, E, e) or non-Rh antigens (e.g., Kell, Duffy) can also cause isoimmunization, but RhD is the most common.

Epidemiology

Incidence: Before routine RhIg prophylaxis, Rh isoimmunization occurred in 10–15% of Rh-incompatible pregnancies. With prophylaxis, the incidence has decreased to <0.1–0.2%.

Population Variation: Higher prevalence of Rh-negative status in Caucasian populations (15–17%) compared to African (5%) or Asian (1%) populations.

HDFN: Accounts for ~1–2% of neonatal jaundice cases in developed countries with effective prophylaxis; remains a major issue in low-resource settings with limited access to RhIg.

Clinical Features

Maternal: Rh isoimmunization is typically asymptomatic in the mother.

Detected through routine prenatal blood group screening or complications in the fetus/newborn.

Rarely, maternal complications (e.g., mirror syndrome, a rare condition mimicking preeclampsia due to severe fetal hydrops) may occur.

Fetal

Mild HDFN: Mild anemia (hemoglobin 10–13 g/dL), minimal jaundice, no significant sequelae.

Moderate HDFN: Moderate anemia (hemoglobin 7–10 g/dL), hepatosplenomegaly, jaundice, and risk of kernicterus if untreated.

Severe HDFN: Severe anemia (hemoglobin <7 g/dL). Hydrops fetalis: Generalized edema, ascites, pleural/pericardial effusions, heart failure. Polyhydramnios due to fetal swallowing difficulties. Stillbirth or intrauterine fetal demise in extreme cases.

Neonatal

Hemolytic anemia: Low hemoglobin at birth, pallor, and tachycardia.

Neonatal jaundice: Early-onset, rapidly rising bilirubin levels due to hemolysis.

Kernicterus: Rare but severe; bilirubin deposition in the brain causes neurological damage (e.g., seizures, hearing loss, cerebral palsy).

Hepatosplenomegaly: From extramedullary hematopoiesis.

Diagnosis

Antenatal Screening

Routine Blood Testing (first prenatal visit):

Maternal blood group and Rh status (ABO and RhD typing).

Antibody screen (indirect Coombs test) to detect anti-D or other alloantibodies.

Paternal Rh Status: If the father is Rh-positive, determine zygosity (homozygous D/D or heterozygous D/d) to assess fetal Rh risk (100% Rh-positive if homozygous, 50% if heterozygous).

Fetal Rh Genotyping: Non-invasive cell-free fetal DNA (cffDNA) testing from maternal blood (after 10 weeks gestation) to determine fetal RhD status in sensitized mothers or high-risk cases.

In Sensitized Pregnancies

Antibody Titers

Measure anti-D antibody titers (e.g., 1:8, 1:16) every 2–4 weeks in sensitized Rh-negative mothers.

Critical titer: Typically 1:16 to 1:32 (lab-specific); titers above this indicate increased risk of HDFN, warranting further evaluation.

Middle Cerebral Artery (MCA) Doppler Ultrasound

Measures peak systolic velocity (PSV) to assess fetal anemia.

MCA-PSV >1.5 multiples of the median (MoM) suggests moderate to severe anemia.

Performed every 1–2 weeks from 18–35 weeks in sensitized pregnancies with high titers.

Amniocentesis (if needed): Measures amniotic fluid bilirubin (via ΔOD450) to assess hemolysis severity. Largely replaced by MCA Doppler due to invasiveness.

Cordocentesis: Direct fetal blood sampling to measure hemoglobin and hematocrit in severe cases (rarely used due to risks).

Postnatal Diagnosis

Cord blood testing

Direct Coombs test (positive in HDFN due to maternal antibodies on fetal RBCs).

Hemoglobin and hematocrit (low in anemia).

Bilirubin levels (elevated in hemolysis).

Blood group and Rh status.

Neonatal assessment: Physical exam for jaundice, pallor, hepatosplenomegaly, or hydrops.

Management

Prevention of Rh Isoimmunization

1. Rh Immunoglobulin (RhIg) Prophylaxis

Standard dose: 300 µg (covers 30 mL of fetal blood or 15 mL of Rh-positive RBCs).

Routine administration

At 28 weeks gestation (reduces sensitization risk from spontaneous FMH).

Within 72 hours post-delivery if the neonate is Rh-positive.

Additional indications (300 µg RhIg for each event)

Miscarriage, abortion, or ectopic pregnancy (>12 weeks).

Amniocentesis, chorionic villus sampling, or cordocentesis.

External cephalic version, trauma, or placental abruption.

Any suspected FMH event (e.g., vaginal bleeding, invasive procedures).

Kleihauer-Betke Test or Flow Cytometry: Quantifies FMH volume to determine if additional RhIg doses are needed (e.g., 300 µg per 30 mL fetal blood).

2. Counseling

Educate Rh-negative women on the importance of RhIg prophylaxis.

Discuss paternal Rh status and fetal Rh testing options.

Management of Sensitized Pregnancies

1. Monitoring

Antibody titers: Check every 2–4 weeks; refer to maternal-fetal medicine if titers exceed critical threshold (e.g., 1:16–1:32).

MCA Doppler: Start at 18 weeks for high-risk cases (titers ≥1:16 or history of severe HDFN); repeat every 1–2 weeks until 35 weeks.

Fetal ultrasound: Assess for hydrops (edema, ascites, effusions), polyhydramnios, or growth issues.

2. Intrauterine Transfusion (IUT)

Indicated for severe fetal anemia (MCA-PSV >1.5 MoM or hydrops).

Performed via cordocentesis (intravascular) or intraperitoneal transfusion.

Uses Rh-negative, cross-matched, irradiated packed RBCs.

Timing: As early as 18–20 weeks, repeated every 2–4 weeks until 34–35 weeks.

Risk: Fetal loss (1–2% per procedure), infection, preterm labor, or worsening sensitization.

3. Delivery Planning

Timing

Mild/moderate HDFN: Deliver at 37–38 weeks.

Severe HDFN or IUT: Deliver at 34–37 weeks, depending on fetal status.

Hydrops or worsening anemia: May require earlier delivery (with neonatal intensive care support).

Mode of delivery

Vaginal delivery preferred unless obstetric indications for cesarean (e.g., hydrops, fetal distress).

Ensure delivery in a facility with neonatal intensive care unit (NICU) capabilities.

Intrapartum: Monitor for fetal distress; avoid procedures increasing FMH (e.g., manual placental removal).

4. Corticosteroids: Administer betamethasone (12 mg IM, two doses 24 hours apart) at 24–34 weeks if preterm delivery is anticipated to enhance fetal lung maturity.

Neonatal Management

Mild HDFN

Monitor bilirubin levels and treat with phototherapy for jaundice.

Check hemoglobin and hematocrit; supplement with folic acid to support erythropoiesis.

Moderate/Severe HDFN

Exchange transfusion: Indicated for severe anemia (Hb <10 g/dL) or rapidly rising bilirubin (>0.5–1 mg/dL/hour) to prevent kernicterus.

Phototherapy: Standard for neonatal jaundice.

Intravenous immunoglobulin (IVIG): Reduces hemolysis in severe cases by blocking Fc receptors (0.5–1 g/kg).

Erythropoietin: Considered for persistent anemia post-exchange transfusion.

Monitoring: Serial bilirubin and hemoglobin levels, neurological assessment for kernicterus risk.

Postpartum Management

Administer RhIg within 72 hours post-delivery if the neonate is Rh-positive and the mother is not sensitized.

Monitor for postpartum hemorrhage (increased risk in severe HDFN).

Counsel on future pregnancies, as sensitization persists lifelong, increasing HDFN risk in subsequent Rh-positive pregnancies.

Complications

Maternal

Mirror syndrome: Rare, preeclampsia-like syndrome associated with severe fetal hydrops.

Psychological stress: From fetal monitoring, interventions, or poor outcomes.

Increased cesarean delivery: Due to fetal distress or hydrops.

Fetal/Neonatal

Fetal anemia: Mild to severe, leading to growth restriction or heart failure.

Hydrops fetalis: Generalized edema, ascites, effusions, and high mortality risk.

Stillbirth: Due to severe anemia or hydrops.

Neonatal jaundice: Risk of kernicterus if untreated.

Long-term sequelae: Neurodevelopmental delays, hearing loss, or cerebral palsy from kernicterus.

IUT-related risks: Infection, preterm labor, fetal loss.

Pregnancy Outcomes

Untreated severe HDFN: High risk of fetal/neonatal mortality (20–50%).

With modern management (RhIg, IUT, neonatal care): Excellent outcomes, with >90% survival in specialized centers.

Prognosis

Unsensitized Rh-negative mothers: Routine RhIg prophylaxis prevents sensitization in >99% of cases.

Sensitized mothers: Prognosis depends on antibody titers, fetal monitoring and timely interventions

Mild HDFN: Good outcome with phototherapy and monitoring.

Moderate/severe HDFN: High survival with IUT and neonatal care, but long-term neurological risks, if kernicterus occurs.

Prevention

RhIg Prophylaxis

Routine at 28 weeks and post-delivery for Rh-negative women with Rh-positive fetuses.

Additional doses for sensitizing events (e.g., miscarriage, trauma, invasive procedures).

Antenatal Screening

Universal blood group and antibody screening at first prenatal visit.

Repeat antibody screen at 28 weeks before RhIg administration in Rh-negative women.

Fetal RhD Genotyping: Non-invasive cffDNA testing to avoid unnecessary RhIg in Rh-negative fetuses.

Education: Counsel Rh-negative women on the importance of RhIg and reporting potential sensitizing events.

Key Points

Rh isoimmunization occurs when an Rh-negative mother develops anti-D antibodies after exposure to Rh-positive fetal RBCs, leading to HDFN in subsequent pregnancies.

Pathophysiology: Maternal IgG antibodies cross the placenta, causing fetal hemolysis, anemia, hydrops and neonatal jaundice.

Diagnosis: Routine blood group/antibody screening, antibody titers, MCA Doppler for fetal anemia and fetal RhD genotyping.

Prevention: RhIg prophylaxis at 28 weeks, post-delivery, and after sensitizing events reduces sensitization risk to <0.2%.

Management: Monitor titers and MCA Doppler in sensitized pregnancies; use IUT for severe anemia; deliver in NICU-equipped facilities for moderate/severe HDFN.

Complications: Fetal hydrops, stillbirth, neonatal jaundice, kernicterus; maternal mirror syndrome (rare).

Prognosis: Excellent with prophylaxis and modern management; untreated severe cases carry high mortality.

8.6 Gastrointestinal Disorders

(*Mi'di Mi'wi Amrad*)

Introduction: Gastrointestinal (GI) disorders in pregnancy are common due to physiological changes, hormonal influences and mechanical effects of the gravid uterus. These disorders range from benign, pregnancy-specific conditions to exacerbations of pre-existing diseases or new-onset pathologies. They can significantly impact maternal and fetal health, requiring careful diagnosis and management to balance maternal symptom relief with fetal safety.

Physiological Changes in Pregnancy Affecting the Gastrointestinal System

Hormonal Effects

Progesterone: Relaxes smooth muscle, reducing lower esophageal sphincter (LES) tone and slowing gastric emptying and intestinal motility, leading to gastroesophageal reflux disease (GERD), nausea/vomiting and constipation.

Estrogen: May contribute to cholestasis by altering bile composition and transport.

Mechanical Effects

The enlarging uterus compresses the stomach, intestines and liver, exacerbating GERD, constipation and hemorrhoids.

Increased intra-abdominal pressure promotes reflux and venous stasis (hemorrhoids).

Metabolic Changes: Increased metabolic demands and altered liver function (e.g., elevated alkaline phosphatase) can affect GI function.

Placental hormones (e.g., human placental lactogen) contribute to insulin resistance, impacting carbohydrate metabolism and appetite regulation.

Common Gastrointestinal Disorders in Pregnancy

1. Nausea and Vomiting of Pregnancy (NVP) and Hyperemesis Gravidarum (HG)

Definition

NVP: Common nausea and/or vomiting, typically in the first trimester, affecting 50–80% of pregnant women.

HG: Severe, persistent vomiting causing dehydration, weight loss (>5% of pre-pregnancy weight), and metabolic disturbances, affecting 0.3–2% of pregnancies.

Etiology

Hormonal (elevated hCG, estrogen, progesterone).

Delayed gastric emptying.

Possible Helicobacter pylori infection or psychological factors (e.g., stress).

Risk factors: Multiparity, multiple gestation, molar pregnancy, history of HG or motion sickness.

Clinical Features

NVP: Mild to moderate nausea, occasional vomiting, no significant dehydration or weight loss.

HG: Persistent vomiting, dehydration (dry mucous membranes, tachycardia), weight loss, ketonuria, electrolyte imbalances (hypokalemia, hyponatremia), and possible jaundice or neurological symptoms (e.g., Wernicke's encephalopathy from thiamine deficiency).

Diagnosis

NVP: Clinical diagnosis; rule out other causes (e.g., gastroenteritis, appendicitis).

HG: Weight loss >5%, ketonuria, abnormal electrolytes, elevated liver enzymes, or suppressed TSH (transient thyrotoxicosis).

Labs: CBC, electrolytes, liver function tests (LFTs), renal function, urinalysis, thyroid function tests.

Ultrasound to exclude molar pregnancy or multiples.

Management

NVP

Non-pharmacological: Small, frequent, bland meals; avoid triggers (odors, fatty foods); ginger (1–2 g daily); acupressure (P6 wrist point).

Pharmacological: Pyridoxine (vitamin B6, 10–25 mg 2–3 times daily), doxylamine (12.5–25 mg at bedtime), dimenhydrinate, or ondansetron (4–8 mg every 8 hours).

HG

Hospitalization for IV fluids (normal saline or Ringer's lactate), thiamine (100 mg IV daily for 2–3 days), and antiemetics (metoclopramide, ondansetron, or corticosteroids for refractory cases).

Correct electrolytes; consider enteral or parenteral nutrition if oral intake is inadequate.

Treat H. pylori if positive (e.g., amoxicillin, clarithromycin, proton pump inhibitor).

Monitoring: Regular weight, fluid status, and fetal growth assessments.

Complications

NVP: Minimal; may progress to HG if untreated.

HG: Dehydration, electrolyte imbalances, Wernicke's encephalopathy, Mallory-Weiss tears, preterm birth, or intrauterine growth restriction (IUGR).

Prognosis: NVP resolves by 16–20 weeks; HG may persist longer but improves with treatment; recurrence risk in future pregnancies is high (15–80% for HG).

2. Gastroesophageal Reflux Disease (GERD)

Definition

Reflux of gastric contents into the esophagus due to reduced LES tone and increased intra-abdominal pressure, affecting 30–50% of pregnant women.

Etiology

Progesterone-mediated LES relaxation.

Mechanical compression by the gravid uterus.

Risk factors: Multiparity, obesity, pre-existing GERD, or hiatal hernia.

Clinical Features

Heartburn, regurgitation, epigastric pain, or dysphagia.

Worse in the third trimester, after meals, or when lying supine.

Rare complications: Esophagitis, hematemesis (Mallory-Weiss tear), or aspiration.

Diagnosis: Clinical, based on symptoms; endoscopy rarely needed unless severe (e.g., bleeding, persistent symptoms).

Management

Non-pharmacological

Elevate head of bed (15–30 cm).

Small, frequent meals; avoid triggers (spicy, fatty foods, caffeine, chocolate).

Avoid lying down within 2–3 hours post-meal.

Pharmacological

Step 1: Antacids (calcium carbonate, magnesium hydroxide) or alginates (e.g., Gaviscon) as needed.

Step 2: H2-receptor antagonists (e.g., ranitidine 150 mg twice daily; note: ranitidine use limited due to safety concerns in some regions).

Step 3: Proton pump inhibitors (PPIs) (e.g., omeprazole 20–40 mg daily) for refractory cases; safe in pregnancy.

Monitoring: Symptom resolution; assess for complications like esophagitis.

Complications: Esophagitis, Barrett's esophagus (rare), or aspiration pneumonia.

Prognosis: Symptoms typically resolve post-delivery; recurrence common in subsequent pregnancies.

3. Constipation

Definition

Infrequent or difficult bowel movements, affecting 25–40% of pregnant women.

Etiology

Progesterone-induced slowed intestinal motility.

Gravid uterus compressing the colon.

Reduced physical activity, dietary changes, or iron supplementation.

Risk factors: Multiparity, sedentary lifestyle, low-fiber diet.

Clinical Features

Hard stools, straining, infrequent bowel movements (<3/week).

Abdominal discomfort, bloating, or rectal pain.

Diagnosis: Clinical, based on Rome IV criteria (e.g., straining, hard stools, sensation of incomplete evacuation).

Management

Non-pharmacological

High-fiber diet (25–30 g/day; e.g., fruits, vegetables, whole grains).

Adequate hydration (2–3 L/day).

Regular exercise (e.g., walking 30 min/day).

Pharmacological

Bulk-forming laxatives: Psyllium or methylcellulose (safe, first-line).

Osmotic laxatives: Lactulose or polyethylene glycol (safe, second-line).

Stimulant laxatives: Bisacodyl or senna (short-term use only; avoid in third trimester due to preterm labor risk).

Avoid mineral oil (reduces fat-soluble vitamin absorption).

Monitoring: Bowel habits; assess for complications like hemorrhoids.

Complications: Hemorrhoids, anal fissures, or fecal impaction (rare).

Prognosis: Improves post-delivery; lifestyle changes reduce recurrence.

4. Hemorrhoids

Definition: Swollen rectal veins due to increased intra-abdominal pressure and venous stasis, affecting 25–35% of pregnant women, especially in the third trimester.

Etiology

Progesterone-induced venous relaxation.

Gravid uterus causing pelvic venous compression.

Constipation and straining during defecation.

Risk factors: Multiparity, prolonged second stage of labor, obesity.

Clinical Features

Perianal pain, itching, or bleeding (bright red blood on wiping).

Prolapsed or thrombosed hemorrhoids (painful mass).

Diagnosis: Clinical; external hemorrhoids visible on inspection; internal hemorrhoids may require anoscopy (rare in pregnancy).

Management

Non-pharmacological

Treat constipation (high-fiber diet, hydration, laxatives).

Sitz baths (warm water, 10–15 min, 2–3 times daily).

Avoid prolonged sitting or straining.

Pharmacological

Topical anesthetics (e.g., lidocaine) or hydrocortisone cream (short-term, <7 days).

Witch hazel pads for symptomatic relief.

Surgical

Thrombosed hemorrhoids may require incision and drainage under local anesthesia.

Hemorrhoidectomy rarely performed in pregnancy; deferred to postpartum.

Complications: Thrombosis, severe pain, or bleeding; anemia (rare).

Prognosis: Most resolve post-delivery; recurrence common in subsequent pregnancies.

5. Intrahepatic Cholestasis of Pregnancy (ICP)

Definition: A pregnancy-specific liver disorder characterized by pruritus and elevated bile acids, typically in the second or third trimester, affecting 0.1–2% of pregnancies.

Etiology

Hormonal (estrogen, progesterone) disruption of bile transport.

Genetic predisposition (e.g., ABCB4 gene mutations).

Risk factors: Multiple gestation, family history, prior ICP, or chronic liver disease.

Clinical Features

Generalized pruritus (worse on palms/soles, nocturnal).

Jaundice (10–20% of cases).

No rash (unlike other pruritic conditions).

Elevated serum bile acids (>10 µmol/L) and transaminases (ALT/AST).

Diagnosis

Total bile acids >10 µmol/L (diagnostic); fasting levels preferred.

Elevated LFTs (ALT/AST 2–10 times normal); normal or mildly elevated bilirubin.

Rule out other causes (e.g., viral hepatitis, gallstones) with ultrasound, viral serologies.

Management

Ursodeoxycholic acid (UDCA): 10–15 mg/kg/day (first-line; reduces bile acids, pruritus, and fetal risk).

Antihistamines: Hydroxyzine or chlorpheniramine for symptomatic relief of pruritus.

Vitamin K: 10 mg daily if jaundice or prolonged prothrombin time (to prevent bleeding).

Fetal monitoring: Non-stress test (NST) or biophysical profile from diagnosis due to risk of stillbirth.

Delivery: Plan delivery at 36–37 weeks (earlier if severe, e.g., bile acids >100 µmol/L).

Complications

Maternal: Fat malabsorption, vitamin K deficiency, increased postpartum hemorrhage risk.

Fetal: Preterm birth, fetal distress, stillbirth (risk increases with bile acids >40 µmol/L).

Prognosis: Symptoms resolve post-delivery; recurrence risk in future pregnancies is 60–90%.

6. Acute Fatty Liver of Pregnancy (AFLP)

Definition: A rare, life-threatening condition in the third trimester characterized by microvesicular fatty infiltration of the liver, leading to acute liver failure.

Etiology

Associated with fetal long-chain 3-hydroxyacyl-CoA dehydrogenase (LCHAD) deficiency.

Risk factors: Nulliparity, multiple gestation, male fetus, or pre-eclampsia.

Clinical Features

Nausea, vomiting, abdominal pain, jaundice.

Signs of liver failure: Hypoglycemia, coagulopathy, encephalopathy.

Often overlaps with HELLP syndrome or pre-eclampsia.

Diagnosis

Swansea criteria: Includes vomiting, abdominal pain, elevated transaminases, hyperbilirubinemia, leukocytosis, hypoglycemia, coagulopathy, or renal impairment.

Labs: Elevated ALT/AST, bilirubin, low glucose, prolonged prothrombin time, renal dysfunction.

Imaging: Ultrasound/CT to rule out other causes (e.g., gallstones); liver biopsy (rarely needed) shows microvesicular steatosis.

Management

Immediate delivery (vaginal or cesarean, based on maternal/fetal status).

Supportive care: IV fluids, glucose infusion (to correct hypoglycemia), fresh frozen plasma for coagulopathy.

ICU monitoring for liver failure or multi-organ dysfunction.

Genetic testing for LCHAD deficiency in mother and neonate.

Complications

Maternal: Liver failure, disseminated intravascular coagulation (DIC), renal failure, death (rare with prompt delivery).

Fetal: Stillbirth, prematurity, neonatal LCHAD deficiency.

Prognosis: Maternal mortality <5% with early delivery; recurrence risk low unless genetic predisposition.

7. Inflammatory Bowel Disease (IBD)

Definition: Includes Crohn's disease and ulcerative colitis, chronic inflammatory conditions of the GI tract that may be active or quiescent during pregnancy.

Etiology

Autoimmune; exacerbated by stress, infections, or medication non-compliance.

Pregnancy does not significantly alter disease course; active disease at conception increases flare risk.

Clinical Features

Diarrhea (bloody in ulcerative colitis), abdominal pain, weight loss, fatigue.

Extraintestinal manifestations: Arthritis, uveitis, or skin lesions (e.g., erythema nodosum).

Diagnosis

Based on pre-pregnancy history or new symptoms.

Labs: Anemia, elevated inflammatory markers (CRP, ESR), fecal calprotectin.

Endoscopy/sigmoidoscopy (if needed) safe in pregnancy; avoid in active flare unless critical.

Management

Maintain remission: Continue pre-pregnancy medications (most are safe):

5-ASA drugs (e.g., mesalamine): Safe, continue for ulcerative colitis or Crohn's.

Corticosteroids: Prednisone or budesonide for flares; safe in low doses.

Immunomodulators: Azathioprine/6-mercaptopurine safe if already stable; avoid starting in pregnancy.

Biologics: Anti-TNF agents (e.g., infliximab, adalimumab) safe; continue through pregnancy, stop in third trimester if possible to reduce neonatal exposure.

Methotrexate: Contraindicated (teratogenic); discontinue preconception.

Flare management: Corticosteroids, hospitalization if severe, nutritional support.

Fetal monitoring: Increased risk of preterm birth or IUGR with active disease.

Delivery: Vaginal delivery preferred; cesarean for perianal Crohn's or obstetric indications.

Complications

Maternal: Malnutrition, anemia, bowel obstruction, or perforation (rare).

Fetal: Preterm birth, low birth weight, miscarriage (with active disease).

Prognosis: Good with controlled disease; active IBD increases adverse outcomes.

8. Other GI Disorders

Appendicitis

Incidence: 0.05–0.1% of pregnancies, most common in second trimester.

Symptoms: Right lower quadrant pain (may shift upward due to uterine displacement), nausea, fever.

Diagnosis: Clinical, ultrasound, or MRI; leukocytosis unreliable in pregnancy.

Management: Appendicectomy (laparoscopic preferred before third trimester); antibiotics for non-perforated cases.

Complications: Preterm labor, perforation, peritonitis, fetal loss (higher with perforation).

Cholecystitis/Gallstones

Incidence: 0.05–0.3% of pregnancies; gallstones common due to altered bile composition.

Symptoms: Right upper quadrant pain, nausea, vomiting, fever (if acute).

Diagnosis: Ultrasound (first-line); elevated LFTs or bilirubin in severe cases.

Management: Conservative (hydration, pain control) for mild cases; cholecystectomy (second trimester safest) for recurrent or complicated cases.

Complications: Pancreatitis, cholangitis, preterm labor.

Peptic Ulcer Disease

Rare in pregnancy due to reduced gastric acid secretion.

Symptoms: Epigastric pain, nausea, hematemesis (rare).

Management: Antacids, H2-receptor antagonists, or PPIs; treat H. pylori post-delivery.

Complications: Bleeding, perforation (rare).

Pancreatitis

Incidence: 0.02–0.1%; often due to gallstones or hypertriglyceridemia.

Symptoms: Epigastric pain radiating to back, nausea, vomiting.

Diagnosis: Elevated amylase/lipase, ultrasound for gallstones.

Management: Supportive (IV fluids, pain control, nil per os); treat underlying cause (e.g., cholecystectomy, lipid-lowering).

Complications: Preterm labor, maternal/fetal mortality (rare).

Diagnosis of GI Disorders

History: Assess onset, duration and triggers of symptoms (e.g., nausea, pain, bowel changes).

Physical Examination: Check for abdominal tenderness, jaundice, dehydration, or perianal findings.

Investigation

Labs: CBC, electrolytes, LFTs, amylase/lipase, bile acids, inflammatory markers, *H. pylori testing (stool antigen, serology).

Imaging: Ultrasound (first-line, safe); MRI for complex cases; avoid CT due to radiation unless critical.

Endoscopy: Safe if indicated (e.g., bleeding, severe GERD, suspected IBD flare); use minimal sedation (e.g., meperidine, propofol).

Differential Diagnosis

Obstetric: Pre-eclampsia/HELLP, AFLP, placental abruption.

Non-obstetric: Appendicitis, cholecystitis, pancreatitis, viral hepatitis, or gastroenteritis.

Complications

Maternal

Dehydration, malnutrition, or electrolyte imbalances (HG, IBD).

Liver failure or coagulopathy (AFLP, severe ICP).

Hemorrhage (peptic ulcer, hemorrhoids).

Perforation or peritonitis (appendicitis, IBD).

Fetal

Preterm birth (HG, ICP, AFLP, IBD flares).

IUGR or low birth weight (HG, IBD).

Stillbirth (ICP, AFLP).

Neonatal jaundice or respiratory distress (preterm delivery).

Prognosis

Most GI disorders (e.g., NVP, GERD, constipation, hemorrhoids) resolve post-delivery with appropriate management.

HG and ICP carry higher risks but improve with treatment; recurrence is common.

AFLP is life-threatening but rare; prompt delivery improves outcomes.

IBD outcomes depend on disease control; quiescent disease has near-normal pregnancy outcomes.

Prevention

Antenatal Screen for H. pylori or pre-existing GI conditions in high-risk women.

Counsel on healthy diet, weight management, and exercise to reduce GERD, constipation, or gallstone risk.

Lifestyle

High-fiber diet and hydration for constipation/hemorrhoids.

Avoid GERD triggers (e.g., spicy foods, large meals).

IBD Management: Optimize therapy preconception to maintain remission.

ICP Prevention: Early UDCA in women with prior ICP or high-risk profiles.

Key Points

GI disorders in pregnancy are influenced by hormonal (progesterone, estrogen) and mechanical (uterine compression) changes, leading to NVP/HG, GERD, constipation, hemorrhoids, ICP, AFLP, and IBD flares.

NVP/HG: Common; HG requires hospitalization for IV fluids, antiemetics, and thiamine to prevent complications like Wernicke's encephalopathy.

GERD: Managed with lifestyle changes, antacids, H2-blockers, or PPIs.

Constipation/Hemorrhoids: Treat with fiber, hydration, and laxatives; surgical intervention rare.

ICP: Pruritus with elevated bile acids; UDCA and early delivery reduce stillbirth risk.

AFLP: Life-threatening; requires immediate delivery and supportive care.

IBD: Continue safe medications (5-ASA, biologics); flares increase preterm birth risk.

Diagnosis: Relies on clinical assessment, labs, and safe imaging (ultrasound, MRI); endoscopy rarely needed.

Complications: Include preterm birth, IUGR, stillbirth, and maternal liver failure; timely management improves outcomes.

Prevention: Focuses on nutrition, preconception optimization, and avoiding triggers.

8.7 Hepatic, Biliary and Pancreatic Disorders

(*Kabisi, marari aur banqarasi Amrad*)

Introduction

Hepatic, biliary, and pancreatic disorders in pregnancy encompass a spectrum of conditions ranging from pregnancy-specific disorders to exacerbations of pre-existing diseases or new-onset pathologies. These disorders are influenced by physiological changes in pregnancy, such as hormonal fluctuations, altered bile metabolism, and increased metabolic demands. They can significantly impact maternal and fetal health, requiring careful diagnosis and management to balance maternal well-being with fetal safety.

Physiological Changes in Pregnancy

Hepatic Changes

Increased estrogen and progesterone: Alter bile composition and transport, increasing the risk of cholestasis and gallstone formation.

Elevated liver enzymes: Alkaline phosphatase (ALP) increases 2–4-fold due to placental production; aspartate aminotransferase (AST) and alanine aminotransferase (ALT) remain normal or slightly elevated.

Increased plasma volume and cardiac output: Affect hepatic blood flow, potentially masking early liver dysfunction.

Reduced albumin: Due to hemodilution, leading to lower total protein levels but normal function.

Biliary Changes

Progesterone: Reduces gallbladder motility, promoting bile stasis and gallstone formation.

Estrogen: Increases cholesterol saturation in bile, contributing to sludge or gallstones.

Pancreatic Changes

Insulin resistance: Induced by placental hormones (e.g., human placental lactogen), increasing pancreatic workload.

Mechanical compression: The gravid uterus may compress pancreatic ducts, though this is rare.

Metabolic Demand: Increased lipid and glucose metabolism can exacerbate underlying conditions (e.g., hypertriglyceridemia-induced pancreatitis).

Common Hepatic, Biliary and Pancreatic Disorders in Pregnancy

1. Intrahepatic Cholestasis of Pregnancy (ICP)

Definition

A pregnancy-specific liver disorder characterized by pruritus and elevated serum bile acids, typically in the second or third trimester, affecting 0.1–2% of pregnancies.

Etiology

Hormonal: Estrogen and progesterone disrupt bile transport, increasing bile acid accumulation.

Genetic: Mutations in bile acid transporter genes (e.g., ABCB4, ABCB11) increase susceptibility.

Risk factors: Multiple gestation, family history, prior ICP, chronic liver disease, or advanced maternal age.

Pathophysiology

Impaired bile acid excretion leads to elevated serum bile acids, causing pruritus and potential hepatotoxicity.

Increased bile acids cross the placenta, increasing fetal risk of complications.

Clinical Features

Generalized pruritus, worse on palms and soles, often nocturnal.

Jaundice (10–20% of cases), typically mild.

No rash (distinguishes from dermatologic conditions).

Elevated serum bile acids (>10 µmol/L), transaminases (ALT/AST 2–10 times normal), and occasionally bilirubin.

Diagnosis

Serum bile acids: >10 µmol/L (diagnostic); fasting levels preferred; severe ICP if >40 µmol/L.

Liver function tests (LFTs): Elevated ALT/AST; normal or mildly elevated bilirubin and ALP (placental ALP masks hepatic contribution).

Exclusion of other causes: Viral hepatitis (serologies), gallstones (ultrasound), autoimmune liver disease (autoantibodies).

Ultrasound: To rule out gallstones or biliary obstruction; liver ultrasound normal in ICP.

Management

Ursodeoxycholic acid (UDCA): First-line; 10–15 mg/kg/day (typically 600–1,200 mg daily in divided doses). Reduces bile acids, pruritus, and fetal risks.

Antihistamines: Hydroxyzine (25–50 mg at night) or chlorpheniramine for symptomatic pruitus relief.

Vitamin K: 10 mg daily orally if jaundice or prolonged prothrombin time to prevent bleeding.

Fetal monitoring: Non-stress test (NST) or biophysical profile weekly from diagnosis due to stillbirth risk.

Delivery

Mild ICP (bile acids 10–40 µmol/L): Deliver at 37–38 weeks.

Severe ICP (bile acids >40 µmol/L): Deliver at 36–37 weeks or earlier if fetal distress.

Vaginal delivery preferred unless obstetric indications for cesarean.

Monitoring: Weekly bile acids and LFTs; fetal surveillance via NST or ultrasound.

Complications

Maternal: Fat malabsorption, vitamin K deficiency (increased postpartum hemorrhage risk), psychological distress from pruritus.

Fetal: Preterm birth (spontaneous or iatrogenic), fetal distress, stillbirth (risk increases with bile acids >40 µmol/L), meconium-stained amniotic fluid.

Prognosis: Symptoms resolve within 2–4 weeks post-delivery; recurrence risk in future pregnancies is 60–90%.

2. Acute Fatty Liver of Pregnancy (AFLP)

Definition

A rare, life-threatening liver disorder in the third trimester (rarely late second trimester) characterized by microvesicular fatty infiltration of hepatocytes, leading to acute liver failure.

Incidence: 0.01–0.05% of pregnancies.

Etiology

Associated with fetal long-chain 3-hydroxyacyl-CoA dehydrogenase (LCHAD) deficiency, impairing fatty acid oxidation.

Risk factors: Nulliparity, multiple gestation, male fetus, pre-eclampsia, or obesity.

Pathophysiology

Impaired maternal and fetal fatty acid oxidation leads to accumulation of toxic metabolites in the liver.

Results in microvesicular steatosis, hepatocyte necrosis, and liver dysfunction.

Clinical Features

Nausea, vomiting, right upper quadrant or epigastric pain.

Jaundice, hypoglycemia, encephalopathy (confusion, lethargy).

Signs of liver failure: Coagulopathy, ascites, or renal impairment.

Often overlaps with pre-eclampsia or HELLP syndrome.

Diagnosis

Swansea criteria (≥6 required for diagnosis):

Vomiting, abdominal pain, polydipsia/polyuria.

Elevated transaminases (ALT/AST >200 IU/L), bilirubin, or uric acid.

Leukocytosis, hypoglycemia, prolonged prothrombin time.

Renal impairment, ascites, or encephalopathy.

Microvesicular steatosis on liver biopsy (rarely performed).

Labs: Elevated ALT/AST (300–1,000 IU/L), bilirubin, low glucose (<70 mg/dL), prolonged INR, low fibrinogen, elevated creatinine.

Imaging: Ultrasound or CT to exclude other causes (e.g., gallstones, thrombosis); liver biopsy (rare) confirms microvesicular steatosis.

Differential diagnosis: HELLP syndrome, viral hepatitis, drug-induced liver injury, or thrombotic microangiopathies.

Management

Immediate delivery: Vaginal or cesarean based on maternal/fetal status; critical for maternal and fetal survival.

Supportive care

IV fluids and dextrose (to correct hypoglycemia).

Fresh frozen plasma or cryoprecipitate for coagulopathy.

Vitamin K (10 mg IV) if bleeding risk.

Monitor in ICU for liver failure, renal dysfunction, or encephalopathy.

Genetic testing: Screen mother and neonate for LCHAD deficiency.

Fetal monitoring: NST or biophysical profile to assess fetal status pre-delivery.

Complications

Maternal: Liver failure, disseminated intravascular coagulation (DIC), renal failure, encephalopathy, death (1–5% with modern care).

Fetal: Stillbirth, prematurity, neonatal LCHAD deficiency (requires dietary management).

Prognosis: Maternal mortality <5% with prompt delivery; fetal mortality 10–20%; recurrence risk low unless genetic predisposition.

3. HELLP Syndrome (Hemolysis, Elevated Liver enzymes, Low Platelets)

Definition

A severe form of pre-eclampsia characterized by hemolysis, elevated liver enzymes and thrombocytopenia, typically in the third trimester or early postpartum.

Incidence: 0.1–0.6% of pregnancies; 10–20% of pre-eclampsia cases.

Etiology

Associated with placental dysfunction and endothelial activation.

Risk factors: Pre-eclampsia, nulliparity, advanced maternal age, multiple gestation, or history of hypertension.

Pathophysiology

Microangiopathic hemolytic anemia due to endothelial damage.

Hepatic sinusoidal obstruction and periportal necrosis cause elevated transaminases.

Platelet consumption leads to thrombocytopenia.

Clinical Features

Right upper quadrant or epigastric pain, nausea, vomiting.

Headache, visual changes, or hypertension (if pre-eclampsia present).

Jaundice (10–20%), edema, or signs of liver dysfunction.

Diagnosis

Criteria (Tennessee or Mississippi classification):

Hemolysis: Elevated lactate dehydrogenase (LDH >600 IU/L), schistocytes on peripheral smear, low haptoglobin.

Elevated liver enzymes: AST/ALT >70 IU/L.

Low platelets: <100,000/μL.

Labs: CBC (thrombocytopenia, anemia), LFTs, LDH, bilirubin, coagulation profile, renal function.

Imaging: Ultrasound or CT to rule out hepatic hematoma or rupture (rare).

Differential diagnosis: AFLP, thrombotic thrombocytopenic purpura (TTP), hemolytic uremic syndrome (HUS), or viral hepatitis.

Management

Delivery: Only definitive treatment; timing depends on gestational age and severity:

≥34 weeks or fetal/maternal compromise: Immediate delivery.

24–34 weeks: Corticosteroids (betamethasone 12 mg IM, two doses 24 hours apart) for fetal lung maturity, then deliver within 24–48 hours.

Supportive care

Magnesium sulfate for seizure prophylaxis (pre-eclampsia).

Antihypertensives (e.g., labetalol, hydralazine) for blood pressure >160/110 mmHg.

Transfusion (platelets, packed RBCs) for severe thrombocytopenia (<20,000/μL) or bleeding.

Monitor for hepatic hematoma or rupture (rare, requires urgent surgery).

Fetal monitoring: NST, biophysical profile, or Doppler ultrasound.

Complications

Maternal: Hepatic hematoma/rupture, DIC, renal failure, pulmonary edema, death (<1% with modern care).

Fetal: Preterm birth, IUGR, stillbirth, neonatal thrombocytopenia.

Prognosis: Maternal recovery within days to weeks post-delivery; recurrence risk 5–25% in future pregnancies.

4. Cholecystitis and Gallstones (Cholelithiasis)

Definition

Gallstones (cholelithiasis) are common in pregnancy (3–12%), with acute cholecystitis (inflammation of the gallbladder) occurring in 0.05–0.3% of pregnancies.

Etiology

Increased cholesterol saturation and reduced gallbladder motility due to estrogen and progesterone.

Risk factors: Obesity, multiparity, diabetes, rapid weight gain, or family history of gallstones.

Pathophysiology

Gallstones (cholesterol or pigment) obstruct the cystic duct, causing bile stasis, inflammation, or infection (acute cholecystitis).

Complications include gallbladder perforation, cholangitis, or pancreatitis.

Clinical Features

Right upper quadrant pain (colicky or constant), nausea, vomiting, fever (in cholecystitis).

Murphy's sign (pain on palpation under right costal margin during inspiration) in acute cholecystitis.

Symptoms often postprandial, triggered by fatty meals.

Diagnosis

Ultrasound: First-line; detects gallstones, gallbladder wall thickening, or pericholecystic fluid.

Labs: Leukocytosis, elevated ALP (normal in pregnancy), mild elevation of ALT/AST or bilirubin in cholecystitis.

MRI: If ultrasound inconclusive; avoids radiation.

Differential diagnosis: Appendicitis, pancreatitis, hepatitis, or pre-eclampsia.

Management

Conservative (mild cases)

IV fluids, pain control (e.g., acetaminophen, opioids if needed), and antibiotics (e.g., ceftriaxone + metronidazole) for cholecystitis. NPO initially, then low-fat diet.

Surgical

Cholecystectomy (laparoscopic preferred) for recurrent or complicated cholecystitis (e.g., perforation, cholangitis).

Second trimester safest; third trimester may require open surgery.

Endoscopic retrograde cholangiopancreatography (ERCP): For choledocholithiasis (common bile duct stones); radiation minimized with shielding.

Fetal monitoring: NST or ultrasound if preterm labor risk.

Complications

Maternal: Pancreatitis, cholangitis, gallbladder perforation, or sepsis.

Fetal: Preterm labor, fetal distress, or stillbirth (rare with prompt treatment).

Prognosis: Good with timely intervention; recurrence risk high if cholecystectomy deferred to postpartum.

5. Pancreatitis

Definition

Acute inflammation of the pancreas, occurring in 0.02–0.1% of pregnancies, often due to gallstones or hypertriglyceridemia.

Etiology

Gallstones: Most common cause (60–70% of cases), due to bile stasis and sludge.

Hypertriglyceridemia: Pregnancy-induced lipid changes (triglycerides >1,000 mg/dL); associated with obesity or diabetes.

Other causes: Alcohol (rare in pregnancy), medications, hypercalcemia, or idiopathic.

Risk factors: Obesity, gestational diabetes, or history of pancreatitis.

Pathophysiology

Pancreatic duct obstruction or autodigestion leads to inflammation, edema, or necrosis.

Systemic inflammatory response syndrome (SIRS) in severe cases causes multi-organ dysfunction.

Clinical Features

Epigastric pain radiating to the back, nausea, vomiting, fever.

Tachycardia, abdominal tenderness, or guarding in severe cases.

Diagnosis

Labs: Elevated amylase and lipase (>3 times upper limit), leukocytosis, elevated LFTs or bilirubin (if gallstone-related).

Imaging: Ultrasound to detect gallstones; MRI or CT (if critical) for pancreatic necrosis or complications.

Differential diagnosis: Cholecystitis, appendicitis, peptic ulcer disease, pre-eclampsia, or AFLP.

Management

Conservative

NPO, IV fluids, and pain control (e.g., fentanyl, avoid morphine due to sphincter of Oddi spasm).

Antibiotics if infection suspected (e.g., imipenem for necrotizing pancreatitis).

Lipid-lowering (e.g., gemfibrozil) for hypertriglyceridemia-induced cases.

Interventional

ERCP for gallstone pancreatitis with cholangitis or bile duct obstruction.

Cholecystectomy (post-resolution or postpartum) to prevent recurrence.

Plasmapheresis or insulin infusion for severe hypertriglyceridemia (>2,000 mg/dL).

Fetal monitoring: NST or biophysical profile due to preterm labor risk.

Delivery: Considered only if maternal/fetal compromise or near term.

Complications

Maternal: Pancreatic necrosis, pseudocyst, abscess, or multi-organ failure.

Fetal: Preterm birth, fetal distress, or stillbirth (5–10% in severe cases).

Prognosis: Maternal mortality <1% with modern care; recurrence risk high if gallstones untreated.

6. Viral Hepatitis

Definition

Hepatitis A, B, C, D, or E infection affecting the liver, with hepatitis B and C most relevant in pregnancy due to vertical transmission risk.

Etiology

Hepatitis A (HAV): Fecal-oral transmission; rare in pregnancy.

Hepatitis B (HBV): Bloodborne, sexual, or perinatal transmission; prevalent in endemic areas.

Hepatitis C (HCV): Bloodborne; less common vertical transmission.

Hepatitis E (HEV): Fecal-oral; severe in pregnancy, especially in third trimester (endemic areas).

Clinical Features

Fatigue, nausea, jaundice, right upper quadrant pain.

Acute hepatitis: Fever, elevated transaminases, bilirubin.

Chronic HBV/HCV: Often asymptomatic, detected via screening.

HEV: Fulminant hepatitis in pregnancy (20–30% mortality in third trimester).

Diagnosis

Serologies: HAV IgM, HBsAg, anti-HBc, anti-HCV, HEV IgM.

Labs: Elevated ALT/AST, bilirubin; HBV DNA or HCV RNA for chronic infection.

Ultrasound: To exclude gallstones or biliary obstruction.

Management

HAV/HEV: Supportive (hydration, rest); HAV vaccine or immunoglobulin post-exposure; no specific therapy for HEV.

HBV: Antiviral therapy (e.g., tenofovir) for high viral load (>200,000 IU/mL) in third trimester to reduce vertical transmission.

Neonatal prophylaxis: Hepatitis B immunoglobulin (HBIG) and HBV vaccine within 12 hours of birth.

HCV: No antiviral therapy in pregnancy; monitor LFTs; treat postpartum.

Fetal monitoring: Assess for IUGR or preterm labor in acute hepatitis.

Delivery: Vaginal delivery safe; cesarean not indicated unless obstetric reasons.

Complications

Maternal: Fulminant hepatitis (HEV), chronic liver disease (HBV/HCV).

Fetal: Vertical transmission (HBV: 10–90% without prophylaxis; HCV: 5–10%; HAV/HEV

rare), preterm birth, or IUGR.

Prognosis: Good for HAV/HBV with management; HEV severe in pregnancy; HCV managed postpartum.

Diagnosis of Hepatic, Biliary and Pancreatic Disorders

History: Assess for nausea, vomiting, pruritus, abdominal pain, jaundice or risk factors (e.g., obesity, gallstones, viral exposure).

Physical Examination: Check for jaundice, right upper quadrant tenderness, Murphy's sign, or signs of liver failure (e.g., encephalopathy, ascites).

Investigations

Laboratory tests:

LFTs (ALT, AST, ALP, bilirubin), bile acids (ICP), amylase/lipase (pancreatitis).

CBC (hemolysis, thrombocytopenia), coagulation profile (INR, fibrinogen).

Viral serologies (HAV, HBV, HCV, HEV).

Glucose, renal function, or triglycerides for AFLP or pancreatitis.

Imaging

Ultrasound: First-line for gallstones, liver, or pancreatic pathology; safe in pregnancy.

MRI: For complex cases (e.g., pancreatitis, hepatic hematoma).

CT: Avoid unless critical (radiation risk).

Invasive tests: Liver biopsy (rare, for AFLP or unclear etiology); ERCP for biliary obstruction.

Differential Diagnosis

Obstetric: Pre-eclampsia/HELLP, AFLP, ICP.

Non-obstetric: Viral hepatitis, cholecystitis, pancreatitis, drug-induced liver injury, or autoimmune hepatitis.

Complications

Maternal

Liver failure (AFLP, severe HEV).

Coagulopathy or DIC (AFLP, HELLP).

Renal failure, encephalopathy, or sepsis (AFLP, pancreatitis).

Postpartum hemorrhage (ICP, AFLP).

Fetal

Preterm birth (ICP, AFLP, HELLP, pancreatitis).

IUGR or low birth weight (HELLP, viral hepatitis).

Stillbirth (ICP, AFLP, severe HEV).

Vertical transmission (HBV, HCV).

Neonatal jaundice or thrombocytopenia (HELLP).

Prognosis

ICP: Resolves post-delivery; high recurrence risk (60–90%); fetal risks minimized with early delivery.

AFLP: Maternal mortality <5% with prompt delivery; fetal mortality 10–20%; recurrence rare unless genetic.

HELLP: Resolves post-delivery; maternal mortality <1%; recurrence risk 5–25%.

Cholecystitis: Good with timely intervention; recurrence high if untreated.

Pancreatitis: Maternal mortality <1%; fetal loss 5–10% in severe cases.

Viral Hepatitis: HAV/HEV resolve acutely; HBV/HCV managed to prevent transmission; HEV severe in pregnancy.

Prevention

Antenatal

Routine HBV screening at first prenatal visit; vaccinate seronegative women postpartum.

Counsel on low-fat diet to reduce gallstone risk in high-risk women (obesity, diabetes).

UDCA prophylaxis in women with prior ICP history.

Monitor triglycerides in women with gestational diabetes or obesity to prevent pancreatitis.

Lifestyle

Maintain healthy weight and diet to reduce gallstone and pancreatitis risk.

Avoid alcohol and hepatotoxic drugs.

Public Health

HBV vaccination programs and neonatal prophylaxis in endemic areas.

Access to safe water to prevent HAV/HEV in endemic regions.

Key Points

Hepatic, biliary, and pancreatic disorders in pregnancy include ICP, AFLP, HELLP, cholecystitis, pancreatitis, and viral hepatitis, driven by hormonal and mechanical changes.

ICP: Pruritus with elevated bile acids; treat with UDCA and early delivery to reduce stillbirth risk.

AFLP: Rare, life-threatening; requires immediate delivery and ICU care for liver failure.

HELLP: Severe pre-eclampsia variant; delivery is definitive treatment; monitor for hepatic hematoma.

Cholecystitis: Gallstones common; manage conservatively or with cholecystectomy (second trimester safest).

Pancreatitis: Often gallstone- or triglyceride-related; treat with supportive care, ERCP if needed.

Viral Hepatitis: HBV/HCV pose vertical transmission risk; neonatal prophylaxis critical for HBV.

Diagnosis: Relies on labs (LFTs, bile acids, amylase/lipase) and ultrasound; MRI for complex cases.

Complications: Preterm birth, stillbirth, maternal liver failure, or coagulopathy; timely intervention improves outcomes.

Prevention: Includes HBV screening, dietary counseling, and early UDCA for ICP recurrence.

8.8 Cardiovascular Disorders

(*Qalbi 'Uruqi amrad*)

Cardiovascular disorders in pregnancy encompass a spectrum of conditions, including pre-existing heart diseases, pregnancy-specific conditions, and new-onset cardiovascular complications. Pregnancy imposes significant hemodynamic changes that can exacerbate underlying cardiac conditions or unmask previously undiagnosed ones, potentially leading to maternal and fetal morbidity or mortality. Effective management requires a multidisciplinary approach involving obstetricians, cardiologists, and maternal-fetal medicine specialists to optimize outcomes.

Physiological Changes in Pregnancy Affecting the Cardiovascular System

Hemodynamic Changes

Increased cardiac output (CO): CO increases by 30–50% (from 4–5 L/min to 6–8 L/min) by the second trimester due to increased stroke volume and heart rate (10–20 bpm increase).

Increased plasma volume: Expands by 40–50% (1–2 L), peaking at 28–34 weeks, leading to hemodilution and physiological anemia.

Decreased systemic vascular resistance (SVR): Progesterone-mediated vasodilation reduces SVR by 20–30%, lowering blood pressure (BP) in the first and second trimesters.

Increased heart rate: Rises by 10–20 bpm to accommodate increased CO.

Mechanical effects: The gravid uterus elevates the diaphragm, causing a leftward shift of the heart and mild cardiomegaly on imaging.

Labor and delivery: CO peaks during labor (up to 80% increase) and immediately postpartum due to autotransfusion of 500–1,000 mL blood from uterine contraction, increasing preload.

Coagulation Changes

Hypercoagulable state due to increased clotting factors (e.g., fibrinogen, factors VII, VIII, X) and decreased fibrinolysis, increasing thromboembolism risk.

Cardiac Examination Findings

Normal findings: Systolic flow murmur (due to increased CO), S3 gallop, mild peripheral edema, or jugular venous distension.

Abnormal findings requiring evaluation: Diastolic murmurs, S4 gallop, severe dyspnea, or cyanosis.

Classification of Cardiovascular Disorders in Pregnancy

Cardiovascular disorders in pregnancy can be classified as

1. Pre-existing Conditions: Congenital heart disease, valvular heart disease, cardiomyopathy, or ischemic heart disease.
2. Pregnancy-Specific Conditions: Peripartum cardiomyopathy, hypertensive disorders (e.g., pre-eclampsia), or thromboembolism.
3. New-Onset or Exacerbated Conditions: Arrhythmias, aortic dissection, or myocardial infarction.

Common Cardiovascular Disorders in Pregnancy

1. Congenital Heart Disease (CHD)

Structural heart defects present at birth, increasingly seen in pregnancy due to improved survival from corrective surgeries.

Common Types

Septal defects: Atrial septal defect (ASD), ventricular septal defect (VSD).

Cyanotic defects: Tetralogy of Fallot, transposition of great arteries (repaired).

Obstructive lesions: Aortic stenosis, pulmonary stenosis, coarctation of aorta.

Etiology

Genetic or environmental; most women with corrected CHD tolerate pregnancy well, but uncorrected or severe lesions pose high risks.

Clinical Features

Symptoms: Dyspnea, fatigue, palpitations, or cyanosis (in uncorrected cyanotic CHD).

Signs: Murmurs, clubbing, or right ventricular heave (depending on lesion).

Risk stratification: Modified WHO (mWHO) classification (I–IV) predicts maternal cardiac risk:

mWHO I–II: Low/moderate risk (e.g., repaired ASD, mild aortic stenosis).

mWHO III–IV: High risk (e.g., pulmonary hypertension, severe aortic stenosis, Marfan syndrome with aortic root dilation).

Diagnosis

Echocardiography: Assesses lesion severity, ventricular function, and pulmonary pressures.

Electrocardiogram (ECG): Detects arrhythmias or chamber hypertrophy.

Cardiac MRI: For complex CHD if echocardiography is inconclusive (avoid gadolinium unless critical).

Management

Preconception counselling: Assess mWHO class; avoid pregnancy in mWHO IV (e.g., Eisenmenger syndrome, severe pulmonary hypertension) due to 30–50% maternal mortality.

Antenatal

Multidisciplinary care with cardiologist and maternal-fetal medicine specialist.

Monitor for heart failure, arrhythmias, or thromboembolism.

Low-risk CHD: Routine prenatal care with periodic echocardiography.

High-risk CHD: Frequent monitoring (every 1–2 weeks), restrict physical activity, and manage volume status (e.g., diuretics for heart failure).

Medications

β-Blockers (e.g., metoprolol) for arrhythmias or aortic root protection (Marfan syndrome).

Anticoagulation (low-molecular-weight heparin, LMWH) for mechanical valves or atrial fibrillation. Avoid ACE inhibitors, ARBs, or spironolactone (teratogenic).

Delivery

Vaginal delivery preferred for mWHO I–II; cesarean for mWHO III–IV or obstetric indications.

Epidural anesthesia to minimize hemodynamic stress.

Monitor in high-dependency unit for high-risk cases.

Postpartum: Highest risk period (first 7–10 days) due to autotransfusion; monitor for heart failure or thromboembolism.

Complications

Maternal: Heart failure, arrhythmias, thromboembolism, or aortic dissection (Marfan syndrome).

Fetal: Preterm birth, IUGR, or congenital heart defects (3–5% risk in offspring).

Prognosis: Good for corrected or mild CHD; high-risk lesions require specialized care.

2. Valvular Heart Disease

Dysfunction of cardiac valves (e.g., mitral/aortic stenosis or regurgitation) from rheumatic heart disease, congenital anomalies, or degenerative causes.

Common Conditions

Mitral stenosis: Most common in developing countries (rheumatic etiology); pregnancy increases risk of pulmonary edema due to increased CO and left atrial pressure.

Aortic stenosis: Congenital or degenerative; severe cases (valve area <1 cm^2) poorly tolerate pregnancy.

Regurgitant lesions: Mitral or aortic regurgitation generally better tolerated.

Prosthetic valves: Mechanical valves require anticoagulation; bioprosthetic valves have lower thromboembolism risk.

Clinical Features

Symptoms: Dyspnea, chest pain, syncope, or heart failure (severe stenosis).

Signs: Murmurs (e.g., diastolic rumble in mitral stenosis, systolic murmur in aortic stenosis), pulmonary edema, or atrial fibrillation.

Diagnosis

Echocardiography: Assesses valve area, gradient, regurgitation, and ventricular function.

ECG: Detects atrial fibrillation or hypertrophy.

Brain natriuretic peptide (BNP): Elevated in heart failure.

Management

Preconception: Valve repair/replacement for severe lesions; counsel on anticoagulation risks for mechanical valves.

Antenatal

Mild/moderate lesions: Monitor with echocardiography every trimester.

Severe stenosis: Restrict activity, use diuretics (e.g., furosemide) or β-blockers for heart failure or arrhythmias.

Mechanical valves: LMWH (e.g., enoxaparin, dose-adjusted for anti-Xa levels 0.8–1.2 IU/mL) in first trimester and after 36 weeks; warfarin (5–7.5 mg daily) in second/third trimesters if stable.

Delivery

Vaginal delivery with epidural for mild/moderate lesions.

Cesarean for severe lesions, heart failure, or anticoagulation complications.

Invasive hemodynamic monitoring in high-risk cases.

Postpartum: Monitor for heart failure; adjust anticoagulation.

Complications

Maternal: Pulmonary edema, atrial fibrillation, thromboembolism, or valve thrombosis.

Fetal: Preterm birth, IUGR, or fetal loss (higher with severe lesions or anticoagulation).

Prognosis: Good for mild lesions; severe mitral/aortic stenosis carries 5–10% maternal mortality risk without intervention.

3. Peripartum Cardiomyopathy (PPCM)

Heart failure with left ventricular systolic dysfunction (ejection fraction <45%) in the last month of pregnancy or within 5 months postpartum, without other identifiable causes.

Incidence: 1:1,000–4,000 pregnancies; higher in African descent, multiple gestation, or pre-eclampsia.

Etiology

Unknown; possible contributors include oxidative stress, prolactin cleavage, or genetic predisposition.

Risk factors: Advanced maternal age, multiparity, pre-eclampsia, hypertension, or African ancestry.

Clinical Features

Dyspnea, orthopnea, paroxysmal nocturnal dyspnea, edema.

Signs: Tachycardia, pulmonary rales, elevated jugular venous pressure, or S3 gallop.

Diagnosis

Echocardiography: Left ventricular ejection fraction (LVEF) <45%, dilated left ventricle.

BNP: Elevated in heart failure.

ECG: Non-specific; may show tachycardia or left ventricular hypertrophy.

Rule out other causes (e.g., ischemic heart disease, myocarditis) with cardiac MRI or coronary angiography (rare).

Management

Antenatal

Treat heart failure: Diuretics (furosemide), β-blockers (metoprolol), or digoxin (safe in pregnancy).

Avoid ACE inhibitors/ARBs (teratogenic); use hydralazine/nitrates for afterload reduction.

Anticoagulation (LMWH) if LVEF <30% or atrial fibrillation due to thromboembolism risk.

Delivery

Vaginal delivery with epidural if stable; cesarean for hemodynamic instability.

Early delivery (34–36 weeks) if severe heart failure.

Postpartum

Continue heart failure therapy; ACE inhibitors (e.g., enalapril) safe in breastfeeding.

Bromocriptine (2.5 mg twice daily for 2–8 weeks) experimental to suppress prolactin (potential benefit in PPCM).

Monitor LVEF at 3–6 months; 50% recover normal function within 6–12 months.

Counseling: Avoid future pregnancies if LVEF remains <50% due to 20–50% recurrence risk.

Complications

Maternal: Heart failure, arrhythmias, thromboembolism, or death (5–10% in severe cases).

Fetal: Preterm birth, IUGR, or stillbirth (rare).

Prognosis: 50–80% recover LVEF within 6 months; persistent dysfunction increases mortality risk.

4. Hypertensive Disorders

Includes chronic hypertension, gestational hypertension, pre-eclampsia, and eclampsia, which can mimic or exacerbate cardiac conditions.

Incidence: 6–8% of pregnancies; pre-eclampsia affects 3–5%.

Etiology

Chronic hypertension: Pre-existing BP ≥140/90 mmHg.

Gestational hypertension: New-onset BP ≥140/90 mmHg after 20 weeks without proteinuria.

Pre-eclampsia: BP ≥140/90 mmHg after 20 weeks with proteinuria (≥300 mg/24h) or end-organ dysfunction (e.g., elevated LFTs, thrombocytopenia, renal impairment).

Risk factors: Nulliparity, obesity, diabetes, or family history.

Clinical Features

Hypertension, edema, headache, visual changes, epigastric pain.

Severe pre-eclampsia: BP ≥160/110 mmHg, oliguria, pulmonary edema, or seizures (eclampsia).

Diagnosis

BP measurement, urinalysis (protein/creatinine ratio), labs (LFTs, platelets, creatinine).

Echocardiography if heart failure suspected (e.g., pulmonary edema).

Management

Chronic hypertension: Methyldopa, labetalol, or nifedipine; target BP <140/90 mmHg.

Pre-eclampsia

Magnesium sulfate for seizure prophylaxis (4–6 g IV bolus, 1–2 g/h maintenance).

Antihypertensives (labetalol, hydralazine, nifedipine) for BP ≥160/110 mmHg.

Delivery: Only definitive treatment; ≥37 weeks for mild cases, 34–36 weeks for severe cases.

Fetal monitoring: NST, biophysical profile, or Doppler ultrasound for IUGR.

Complications

Maternal: Pulmonary edema, stroke, renal failure, HELLP syndrome, or eclampsia.

Fetal: IUGR, preterm birth, stillbirth.

Prognosis: Resolves post-delivery; chronic hypertension increases future cardiovascular risk.

5. Thromboembolic Disease

Includes deep vein thrombosis (DVT) and pulmonary embolism (PE), with pregnancy increasing risk 5–10-fold due to hypercoagulability.

Incidence: 0.1–0.2% of pregnancies; postpartum period highest risk.

Etiology

Virchow's triad: Hypercoagulability (increased clotting factors), venous stasis (uterine compression), and endothelial injury (delivery, cesarean).

Risk factors: Obesity, immobility, cesarean delivery, thrombophilia, or smoking.

Clinical Features

DVT: Unilateral leg swelling, pain, or warmth.

PE: Dyspnea, chest pain, tachycardia, hypoxia, or sudden collapse.

Diagnosis

DVT: Compression ultrasound (first-line); D-dimer unreliable in pregnancy.

PE: Ventilation-perfusion (V/Q) scan or CT pulmonary angiography (CTPA); low radiation risk to fetus with shielding.

ECG: Sinus tachycardia, S1Q3T3 pattern (rare).

Management

Anticoagulation: LMWH (e.g., enoxaparin 1 mg/kg twice daily, adjusted for anti-Xa levels) preferred; safe in pregnancy. Unfractionated heparin (UFH) for renal impairment or near delivery.

Warfarin avoided in pregnancy (teratogenic) but safe postpartum.

Continue anticoagulation for 6 weeks postpartum or longer if thrombophilia.

Thrombolysis: Reserved for life-threatening PE (e.g., hemodynamic instability); consult specialists.

Inferior vena cava filter: For recurrent PE despite anticoagulation.

Delivery: Stop LMWH 24 hours before planned delivery; switch to UFH if near term.

Complications

Maternal: Post-thrombotic syndrome, recurrent thromboembolism, or death (PE).

Fetal: Minimal direct risk; preterm delivery if maternal instability.

Prognosis: Good with prompt anticoagulation; recurrence risk 5–10% in future pregnancies.

6. Arrhythmias

Abnormal heart rhythms, often exacerbated by pregnancy's hemodynamic stress.

Common Types

Supraventricular tachycardia (SVT), atrial fibrillation (AF), or premature ventricular contractions (PVCs).

Ventricular tachycardia (VT) rare but serious, often in structural heart disease.

Clinical Features: Palpitations, dizziness, syncope, or heart failure (in severe cases).

Diagnosis

ECG: Confirms rhythm (e.g., narrow QRS in SVT, irregular in AF).

Echocardiography: To assess structural heart disease.

Holter monitor: For intermittent symptoms.

Management

Benign arrhythmias (e.g., PVCs): Reassurance, avoid stimulants (caffeine).

SVT: Vagal maneuvers, adenosine (6–12 mg IV, safe in pregnancy), or β-blockers (metoprolol).

AF: Rate control (β-blockers, digoxin); anticoagulation (LMWH) if persistent.

VT: Antiarrhythmics (e.g., lidocaine), cardioversion if unstable; implantable cardioverter-defibrillator (ICD) management if pre-existing.

Complications: Heart failure, thromboembolism (AF), or fetal distress (severe arrhythmias).

Prognosis: Excellent for benign arrhythmias; structural heart disease worsens outcomes.

7. Myocardial Infarction (MI) and Coronary Artery Disease

Rare in pregnancy (1:10,000–30,000), but incidence rising due to older maternal age and cardiovascular risk factors.

Etiology

Coronary atherosclerosis (older women, diabetes, smoking).

Coronary artery dissection (pregnancy-related, due to hormonal weakening of vessel walls).

Coronary spasm or thrombosis.

Clinical Features: Chest pain, dyspnea, nausea, or syncope; may mimic pre-eclampsia.

Diagnosis

ECG: ST-elevation, Q waves, or T-wave changes.

Troponins: Elevated; interpret cautiously as mild elevations occur in pre-eclampsia.

Coronary angiography: Gold standard; low radiation risk with fetal shielding.

Management

Medical: Aspirin (81 mg daily, safe), β-blockers, nitrates; avoid ACE inhibitors.

Interventional: Percutaneous coronary intervention (PCI) preferred over thrombolytics (fetal bleeding risk).

Delivery: Vaginal with epidural if stable; cesarean for acute MI or obstetric indications.

Complications: Heart failure, arrhythmias, maternal death (5–10%), or preterm birth.

Prognosis: Good with timely intervention; recurrence risk depends on risk factors.

Diagnosis of Cardiovascular Disorders

History: Assess for dyspnea, chest pain, palpitations, syncope, or family history of heart disease.

Physical Examination: Check for murmurs, edema, jugular venous distension, or signs of heart failure.

Investigations

ECG: Arrhythmias, ischemia, or hypertrophy.

Echocardiography: Assesses ventricular function, valve pathology, or congenital defects.

BNP: Elevated in heart failure.

Troponin: For suspected MI.

Chest X-ray: For pulmonary edema or cardiomegaly (minimize radiation).

Cardiac MRI: For PPCM or complex CHD (avoid gadolinium).

V/Q scan or CTPA: For suspected PE.

Differential Diagnosis

Obstetric: Pre-eclampsia, amniotic fluid embolism.

Non-cardiac: Pulmonary embolism, pneumonia, or GERD.

Complications

Maternal: Heart failure, arrhythmias, thromboembolism, or stroke, pulmonary edema (pre-eclampsia, PPCM, valvular disease). Maternal death (1–5% in high-risk conditions like PPCM or pulmonary hypertension).

Fetal: Preterm birth, IUGR, or stillbirth, Congenital heart defects (in maternal CHD). Neonatal complications from prematurity or maternal instability.

Prognosis

Low-risk conditions (e.g., repaired CHD, mild valvular disease): Near-normal outcomes with monitoring.

High-risk conditions (e.g., PPCM, severe valvular stenosis, pulmonary hypertension): Significant morbidity/mortality without specialized care.

Hypertensive disorders: Resolve post-delivery; chronic hypertension increases long-term cardiovascular risk.

PPCM: 50–80% recover; persistent dysfunction increases mortality.

Thromboembolism: Excellent with anticoagulation; recurrence risk persists postpartum.

Prevention

Preconception

Optimize cardiac status (e.g., valve repair, control hypertension) in women with known heart disease.

Counsel on pregnancy risks using mWHO classification; avoid pregnancy in mWHO IV.

Screen for cardiovascular risk factors (e.g., diabetes, obesity, smoking).

Antenatal

Routine BP monitoring and early pre-eclampsia screening.

Thromboprophylaxis (LMWH) for high-risk women (e.g., prior DVT, mechanical valves).

Avoid teratogenic drugs (e.g., ACE inhibitors, warfarin in first trimester).

Lifestyle

Encourage healthy weight, diet, and exercise before and during pregnancy.

Smoking cessation and control of diabetes/hypertension.

Public Health

Access to prenatal care and multidisciplinary teams for high-risk pregnancies.

Education on cardiovascular risks and symptoms in pregnancy.

8.9 Renal and Urinary Tract Disorders in Pregnancy

(*Amrad-i-Kulya wa Majra-i-Bawl*)

Renal and urinary tract disorders in pregnancy encompass a range of conditions, from physiological adaptations to pathological states, including urinary tract infections (UTIs), pyelonephritis, nephrolithiasis, and pregnancy-specific disorders such as pre-eclampsia-related renal dysfunction. Pregnancy induces significant renal and hemodynamic changes that can exacerbate pre-existing conditions or unmask new ones, potentially affecting maternal and fetal outcomes. Effective management requires balancing maternal treatment with fetal safety, often involving multidisciplinary care

Physiological Changes in Pregnancy Affecting the Renal and Urinary Systems

Renal Hemodynamics

Increased renal blood flow (RBF): Rises by 50–80% due to increased cardiac output and decreased systemic vascular resistance, peaking in the second trimester.

Increased glomerular filtration rate (GFR): Increases by 40–50% (from 100 to 150 mL/min) by 12–16 weeks, leading to lower serum creatinine (normal: 0.4–0.8 mg/dL in pregnancy) and urea (normal: 10–20 mg/dL).

Proteinuria: Mild increase (<300 mg/24h) due to higher GFR and altered tubular reabsorption; significant proteinuria (>300 mg/24h) suggests pathology.

Urinary Tract Changes

Ureteral dilation (hydronephrosis): Progesterone-mediated smooth muscle relaxation and mechanical compression by the gravid uterus cause dilation, more pronounced on the right side due to uterine dextrorotation.

Bladder changes: Reduced tone and increased capacity; vesicoureteral reflux may occur, increasing UTI risk.

Increased urine volume: Due to higher GFR and fluid intake, leading to dilute urine and lower specific gravity.

Electrolyte and Acid-Base Balance

Sodium retention: Increased by 900–950 mmol to support plasma volume expansion, but aldosterone and progesterone balance prevents edema in normal pregnancy.

Mild respiratory alkalosis: Due to progesterone-driven hyperventilation, reducing serum bicarbonate (18–22 mmol/L).

Increased urinary calcium: Predisposes to nephrolithiasis, balanced by increased citrate excretion.

Coagulation Changes: Hypercoagulable state increases risk of renal vein thrombosis or thromboembolism in predisposed women.

Common Renal and Urinary Tract Disorders in Pregnancy

1. Urinary Tract Infections (UTIs)

Asymptomatic bacteriuria (ASB): Significant bacterial growth ($\geq 10^5$ CFU/mL of a single organism) in urine without symptoms, affecting 2–10% of pregnancies.

Cystitis: Symptomatic lower UTI, affecting 1–2% of pregnancies.

Pyelonephritis: Upper UTI involving the renal pelvis, affecting 0.5–2% of pregnancies.

Etiology

Common pathogens: Escherichia coli (70–80%), Klebsiella, Proteus, or Enterococcus.

Risk factors: Stasis from ureteral dilation, vesicoureteral reflux, glycosuria, reduced bladder tone, or prior UTI history.

Clinical Features

ASB: Asymptomatic; detected via screening.

Cystitis: Dysuria, urgency, frequency, suprapubic pain; no systemic symptoms.

Pyelonephritis: Fever, chills, flank pain, nausea, vomiting, costovertebral angle tenderness; may present with sepsis or preterm labor.

Diagnosis

Urine culture: Gold standard for ASB and symptomatic UTI; clean-catch midstream sample; $\geq 10^5$ CFU/mL confirms diagnosis.

Urinalysis: Pyuria (>10 WBC/hpf), hematuria, or nitrites in symptomatic UTI.

Pyelonephritis: Add blood cultures, CBC (leukocytosis), and inflammatory markers (CRP, ESR); ultrasound to assess for abscess or hydronephrosis.

Management

ASB: Treat to prevent pyelonephritis (20–40% risk if untreated) and preterm birth. Antibiotics (7-day course, safe in pregnancy): Nitrofurantoin (100 mg twice daily), amoxicillin (500 mg three times daily), or cephalexin (500 mg four times daily). Avoid trimethoprim-sulfamethoxazole in first trimester (folate antagonist) or near term (neonatal jaundice risk). Follow-up culture 1–2 weeks post-treatment to confirm eradication.

Cystitis: Similar antibiotics as ASB; 3–7-day course.

Symptomatic relief: Phenazopyridine (short-term, avoid near term).

Pyelonephritis: Hospitalization for IV antibiotics (e.g., ceftriaxone 1–2 g daily or ampicillin/gentamicin until afebrile), then oral antibiotics for 10–14 days. IV fluids for dehydration; monitor for sepsis or preterm labor. Fetal monitoring: Non-stress test (NST) or ultrasound if preterm labor risk. Screening: Routine urine culture at first prenatal visit (12–16 weeks); repeat in high-risk women (e.g., diabetes, recurrent UTI).

Complications

Maternal: Pyelonephritis, sepsis, acute respiratory distress syndrome (ARDS, rare), or renal dysfunction.

Fetal: Preterm birth, low birth weight, or fetal loss (higher with pyelonephritis).

Prognosis: Excellent with early treatment; untreated ASB increases pyelonephritis risk, impacting maternal and fetal outcomes.

2. Nephrolithiasis

Kidney stones, affecting 0.05–0.1% of pregnancies, often presenting in the second or third trimester.

Etiology

Increased urinary calcium and uric acid due to higher GFR; balanced by increased citrate (stone inhibitor).

Risk factors: Prior stones, dehydration, obesity, or hyperparathyroidism.

Pathophysiology: Stones (calcium oxalate/phosphate most common) cause ureteral obstruction, leading to pain, infection, or hydronephrosis.

Clinical Features

Flank pain (colicky), hematuria, nausea, vomiting, or dysuria.

May mimic pyelonephritis or preterm labor.

Diagnosis

Ultrasound: First-line; detects stones, hydronephrosis, or ureteral dilation; sensitivity lower in pregnancy.

Non-contrast C: Second-line if ultrasound inconclusive (low radiation risk with shielding).

Urinalysis: Hematuria, crystals (e.g., calcium oxalate), or pyuria (if concurrent UTI).

Labs: Check renal function, electrolytes, and calcium levels.

Management

Conservative (80–90% pass spontaneously):

Hydration (IV or oral, 2–3 L/day), pain control (acetaminophen, opioids if needed).

Strain urine to confirm stone passage.

Interventional (obstruction, infection, or persistent pain):

Ureteral stent or nephrostomy tube (under ultrasound guidance).

Ureteroscopy with laser lithotripsy (safe in second/third trimester).

Extracorporeal shock wave lithotripsy (ESWL) contraindicated due to fetal risk.

Antibiotics: If concurrent UTI (e.g., nitrofurantoin or cephalexin).

Fetal monitoring: NST or ultrasound if preterm labor risk.

Complications

Maternal: UTI, pyelonephritis, renal obstruction, or acute kidney injury (AKI).

Fetal: Preterm labor or fetal distress (rare).

Prognosis: Good with timely management; recurrence risk high if underlying metabolic cause untreated.

3. Pre-eclampsia-Related Renal Dysfunction

Renal dysfunction in pre-eclampsia, characterized by proteinuria (≥300 mg/24h), reduced GFR, or AKI, typically after 20 weeks gestation.

Incidence: Pre-eclampsia affects 3–5% of pregnancies; renal involvement common in severe cases.

Etiology

Placental dysfunction causes endothelial damage, vasoconstriction, and reduced renal perfusion.

Risk factors: Nulliparity, obesity, chronic hypertension, diabetes, or multiple gestation.

Pathophysiology

Glomerular endotheliosis reduces GFR, causing proteinuria and oliguria.

Systemic vasoconstriction and hypertension exacerbate renal ischemia.

May progress to AKI or overlap with HELLP syndrome.

Clinical Features

Hypertension (BP ≥140/90 mmHg), proteinuria, edema.

Severe pre-eclampsia: BP ≥160/110 mmHg, oliguria (<500 mL/24h), elevated creatinine (>1.1 mg/dL), or epigastric pain.

Diagnosis

Urinalysis: Protein/creatinine ratio ≥0.3 or 24-hour urine protein ≥300 mg.

Labs: Serum creatinine (>1.1 mg/dL or doubling from baseline), LFTs, platelets (for HELLP).

Ultrasound: Assess fetal growth and amniotic fluid; renal ultrasound if AKI suspected.

Management

Mild pre-eclampsia: Monitor BP, proteinuria, and fetal status; deliver at 37–38 weeks.

Severe pre-eclampsia

Magnesium sulfate (4–6 g IV bolus, 1–2 g/h maintenance) for seizure prophylaxis.

Antihypertensives (labetalol, hydralazine, nifedipine) for BP ≥160/110 mmHg.

Delivery: ≥34 weeks or earlier if maternal/fetal compromise.

Corticosteroids (betamethasone) for fetal lung maturity if <34 weeks.

AKI: Fluid management (avoid overload), monitor electrolytes, consider dialysis (rare).

Fetal monitoring: NST, biophysical profile, or Doppler ultrasound for IUGR.

Complications

Maternal: AKI, pulmonary edema, eclampsia, or renal failure (rare).

Fetal: Preterm birth, IUGR, stillbirth.

Prognosis: Resolves post-delivery; persistent proteinuria or hypertension suggests underlying renal disease.

4. Acute Kidney Injury (AKI)

Sudden decline in renal function (increased creatinine or oliguria), rare in pregnancy (0.01–0.02%).

Etiology

Prerenal: Hypovolemia (e.g., hyperemesis gravidarum, hemorrhage), pre-eclampsia.

Intrinsic: Acute tubular necrosis (sepsis, postpartum hemorrhage), glomerulonephritis, or bilateral cortical necrosis (severe pre-eclampsia or placental abruption).

Postrenal: Ureteral obstruction (nephrolithiasis, gravid uterus, rare).

Clinical Features: Oliguria (<500 mL/24h), edema, hypertension, or signs of underlying cause (e.g., sepsis, pre-eclampsia).

Diagnosis

Labs: Elevated creatinine (>1.1 mg/dL or doubling), electrolyte imbalances (hyperkalemia, acidosis), or anemia.

Urinalysis: Hematuria, proteinuria, or casts (e.g., muddy brown casts in ATN).

Ultrasound: Assess for obstruction or hydronephrosis.

Management

Treat underlying cause: IV fluids for hypovolemia, antibiotics for sepsis, delivery for pre-eclampsia.

Supportive care: Correct electrolytes, avoid nephrotoxic drugs (e.g., NSAIDs), monitor fluid balance.

Dialysis: Rarely needed for severe AKI (e.g., hyperkalemia, uremia, or refractory acidosis).

Fetal monitoring: NST or ultrasound for fetal distress.

Complications

Maternal: Chronic kidney disease (CKD), dialysis dependence (rare), or death.

Fetal: Preterm birth, IUGR, or stillbirth.

Prognosis: Good if reversible cause treated promptly; poor if bilateral cortical necrosis.

5. Chronic Kidney Disease (CKD)

Pre-existing renal dysfunction (GFR <60 mL/min or structural damage) persisting ≥3 months, present in 0.1–0.3% of pregnancies.

Etiology

Causes: Diabetic nephropathy, glomerulonephritis, lupus nephritis, polycystic kidney disease, or hypertensive nephropathy.

Risk factors: Pre-pregnancy CKD, hypertension, or proteinuria.

Clinical Features

Asymptomatic in early stages (CKD stages 1–2); hypertension, proteinuria, or edema in advanced stages (3–5).

Symptoms: Fatigue, edema, or uremic symptoms (nausea, pruritus) in severe cases.

Diagnosis

Labs: Elevated creatinine (>1.1 mg/dL), proteinuria (>300 mg/24h), or abnormal electrolytes.

Ultrasound: Assess kidney size (small in CKD, normal/large in diabetic nephropathy).

Staging: Based on GFR (e.g., stage 1: GFR >90 with proteinuria; stage 5: GFR <15 or dialysis).

Management

Preconception: Optimize renal function, control BP (<140/90 mmHg), and reduce proteinuria with ACE inhibitors (top preconception).

Antenatal: Monitor BP, renal function, and proteinuria every 2–4 weeks.

Antihypertensives: Methyldopa, labetalol, or nifedipine (avoid ACE inhibitors/ARBs).

Low-dose aspirin (81 mg daily) to reduce pre-eclampsia risk.

Erythropoietin or iron for anemia; adjust doses for pregnancy GFR.

Delivery: Vaginal delivery preferred; cesarean for obstetric indications.

Fetal monitoring: Serial ultrasounds for IUGR; NST from 32 weeks if CKD stage 3–5.

Complications

Maternal: Pre-eclampsia (20–50% risk), worsening CKD, dialysis need, or hypertension.

Fetal: Preterm birth (50–70%), IUGR, stillbirth (higher in CKD stages 4–5).

Prognosis: Good for CKD stages 1–2; stage 3–5 increases maternal and fetal risks; dialysis-dependent patients have 50% live birth rate.

6. Renal Vein Thrombosis (RVT)

Rare thrombosis of renal veins, often unilateral, associated with pregnancy's hypercoagulable state.

Etiology

Hypercoagulability, venous stasis, or endothelial injury (Virchow's triad).

Risk factors: Nephrotic syndrome, thrombophilia, or dehydration.

Clinical Features: Flank pain, hematuria, oliguria, or hypertension; may be asymptomatic.

Diagnosis

Ultrasound with Doppler: First-line; detects thrombus or reduced renal vein flow.

MRI/CT: If ultrasound inconclusive (minimize radiation).

Labs: Elevated creatinine, proteinuria, or hematuria.

Management

Anticoagulation: LMWH (e.g., enoxaparin, dose-adjusted) for 3–6 months, continued postpartum.

Treat underlying cause (e.g., nephrotic syndrome).

Fetal monitoring for preterm labor risk.

Complications: Renal infarction, AKI, or pulmonary embolism.

Prognosis: Good with anticoagulation; recurrence risk depends on thrombophilia

Diagnosis of Renal and Urinary Tract Disorders

History: Assess for dysuria, flank pain, hematuria, hypertension, edema, or history of renal disease/ UTI.

Physical Examination: Check for costovertebral angle tenderness, edema, BP, or signs of pre-eclampsia (e.g., headache, epigastric pain).

Investigations

Urinalysis: Proteinuria, hematuria, pyuria, or casts.

Urine culture: For ASB or symptomatic UTI.

Labs: Serum creatinine, urea, electrolytes, CBC, LFTs, or coagulation profile (pre-eclampsia, AKI).

Imaging: Ultrasound (renal, ureteral, or fetal); MRI/CT for complex cases (e.g., nephrolithiasis, RVT).

Differential Diagnosis

Obstetric: Pre-eclampsia, HELLP syndrome, acute fatty liver of pregnancy (AFLP).

Non-obstetric: Appendicitis, cholecystitis, pyelonephritis, or glomerulonephritis.

Complications

Maternal: AKI, CKD progression, or dialysis dependence, pre-eclampsia, eclampsia, or pulmonary edema. Sepsis (pyelonephritis) or thromboembolism (RVT).

Fetal: Preterm birth, IUGR, or stillbirth, neonatal complications from prematurity or maternal instability. Congenital anomalies (rare, in severe CKD or teratogenic exposures)

Prognosis

UTIs: Excellent with early treatment; untreated ASB or pyelonephritis increases preterm birth risk.

Nephrolithiasis: Most stones pass spontaneously; good outcomes with intervention if needed.

Pre-eclampsia-related renal dysfunction: Resolves post-delivery; persistent dysfunction suggests underlying CKD.

AKI: Reversible if cause treated promptly; poor prognosis in cortical necrosis.

CKD: Outcomes depend on stage; stages 1–2 have near-normal outcomes, stages 4–5 high-risk.

RVT: Good with anticoagulation; recurrence risk low unless thrombophilia present.

Prevention

Antenatal: Routine urine culture at 12–16 weeks to detect ASB. Low-dose aspirin (81 mg daily) for pre-eclampsia prevention in high-risk women (e.g., CKD, hypertension). Adequate hydration (2–3 L/day) to reduce UTI and nephrolithiasis risk. Thromboprophylaxis (LMWH) for high-risk women (e.g., nephrotic syndrome, prior RVT).

Preconception: Optimize renal function and BP in CKD patients; discontinue teratogenic drugs (e.g., ACE inhibitors). Counsel on pregnancy risks in advanced CKD or dialysis.

Lifestyle: Encourage healthy diet, weight management, and hygiene to prevent UTIs. Avoid dehydration or nephrotoxic drugs (e.g., NSAIDs).

Public Health: Access to prenatal care and screening for ASB in low-resource settings. Education on UTI symptoms and early reporting.

Key Points

Renal and urinary tract disorders in pregnancy include UTIs, nephrolithiasis, pre-eclampsia-related renal dysfunction, AKI, CKD, and RVT, influenced by increased GFR, ureteral dilation, and hypercoagulability.

UTIs: ASB requires treatment to prevent pyelonephritis; cystitis and pyelonephritis treated with safe antibiotics (nitrofurantoin, cephalexin).

Nephrolithiasis: Managed conservatively (hydration, pain control) or with stents/ureteroscopy; ESWL contraindicated.

Pre-eclampsia-related renal dysfunction: Proteinuria and AKI; delivery is definitive treatment.

AKI: Rare; treat underlying cause (e.g., hypovolemia, sepsis); dialysis rarely needed.

CKD: Higher maternal/fetal risks in advanced stages; monitor BP, proteinuria, and fetal growth.

RVT: Anticoagulation with LMWH; rare but serious.

Diagnosis: Relies on urinalysis, culture, renal function tests, and ultrasound; MRI/CT for complex cases.

Complications: Preterm birth, IUGR, stillbirth, or maternal renal failure; timely intervention improves outcomes.

Prevention: Routine ASB screening, hydration, and preconception optimization reduce risks.

8.10 Viral, Bacterial, Parasitic & Protozoal Infestation & Infection in pregnancy

(*Daurane Haml fairoosu, jarasimi, tufeli aur awali ibteka wa ta'diya*)

Bacterial Infections in Pregnancy

Bacterial infections in pregnancy are significant due to their potential to cause maternal morbidity, fetal complications, and adverse pregnancy outcomes. The physiological changes of pregnancy, including immune modulation, increased metabolic demands, and anatomical alterations, predispose pregnant women to certain infections and exacerbate their severity. Prompt diagnosis and management are critical to minimize maternal and fetal risks while ensuring the use of pregnancy-safe antibiotics.

Physiological Changes in Pregnancy Predisposing to Bacterial Infections

Immune Modulation: Pregnancy induces a shift toward a Th2-dominated immune response to prevent fetal rejection, reducing cell-mediated immunity and increasing susceptibility to certain bacterial infections (e.g., Listeria monocytogenes). Decreased phagocytic activity and altered cytokine profiles impair pathogen clearance.

Anatomical Changes: Urinary tract: Ureteral dilation (due to progesterone and uterine compression), vesicoureteral reflux, and glycosuria increase the risk of urinary tract infections (UTIs). Respiratory tract: Diaphragmatic elevation and increased oxygen demand predispose to pneumonia. Gastrointestinal tract: Reduced gastric acidity and motility increase susceptibility to enteric infections (e.g., Listeria, Salmonella).

Hypercoagulable State: Increases risk of septic pelvic thrombophlebitis post-delivery or with chorioamnionitis.

Increased Blood Volume and Cardiac Output: May mask early signs of sepsis (e.g., tachycardia, hypotension) or exacerbate systemic infection.

Common Bacterial Infections in Pregnancy

1. Urinary Tract Infections (UTIs)

Definition: Asymptomatic Bacteriuria (ASB): Significant bacterial growth ($\geq 10^5$ colony-forming units [CFU]/mL of a single organism) in urine without symptoms, affecting 2–10% of pregnancies.

Cystitis: Symptomatic lower UTI, affecting 1–2% of pregnancies.

Pyelonephritis: Upper UTI involving the renal pelvis, affecting 0.5–2% of pregnancies.

Etiology: Common pathogens: Escherichia coli(70–80%), Klebsiella pneumoniae, Proteus mirabilis, Enterococcus faecalis, Staphylococcus saprophyticus.

Risk factors: Ureteral dilation, vesicoureteral reflux, glycosuria, prior UTI, diabetes, or sickle cell trait.

Pathophysiology: Urinary stasis and glycosuria promote bacterial growth. Untreated ASB progresses to pyelonephritis in 20–40% of cases, increasing risks of sepsis and preterm labour.

Clinical Features

ASB: Asymptomatic; detected via screening.

Cystitis: Dysuria, urgency, frequency, suprapubic pain; no fever or systemic symptoms.

Pyelonephritis: Fever (>38°C), chills, flank pain, costovertebral angle tenderness, nausea, vomiting; may present with sepsis or preterm contractions.

Diagnosis

Urine culture: Gold standard; clean-catch midstream sample; $\geq 10^5$ CFU/mL confirms ASB or symptomatic UTI.

Urinalysis: Pyuria (>10 WBC/hpf), haematuria, or nitrites (suggestive of Enterobacteriaceae).

Pyelonephritis: Blood cultures (if septic), CBC (leukocytosis), C-reactive protein (CRP), or erythrocyte sedimentation rate (ESR); renal ultrasound to assess for abscess or hydronephrosis.

Management

ASB: Treat to prevent pyelonephritis and preterm birth. Antibiotics (7-day course, safe in pregnancy): Nitrofurantoin (100 mg twice daily), amoxicillin (500 mg three times daily), or cephalexin (500 mg four times daily). Avoid trimethoprim-sulfamethoxazole in first trimester (folate antagonist) or near term (neonatal jaundice risk). Follow-up urine culture 1–2 weeks post-treatment.

Cystitis: Same antibiotics as ASB; 3–7-day course. Symptomatic relief: Phenazopyridine (100–200 mg three times daily, short-term; avoid near term).

Pyelonephritis: Hospitalization for IV antibiotics: Ceftriaxone (1–2 g daily), cefazolin, or ampicillin/gentamicin until afebrile for 48 hours, then oral antibiotics (e.g., cephalexin) for 10–14 days total. IV fluids for dehydration; monitor for sepsis or preterm labor.

Fetal monitoring: Non-stress test (NST) or ultrasound if preterm labor risk. Screening: Routine urine culture at 12–16 weeks; repeat in high-risk women (e.g., diabetes, recurrent UTI).

Complications

Maternal: Pyelonephritis, sepsis, acute respiratory distress syndrome (ARDS, rare), or acute kidney injury (AKI).

Foetal: Preterm birth, low birth weight, or foetal loss (higher with pyelonephritis).

Prognosis: Excellent with early treatment; untreated ASB increases pyelonephritis risk, impacting outcomes.

2. Chorioamnionitis

Definition: Bacterial infection of the amniotic fluid, membranes, or placenta, typically ascending from the lower genital tract, affecting 1–4% of pregnancies.

Etiology

Polymicrobial: Group B Streptococcus (GBS), E. coli, Bacteroides, Mycoplasma, or Ureaplasma.

Risk factors: Prolonged rupture of membranes (PROM), preterm labor, multiple vaginal examinationss, or bacterial vaginosis.

Pathophysiology

Ascending bacteria cause inflammation of chorioamniotic membranes, leading to cytokine release, prostaglandin production, and preterm labor or membrane rupture.

Can progress to maternal or fetal sepsis if untreated.

Clinical Features

Maternal fever (>38°C), uterine tenderness, foul-smelling amniotic fluid, or tachycardia (maternal or fetal).

Preterm labor, PROM, or leukocytosis.

Diagnosis

Clinical: Fever plus ≥1 of uterine tenderness, maternal/fetal tachycardia, or foul amniotic fluid.

Labs: Leukocytosis (>15,000/µL), elevated CRP; amniotic fluid culture (via amniocentesis, rarely needed).

Ultrasound: Assess for placental abnormalities or fetal distress.

Management

Antibiotics: Broad-spectrum IV antibiotics (e.g., ampicillin 2 g every 6 hours + gentamicin 1.5 mg/kg every 8 hours) until delivery; add clindamycin (900 mg every 8 hours) if cesarean planned.

Delivery: Expedite delivery (vaginal preferred) after antibiotics initiated; cesarean for obstetric indications.

Supportive care: Antipyretics (acetaminophen), IV fluids; monitor for sepsis.

Complications

Maternal: Sepsis, endometritis, postpartum hemorrhage, or septic pelvic thrombophlebitis.

Fetal: Neonatal sepsis, pneumonia, meningitis, or cerebral palsy (from preterm birth or hypoxia).

Prognosis: Good with prompt antibiotics and delivery; delayed treatment increases neonatal morbidity.

3. Group B Streptococcus (GBS) Colonization and Infection

Definition: Colonization of the genital or rectal tract by Streptococcus agalactiae (GBS), present in 10–30% of pregnant women; can cause maternal or neonatal infection.

Etiology

GBS is a gram-positive coccus, part of normal vaginal/rectal flora in many women.

Risk factors for neonatal infection: GBS colonization, PROM, preterm labor, maternal fever, or prior GBS-infected infant.

Pathophysiology

Vertical transmission during labor causes early-onset neonatal GBS disease (sepsis, pneumonia, meningitis).

Maternal infections include chorioamnionitis, endometritis, or UTI.

Clinical Features

Maternal: Asymptomatic colonization; symptomatic if UTI, chorioamnionitis, or endometritis (fever, uterine tenderness).

Neonatal: Early-onset (0–6 days): Sepsis, respiratory distress; late-onset (7–90 days): Meningitis, bacteremia.

Diagnosis

Screening: Universal vaginal-rectal swab culture at 36–38 weeks (or earlier if preterm labor).

Maternal infection: Urine culture (for UTI), amniotic fluid culture, or blood cultures (if septic).

Neonatal: Blood/CSF cultures, chest X-ray if symptomatic.

Management

Intrapartum antibiotic prophylaxis (IAP):

Indications: Positive GBS culture, prior GBS-infected infant, GBS bacteriuria, or unknown GBS status with risk factors (PROM ≥18 hours, preterm labor, maternal fever).

Antibiotics: Penicillin G (5 million units IV initial dose, then 2.5–3 million units every 4 hours until delivery); ampicillin alternative.

For penicillin allergy: Cefazolin (if low anaphylaxis risk) or vancomycin/clindamycin (if high risk, based on susceptibility).

Administer ≥4 hours before delivery for optimal efficacy.

Maternal infection: Treat as UTI, chorioamnionitis, or endometritis (see respective sections).

Neonatal: Empiric antibiotics (ampicillin + gentamicin) for suspected sepsis; monitor in NICU.

Complications

Maternal: Chorioamnionitis, endometritis, or sepsis (rare).

Fetal/Neonatal: Early-onset GBS disease (1–2% without IAP), preterm birth, or neurological sequelae.

Prognosis: Excellent with IAP; neonatal GBS disease mortality <5% with treatment.

4. Listeriosis

Definition: Infection with Listeria monocytogenes, a foodborne gram-positive bacillus, rare but severe in pregnancy (20–100 times higher risk than non-pregnant women).

Incidence: 0.1–1 per 10,000 pregnancies; higher in endemic areas.

Etiology

Sources: Contaminated foods (soft cheeses, deli meats, unpasteurized dairy, raw vegetables).

Risk factors: Immunosuppression of pregnancy, poor food hygiene.

Pathophysiology

Listeria crosses the placenta, causing placentitis, fetal infection, or abortion.

Maternal bacteremia can lead to sepsis or meningitis.

Clinical Features

Maternal: Fever, flu-like symptoms (myalgia, malaise), nausea, diarrhea; severe cases may present with sepsis or meningitis.

Fetal: Miscarriage, preterm labor, stillbirth, or neonatal listeriosis (granulomatosis infantiseptica).

Diagnosis

Blood cultures: Gold standard for maternal infection.

Amniotic fluid or placental cultures: If fetal loss or chorioamnionitis suspected.

CSF analysis: If meningitis suspected (lymphocytic pleocytosis, low glucose).

Management

Antibiotics: Ampicillin (2 g IV every 4 hours) + gentamicin (1.5 mg/kg every 8 hours) for synergy; treat for 14–21 days.

Penicillin allergy: Trimethoprim-sulfamethoxazole (avoid in first trimester) or vancomycin.

Fetal monitoring: Ultrasound for fetal viability, NST if preterm labor.

Delivery: Expedite if fetal distress or severe maternal infection; vaginal delivery unless obstetric indications.

Complications

Maternal: Sepsis, meningitis, or multi-organ failure (rare).

Fetal: Miscarriage (20–50% in early pregnancy), stillbirth, preterm birth, or neonatal sepsis (mortality 20–30%).

Prognosis: Maternal recovery good with antibiotics; fetal outcomes poor if infection early or untreated.

5. Postpartum Endometritis

Definition: Infection of the uterine lining post-delivery, affecting 1–3% of vaginal deliveries and 5–15% of cesarean deliveries.

Etiology

Polymicrobial: GBS, E. coli, Bacteroides, Clostridium, or Streptococcus species.

Risk factors: Cesarean delivery, prolonged labor, PROM, multiple vaginal exams, or retained products of conception.

Pathophysiology: Ascending infection from vaginal flora or direct contamination during delivery causes endometrial inflammation, potentially spreading to myometrium or parametrium.

Clinical Features

Fever (>38°C), uterine tenderness, foul-smelling lochia, or tachycardia within 1–7 days postpartum.

Severe cases: Sepsis, pelvic abscess, or septic pelvic thrombophlebitis.

Diagnosis:

Clinical: Fever plus uterine tenderness or foul lochia.

Labs: Leukocytosis, elevated CRP; blood cultures if septic.

Ultrasound: To detect retained products or pelvic abscess.

Management

Antibiotics: Broad-spectrum IV antibiotics (e.g., clindamycin 900 mg every 8 hours + gentamicin 1.5 mg/kg every 8 hours) until afebrile for 48 hours; oral antibiotics not needed if resolved.

Supportive care: IV fluids, antipyretics; evacuate retained products if present.

Monitoring: Assess for sepsis, abscess, or thromboembolism.

Complications

Maternal: Sepsis, pelvic abscess, septic pelvic thrombophlebitis, or infertility (rare).

Neonatal: Minimal direct risk; monitor if maternal sepsis severe.

Prognosis: Excellent with early antibiotics; complications rare with prompt treatment.

6. Pneumonia

Definition: Bacterial infection of the lungs, rare in pregnancy (0.1–0.2%) but more severe due to respiratory changes.

Etiology

Common pathogens: Streptococcus pneumoniae, Haemophilus influenzae, Mycoplasma pneumoniae (atypical), or Staphylococcus aureus (post-influenza).

Risk factors: Asthma, smoking, or immunosuppression.

Pathophysiology: Bacterial invasion of alveoli causes inflammation, consolidation, and impaired gas exchange, exacerbated by pregnancy's reduced functional residual capacity.

Clinical Features

Fever, cough, dyspnea, chest pain, or tachypnea.

Severe cases: Hypoxia, respiratory failure, or sepsis.

Diagnosis

Chest X-ray: Consolidation or infiltrates (low radiation risk with shielding).

Sputum culture, blood cultures, or urinary antigens (S. pneumoniae, Legionella).

Labs: Leukocytosis, elevated CRP, or hypoxemia on arterial blood gas.

Management

Antibiotics: Ceftriaxone (1–2 g IV daily) + azithromycin (500 mg IV daily) for community-acquired pneumonia; vancomycin for MRSA if suspected.

Supportive care: Oxygen therapy, IV fluids; ICU for respiratory failure.

Fetal monitoring: NST or ultrasound for preterm labor or fetal distress.

Complications

Maternal: Respiratory failure, ARDS, or sepsis.

Fetal: Preterm birth, IUGR, or stillbirth (rare).

Prognosis: Good with early treatment; severe cases increase maternal/fetal mortality.

7. Bacterial Vaginosis (BV)

Definition: Overgrowth of anaerobic bacteria in the vagina, not a true infection but associated with adverse pregnancy outcomes, affecting 10–30% of pregnant women.

Etiology

Polymicrobial: Gardnerella vaginalis, Mobiluncus, Bacteroides.

Risk factors: Multiple sexual partners, douching, or smoking.

Pathophysiology: Disruption of vaginal flora (reduced Lactobacillus) increases vaginal pH, promoting anaerobic growth and inflammation, linked to preterm labor.

Clinical Features

Thin, greyish-white vaginal discharge, fishy odor (after KOH whiff test).

Often asymptomatic; detected via screening in high-risk women.

Diagnosis

Amsel criteria (≥3/4): Homogeneous discharge, pH >4.5, positive whiff test, clue cells on wet mount.

Gram stain: Nugent score ≥7 confirms BV.

Management

Symptomatic or high-risk (prior preterm birth):

Metronidazole (500 mg orally twice daily or 250 mg three times daily for 7 days) or clindamycin (300 mg orally twice daily for 7 days).

Avoid vaginal metronidazole gel in first trimester.

Asymptomatic low-risk: Treatment controversial; consider if prior preterm birth.

Follow-up: Repeat testing if symptoms persist.

Complications

Maternal: Increased risk of chorioamnionitis or endometritis.

Fetal: Preterm birth, low birth weight, or PROM.

Prognosis: Good with treatment; reduces preterm birth risk in high-risk women.

Diagnosis of Bacterial Infections

History: Assess for fever, pain, discharge, urinary symptoms, or preterm labor risk factors.

Physical Examination: Check for fever, tachycardia, uterine/flank tenderness, or respiratory signs.

Investigations:

Cultures: Urine (UTI), blood (sepsis, listeriosis), amniotic fluid (chorioamnionitis), vaginal-rectal swab (GBS), or sputum (pneumonia).

Urinalysis: Pyuria, hematuria, or nitrites for UTI; vaginal wet mount for BV.

Labs: CBC (leukocytosis), CRP/ESR, renal/liver function, or blood gas (pneumonia, sepsis).

Imaging: Ultrasound (renal, fetal, or placental), chest X-ray (pneumonia), or MRI/CT (rare, for abscess).

Differential Diagnosis:

Obstetric: Pre-eclampsia, AFLP, or placental abruption.

Non-bacterial: Viral infections (e.g., influenza, CMV), fungal infections, or non-infectious causes (e.g., appendicitis, nephrolithiasis).

Complications

Maternal:

Sepsis, ARDS, or multi-organ failure (pyelonephritis, chorioamnionitis, listeriosis, pneumonia).

Postpartum endometritis, pelvic abscess, or septic thrombophlebitis.

Chronic morbidity (e.g., infertility from endometritis, renal dysfunction from pyelonephritis).

Fetal/Neonatal:

Preterm birth, low birth weight, or PROM (UTI, chorioamnionitis, BV).

Stillbirth or miscarriage (listeriosis, chorioamnionitis).

Neonatal sepsis, pneumonia, or meningitis (GBS, listeriosis).

Long-term neurological sequelae (e.g., cerebral palsy from chorioamnionitis).

Prognosis

UTIs: Excellent with early antibiotic treatment; untreated ASB increases pyelonephritis and preterm birth risk.

Chorioamnionitis: Good with prompt antibiotics and delivery; delayed treatment increases neonatal morbidity.

GBS: Neonatal disease rare (<1%) with IAP; mortality <5% with treatment.

Listeriosis: Maternal recovery good; fetal loss high (20–50%) if early or untreated.

Endometritis: Resolves with antibiotics; complications rare with early treatment.

Pneumonia: Good with timely antibiotics; severe cases increase maternal/fetal mortality.

BV: Treatment reduces preterm birth risk in high-risk women; low-risk asymptomatic cases often resolve spontaneously.

Prevention

Antenatal:

Screening:

Urine culture at 12–16 weeks for ASB.

GBS vaginal-rectal swab at 36–38 weeks.

Screen high-risk women for BV (prior preterm birth).

Vaccinations: Maternal pneumococcal vaccine (pre-pregnancy or postpartum) for high-risk women (e.g., asthma, diabetes).

Hygiene: Educate on perineal hygiene, voiding after intercourse, and avoiding douching to reduce UTI/BV risk.

Preconception:

Treat pre-existing infections (e.g., UTI, BV) before pregnancy.

Optimize chronic conditions (e.g., diabetes) to reduce infection risk.

Lifestyle:

Adequate hydration (2–3 L/day) to prevent UTI and promote urinary flow.

Avoid high-risk foods (e.g., unpasteurized dairy, deli meats) to prevent listeriosis.

Smoking cessation to reduce pneumonia and BV risk.

Intrapartum:

GBS prophylaxis for colonized women or risk factors.

Minimize vaginal exams and monitor for PROM to reduce chorioamnionitis risk.

Public Health

Access to prenatal screening and antibiotics in low-resource settings.

Food safety education to prevent listeriosis (e.g., pasteurization, proper food storage).

Key Points

Bacterial infections in pregnancy include UTIs, chorioamnionitis, GBS, listeriosis, postpartum endometritis, pneumonia, and BV, exacerbated by immune and anatomical changes.

UTIs: ASB requires treatment to prevent pyelonephritis; use nitrofurantoin or cephalexin; pyelonephritis needs IV antibiotics and hospitalization.

Chorioamnionitis: Ascending infection causing preterm labor; treat with broad-spectrum antibiotics.

Parasitic and Protozoal Infestations

Parasitic and protozoal infestations in pregnancy pose unique challenges due to the potential for maternal morbidity, fetal complications, and adverse pregnancy outcomes. The immune modulation of pregnancy, combined with physiological changes, increases susceptibility to certain parasites and alters disease severity. These infections, often transmitted via food, water, vectors, or vertical routes, can lead to miscarriage, preterm birth, congenital anomalies, or neonatal infections. Management requires balancing maternal treatment with fetal safety, using pregnancy-safe antiparasitic agents.

Physiological Changes in Pregnancy Predisposing to Parasitic Infections

Immune Modulation:

Pregnancy shifts immunity toward a T-helper 2 (Th2) response to prevent fetal rejection, reducing Th1-mediated cellular immunity and increasing susceptibility to intracellular parasites (e.g., Toxoplasma gondii, Plasmodium spp.).

Decreased phagocytic activity and altered cytokine profiles impair clearance of certain protozoa.

Hormonal Changes:

Elevated progesterone and estrogen levels may enhance parasite survival by modulating immune responses.

Increased Blood Volume and Hemodynamic Changes:

Increased plasma volume and cardiac output can exacerbate anemia in parasitic infections (e.g., malaria).

Hypercoagulability increases the risk of placental vascular complications in severe infections.

Anatomical Changes:

Gastrointestinal changes (e.g., reduced gastric acidity, slowed motility) increase susceptibility to foodborne parasites (e.g., Toxoplasma, Entamoeba histolytica).

Uterine compression and altered metabolism may influence drug pharmacokinetics, affecting treatment efficacy.

Common Parasitic and Protozoal Infestations in Pregnancy

1. Toxoplasmosis

Definition: Infection caused by Toxoplasma gondii, a protozoan parasite, affecting 0.1–1% of pregnancies in high-prevalence areas.

Etiology

Transmission: Ingestion of undercooked meat containing tissue cysts, contact with cat feces containing oocysts, or contaminated water/soil; rarely transplacental (congenital toxoplasmosis).

Risk factors: Exposure to cats, raw meat consumption, or living in endemic areas (e.g., South America, Europe).

Pathophysiology

Acute infection in immunocompetent women is often asymptomatic or mild; tachyzoites invade tissues, including the placenta.

Transplacental transmission (10–50% risk, higher in third trimester) causes congenital toxoplasmosis, with severity greatest in early pregnancy.

Clinical Features

Maternal: Asymptomatic (60–80%) or flu-like symptoms (fever, myalgia, lymphadenopathy); rarely severe (e.g., encephalitis in immunocompromised).

Fetal/Neonatal: Congenital toxoplasmosis (classic triad: chorioretinitis, hydrocephalus, intracranial calcifications), growth restriction, hepatosplenomegaly, or jaundice.

Diagnosis

Maternal: Serology: IgG (past infection), IgM (acute infection), or IgG avidity (low avidity indicates recent infection).

PCR: Detects Toxoplasma DNA in blood or amniotic fluid (confirms active infection).

Fetal: Amniocentesis (PCR for Toxoplasma DNA after 18 weeks); ultrasound for hydrocephalus, calcifications, or growth restriction.

Neonatal: Cord blood serology, PCR, or ophthalmologic/neurologic evaluation.

Management

Maternal:

Acute infection: Spiramycin (1 g orally three times daily, safe in pregnancy) to reduce placental transmission; does not cross placenta.

Confirmed fetal infection: Pyrimethamine (25–50 mg daily) + sulfadiazine (2–4 g daily) + folinic acid (10–20 mg daily) after first trimester to treat fetal infection; avoid pyrimethamine in first trimester (teratogenic).

Fetal monitoring: Serial ultrasound every 2–4 weeks for anomalies or growth restriction.

Delivery: Vaginal delivery unless obstetric indications; no specific timing unless fetal compromise.

Neonatal: Treat congenital toxoplasmosis with pyrimethamine, sulfadiazine, and folinic acid for 12 months; monitor for chorioretinitis or neurologic sequelae.

Complications

Maternal: Rare (e.g., encephalitis in immunocompromised).

Fetal/Neonatal: Miscarriage, stillbirth, preterm birth, or congenital toxoplasmosis (10–30% of infected fetuses; severe in first trimester).

Prognosis: Maternal recovery good; congenital infection outcomes depend on gestational age at infection (worse in early pregnancy); treatment reduces severity.

2. Malaria

Definition: Infection caused by Plasmodium spp. (P. falciparum, P. vivax, P. ovale, P. malariae), transmitted by Anopheles mosquitoes, affecting pregnant women in endemic areas (e.g., sub-Saharan Africa, Southeast Asia).

Incidence: 10–25% of pregnant women in endemic areas; P. falciparum most severe.

Etiology

Transmission: Mosquito bites; rarely congenital or transfusion-related.

Risk factors: Primigravida, young maternal age, or lack of immunity in endemic areas.

Pathophysiology:

P. falciparum sequesters in the placenta via chondroitin sulfate A binding, causing placental malaria, reduced placental blood flow, and fetal hypoxia.

Increased parasitemia in pregnancy due to immune suppression.

Clinical Features

Maternal: Fever, chills, headache, myalgia, anemia; severe malaria (P. falciparum): Hypoglycemia, renal failure, pulmonary edema, or cerebral malaria.

Fetal: Intrauterine growth restriction (IUGR), preterm birth, or stillbirth.

Diagnosis

Microscopy: Giemsa-stained thick/thin blood smears to identify Plasmodium species and parasitemia level.

Rapid diagnostic tests (RDTs): Detect Plasmodium antigens; useful in resource-limited settings.

PCR: Highly sensitive for low parasitemia; not routinely available.

Labs: Anemia (hemoglobin <10 g/dL), thrombocytopenia, or elevated lactate dehydrogenase (LDH).

Ultrasound: Assess for IUGR or placental abnormalities.

Management

Uncomplicated malaria:

First trimester: Quinine (10 mg/kg three times daily) + clindamycin (300 mg four times daily) for 7 days.

Second/third trimester: Artemisinin-based combination therapy (ACT, e.g., artemether-lumefantrine) preferred; safe after first trimester.

Severe malaria:

IV artesunate (2.4 mg/kg at 0, 12, 24 hours, then daily) until oral therapy tolerated; quinine IV if artesunate unavailable.

Supportive care: IV fluids, glucose for hypoglycemia, oxygen for respiratory distress, or blood transfusion for severe anemia.

Fetal monitoring: NST or ultrasound for IUGR or fetal distress; deliver early if severe maternal/fetal compromise.

Neonatal: Screen for congenital malaria (rare, <5%); treat with chloroquine or ACT.

Complications

Maternal: Severe anemia, acute respiratory distress syndrome (ARDS), renal failure, cerebral malaria, or death (5–20% in severe P. falciparum).

Fetal: Miscarriage, preterm birth, IUGR, stillbirth, or congenital malaria.

Prognosis: Good with prompt treatment; untreated severe malaria has high maternal/fetal mortality.

3. Chagas Disease (American Trypanosomiasis)

Definition: Chronic infection caused by Trypanosoma cruzi, a protozoan parasite, affecting 1–10% of pregnant women in endemic areas (Latin America).

Etiology

Transmission: Vector-borne (triatomine bugs), congenital (5–10% of infected mothers), blood transfusion, or contaminated food.

Risk factors: Living in endemic areas, poor housing conditions, or maternal chronic infection.

Pathophysiology

Acute infection: Trypomastigotes invade tissues, causing fever or lymphadenopathy (rare in pregnancy).

Chronic infection: Asymptomatic or cardiac/gastrointestinal involvement; transplacental transmission causes congenital Chagas disease.

Clinical Features

Maternal: Usually asymptomatic (chronic phase); acute infection (rare) presents with fever, hepatosplenomegaly, or myocarditis.

Fetal/Neonatal: Congenital Chagas (preterm birth, IUGR, hepatosplenomegaly, anemia, or myocarditis).

Diagnosis

Maternal:Serology: IgG for chronic infection; IgM or PCR for acute infection. Microscopy or PCR: Detects trypomastigotes in blood (acute phase).

Fetal/Neonatal: Cord blood PCR, serology, or microscopy; repeat serology at 6–12 months to confirm congenital infection.

Management

Maternal: Avoid treatment in pregnancy (benznidazole, nifurtimox teratogenic); treat postpartum to reduce future congenital transmission.

Neonatal: Benznidazole (5–7 mg/kg/day for 60 days) or nifurtimox for confirmed congenital infection.

Fetal monitoring: Ultrasound for IUGR or fetal anomalies.

Delivery: Vaginal delivery unless obstetric indications.

Complications

Maternal: Cardiomyopathy or megacolon (chronic phase, rare in pregnancy).

Fetal/Neonatal: Preterm birth, IUGR, or congenital infection (5–10% risk).

Prognosis: Maternal prognosis depends on chronic disease stage; congenital infection treatable with good outcomes if diagnosed early.

4. Amoebiasis

Definition: Infection caused by Entamoeba histolytica, a protozoan parasite, rare in pregnancy but significant in endemic areas (e.g., Africa, Asia, Latin America).

Etiology

Transmission: Fecal-oral route via contaminated water/food.

Risk factors: Poor sanitation, travel to endemic areas, or crowding.

Pathophysiology:

Cysts ingested transform into trophozoites, invading intestinal mucosa, causing dysentery or extraintestinal spread (e.g., liver abscess).

Congenital transmission rare; maternal complications impact pregnancy.

Clinical Features

Maternal: Asymptomatic (most cases) or dysentery (bloody diarrhea, abdominal pain, fever); liver abscess (right upper quadrant pain, fever, hepatomegaly).

Fetal: No direct congenital infection; preterm labor or IUGR from severe maternal illness.

Diagnosis

Stool microscopy or antigen detection: Detects E. histolytica cysts/trophozoites.

PCR: Confirms infection in stool or abscess aspirate.

Serology: Positive in invasive disease (e.g., liver abscess).

Ultrasound: For liver abscess (hypoechoic lesion).

Management

Asymptomatic: Paromomycin (25–35 mg/kg/day orally for 7 days, safe in pregnancy).

Invasive (dysentery, liver abscess): Metronidazole (500–750 mg orally three times daily for 7–10 days, safe after first trimester) followed by paromomycin to eliminate cysts.

Fetal monitoring: Ultrasound if preterm labor or IUGR suspected.

Complications

Maternal: Liver abscess, colonic perforation, or sepsis (rare).

Fetal: Preterm birth or IUGR from maternal illness.

Prognosis: Good with treatment; untreated invasive disease increases maternal/fetal morbidity.

5. Hookworm and Other Helminths

Definition: Soil-transmitted helminths (Ancylostoma duodenale, Necator americanus) causing intestinal infection, affecting 20–30% of pregnant women in endemic areas (e.g., sub-Saharan Africa, Asia).

Etiology

Transmission: Skin penetration by larvae in contaminated soil; fecal-oral for other helminths (e.g., Ascaris, Trichuris).

Risk factors: Barefoot walking, poor sanitation, or malnutrition.

Pathophysiology:

Hookworms attach to intestinal mucosa, causing blood loss and anemia.

Maternal anemia exacerbates pregnancy-related anemia, increasing fetal risks.

Clinical Features

Maternal: Asymptomatic or fatigue, pallor, abdominal pain; severe cases: Anemia (hemoglobin <10 g/dL), malnutrition.

Fetal: IUGR, preterm birth, or low birth weight from maternal anemia.

Diagnosis

Stool microscopy: Detects hookworm eggs; Kato-Katz technique for worm burden.

Labs: Eosinophilia, anemia (microcytic, hypochromic).

Management

Anthelmintics: Albendazole (400 mg single dose) or mebendazole (100 mg twice daily for 3 days) after first trimester; safe in pregnancy.

Supportive care: Iron supplementation (60–120 mg daily) and folate for anemia.

Fetal monitoring: Ultrasound for IUGR.

Complications

Maternal: Severe anemia, heart failure, or malnutrition.

Fetal: Preterm birth, IUGR, or stillbirth (rare).

Prognosis: Excellent with treatment; untreated anemia increases maternal/fetal risks.

6. Other Parasitic Infections

Schistosomiasis

Caused by Schistosoma spp.; transmitted via freshwater snails in endemic areas.

Maternal: Hematuria, dysuria, or chronic liver/bladder damage; rare congenital transmission.

Diagnosis: Stool/urine microscopy, serology, or PCR.

Management: Praziquantel (40 mg/kg single dose) after first trimester; safe in pregnancy.

Complications: Anemia, IUGR, or preterm birth.

Leishmaniasis

Caused by Leishmania spp.; visceral (kala-azar) form severe in pregnancy.

Maternal: Fever, hepatosplenomegaly, pancytopenia.

Diagnosis: PCR, serology, or tissue biopsy.

Management: Liposomal amphotericin B (3–5 mg/kg/day for 7–10 days); avoid miltefosine (teratogenic).

Complications: Miscarriage, stillbirth, or congenital leishmaniasis (rare).

Giardiasis

Caused by Giardia lamblia; fecal-oral transmission.

Maternal: Diarrhea, malabsorption, weight loss.

Diagnosis: Stool antigen or microscopy.

Management: Metronidazole (500 mg twice daily for 5–7 days) after first trimester.

Complications: IUGR or preterm birth from maternal malnutrition.

Diagnosis of Parasitic and Protozoal Infestations

History: Assess for fever, diarrhea, travel to endemic areas, food exposure (e.g., raw meat, unpasteurized dairy), or environmental risks (e.g., cats, soil contact).

Physical Examination: Check for fever, pallor, hepatosplenomegaly, lymphadenopathy, or jaundice.

Investigations:

Microscopy: Stool (hookworm, amoebiasis), blood smears (malaria), or amniotic fluid (toxoplasmosis).

Serology: IgG/IgM for toxoplasmosis, Chagas, or leishmaniasis.

PCR: Detects parasite DNA in blood, amniotic fluid, or tissue (toxoplasmosis, malaria, Chagas).

Antigen tests: Rapid tests for malaria or Giardia.

Labs: Anemia, eosinophilia (helminths), or elevated liver enzymes (amoebiasis, malaria).

Imaging: Ultrasound for fetal anomalies (toxoplasmosis), placental changes (malaria), or liver abscess (amoebiasis).

Differential Diagnosis

Obstetric: Pre-eclampsia, acute fatty liver of pregnancy (AFLP), or chorioamnionitis.

Non-parasitic: Viral hepatitis, bacterial infections (e.g., Listeria), or gastroenteritis.

Complications

Maternal:

Anemia (malaria, hookworm), malnutrition (helminths, giardiasis), or organ failure (severe malaria, amoebiasis).

Sepsis or multi-organ dysfunction (severe malaria, leishmaniasis).

Fetal/Neonatal:

Miscarriage, stillbirth, or preterm birth (toxoplasmosis, malaria, Chagas).

IUGR or low birth weight (malaria, hookworm).

Congenital infections (toxoplasmosis, Chagas, leishmaniasis) with long-term sequelae (e.g., chorioretinitis, cardiomyopathy).

Prognosis

Toxoplasmosis: Maternal recovery good; congenital infection severe if untreated, especially in early pregnancy.

Malaria: Good with prompt treatment; untreated P. falciparum has high maternal/fetal mortality.

Chagas: Chronic maternal disease stable; congenital infection treatable if diagnosed early.

Amoebiasis: Resolves with treatment; untreated invasive disease increases morbidity.

Helminths: Excellent with anthelmintics and iron supplementation; untreated anemia worsens outcomes.

Leishmaniasis/Giardiasis: Good with appropriate therapy; untreated visceral leishmaniasis has high mortality.

Prevention

Antenatal Screening: Routine toxoplasmosis serology in high-risk areas; malaria testing in endemic regions.

Prophylaxis: Intermittent preventive treatment for malaria (IPTp) with sulfadoxine-pyrimethamine (three doses after first trimester) in endemic areas.

Education: Avoid raw/undercooked meat (toxoplasmosis), contaminated water/food (amoebiasis, giardiasis), or soil contact (hookworm).

Preconception: Screen and treat chronic infections (e.g., Chagas, schistosomiasis) to reduce congenital transmission. Optimize nutrition and anemia management (hookworm).

Lifestyle:

Use insecticide-treated bed nets and repellents in malaria-endemic areas.

Practice food safety: Cook meat thoroughly, avoid unpasteurized dairy, and wash produce.

Wear shoes in endemic areas to prevent hookworm.

Public Health:

Improve sanitation and water quality to reduce amoebiasis, giardiasis, and helminths.

Vector control (mosquitoes for malaria, triatomine bugs for Chagas).

Access to prenatal care and antiparasitic drugs in low-resource settings.

Key Points

Toxoplasmosis: Foodborne or cat-related; congenital infection causes chorioretinitis, hydrocephalus; treat with spiramycin or pyrimethamine/sulfadiazine.

Malaria: P. falciparum severe; causes placental malaria, IUGR; treat with quinine (first trimester) or ACT (second/third trimester).

Chagas: Chronic infection; congenital transmission (5–10%); treat neonates, defer maternal treatment to postpartum.

Amoebiasis: Dysentery or liver abscess; metronidazole safe after first trimester.

Hookworm: Causes anemia; albendazole safe after first trimester.

Diagnosis: Relies on serology, PCR, microscopy, or antigen tests; ultrasound for fetal monitoring.

Complications: Preterm birth, IUGR, stillbirth, or congenital infections; severe maternal disease (malaria, leishmaniasis) increases mortality.

Prevention: Screening, prophylaxis (malaria), food safety, vector control, and sanitation reduce infection burden.

8.11 Gynecological Disorders in Pregnancy

(*Daurane Haml lahaq hone wale Niswani Amrad*)

Introduction

Gynecological disorders in pregnancy encompass a range of conditions affecting the female reproductive system, including pre-existing gynecological conditions, pregnancy-specific complications, and new-onset disorders. These disorders can significantly impact maternal and fetal health, often complicated by the physiological and anatomical changes of pregnancy. Effective management requires a multidisciplinary approach, balancing maternal treatment with fetal safety, and careful consideration of diagnostic and therapeutic interventions.

Physiological and Anatomical Changes in Pregnancy

Hormonal Changes

Elevated estrogen and progesterone levels promote endometrial growth, cervical softening (Goodell's sign), and increased vaginal discharge, but may exacerbate pre-existing conditions like fibroids or endometriosis.

Human chorionic gonadotropin (hCG) supports pregnancy but can stimulate ovarian cysts or trophoblastic disease.

Anatomical Changes

Uterine enlargement: The gravid uterus compresses pelvic structures, potentially exacerbating prolapse, fibroid symptoms, or adnexal masses.

Cervical changes: Increased vascularity and softening (Hegar's sign) may increase bleeding risk from cervical lesions.

Vascular changes: Increased pelvic blood flow and venous stasis predispose to varicosities or hemorrhage from gynecological lesions.

Immune Modulation

Shift to a Th2-dominated immune response reduces inflammation, potentially masking symptoms of chronic gynecological conditions (e.g., endometriosis) or increasing susceptibility to infections (e.g., bacterial vaginosis).

Coagulation Changes

Hypercoagulable state increases risk of thromboembolism associated with pelvic masses or surgical interventions.

Common Gynecological Disorders in Pregnancy

1. Uterine Fibroids (Leiomyomas)

Definition: Benign smooth muscle tumors of the uterus, present in 2–10% of pregnant women, often asymptomatic but potentially complicating pregnancy.

Etiology

Pre-existing fibroids; estrogen and progesterone stimulate growth during pregnancy.

Risk factors: Advanced maternal age, African descent, obesity, or nulliparity.

Pathophysiology

Fibroids may grow in the first trimester due to hormonal stimulation, causing pain, pressure, or mechanical obstruction.

Degeneration (red/carneous degeneration) occurs due to outgrown blood supply, leading to necrosis and pain.

Clinical Features

Asymptomatic (most cases) or pelvic pain, pressure, or vaginal bleeding.

Complications: Preterm labor, malpresentation, or placental abruption (submucosal fibroids).

Diagnosis

Ultrasound: First-line; identifies fibroid size, location (submucosal, intramural, subserosal), and degeneration (heterogeneous echotexture).

MRI: Rarely needed for complex cases or to differentiate from other masses (e.g., ovarian tumors).

Labs: Monitor for anemia (bleeding) or infection (degeneration).

Management

Asymptomatic: Observation with serial ultrasound to monitor fibroid growth and fetal status.

Symptomatic (pain, degeneration)

Conservative: Analgesics (acetaminophen, opioids if severe), hydration, and rest.

Hospitalization for severe pain, fever, or preterm labor risk.

Tocolytics (e.g., nifedipine) if preterm contractions occur.

Surgical: Myomectomy rarely performed in pregnancy due to bleeding risk; reserved for torsion of pedunculated fibroids or intractable pain.

Delivery: Vaginal delivery preferred; cesarean if fibroids obstruct the birth canal (e.g., cervical fibroids) or cause malpresentation.

Fetal monitoring: Ultrasound for growth restriction or malpresentation; non-stress test (NST) if preterm labor suspected.

Complications

Maternal: Pain, preterm labor, placental abruption, or postpartum hemorrhage (PPH).

Fetal: Preterm birth, intrauterine growth restriction (IUGR), or malpresentation.

Prognosis: Most fibroids remain asymptomatic; complications rare with monitoring; fibroids often regress postpartum.

2. Ovarian Cysts and Masses

Definition: Benign or malignant adnexal masses, including functional cysts, dermoids, or rarely ovarian cancer, found in 1–4% of pregnancies.

Etiology

Functional cysts: Corpus luteum cysts or follicular cysts (common in first trimester due to hCG stimulation).

Benign tumors: Dermoid cysts (teratomas), cystadenomas.

Malignant: Rare (1:10,000–50,000 pregnancies); includes germ cell tumors or epithelial ovarian cancer.

Risk factors: Advanced maternal age, history of ovarian cysts, or infertility treatment.

Pathophysiology

Cysts may grow due to hormonal stimulation, cause pain (rupture, torsion), or compress pelvic structures.

Malignant masses may metastasize, complicating pregnancy management.

Clinical Features

Asymptomatic (most functional cysts) or pelvic pain, pressure, or acute abdomen (torsion, rupture).

Malignant masses: Abdominal distension, weight loss, or ascites (rare).

Diagnosis

Ultrasound: First-line; distinguishes simple cysts (functional) from complex masses (dermoids, malignancy); features of malignancy include solid components, septations, or ascites.

MRI: For complex masses or suspected malignancy (avoid gadolinium).

Tumor markers: CA-125 mildly elevated in pregnancy (normal <35 U/mL); avoid as sole diagnostic tool.

Laparoscopy/Laparotomy: Diagnostic if imaging inconclusive or malignancy suspected.

Management

Asymptomatic simple cysts (<6 cm): Observation; most resolve by 16–20 weeks.

Symptomatic or large cysts (>6 cm)

Conservative: Analgesics, monitor with ultrasound.

Surgical: Laparoscopy (second trimester preferred) or laparotomy for torsion, rupture, or suspected malignancy.

Malignant masses: Multidisciplinary management; surgery (oophorectomy, staging) in second trimester or postpartum; chemotherapy (e.g., carboplatin) safe after first trimester.

Delivery: Vaginal delivery unless mass obstructs pelvis; cesarean for large masses or malignancy.

Fetal monitoring: Ultrasound for growth or anomalies; NST if preterm labor risk.

Complications

Maternal: Torsion, rupture, hemorrhage, or malignancy.

Fetal: Preterm birth, IUGR, or fetal distress (rare).

Prognosis: Excellent for benign cysts; malignant masses require aggressive management; functional cysts often resolve spontaneously.

3. Cervical Disorders

Definition: Includes cervical incompetence, cervical polyps, or rarely cervical cancer, which can complicate pregnancy.

Etiology

Cervical incompetence: Weakened cervix leading to painless dilation and preterm birth; risk factors include prior cervical surgery (e.g., cone biopsy), trauma, or congenital anomalies.

Cervical polyps: Benign growths due to increased vascularity; may cause bleeding.

Cervical cancer: Rare (1:2,000–10,000 pregnancies); associated with HPV, smoking, or immunosuppression.

Pathophysiology

Cervical incompetence: Inadequate cervical strength leads to premature dilation, PROM, or preterm labor.

Polyps: Increased estrogen causes hyperplastic growth, leading to bleeding or irritation.

Cervical cancer: HPV-driven dysplasia progresses to invasive carcinoma, potentially spreading to lymph nodes or placenta.

Clinical Features

Cervical incompetence: Painless cervical dilation, vaginal pressure, or preterm labor (second trimester).

Cervical polyps: Spotting, postcoital bleeding, or visible mass on speculum exam.

Cervical cancer: Abnormal vaginal bleeding, discharge, pelvic pain, or palpable cervical mass.

Diagnosis

Cervical incompetence: Transvaginal ultrasound (cervical length <25 mm before 24 weeks or funneling); history of prior preterm birth.

Cervical polyps: Speculum exam; biopsy if atypical features.

Cervical cancer: Pap smear (routine screening at first prenatal visit), colposcopy with biopsy if abnormal; MRI for staging.

Management

i. Cervical incompetence

Prophylactic cerclage (12–14 weeks) for prior preterm birth or short cervix (<25 mm).

Emergency cerclage for painless dilation before viability (controversial).

Vaginal progesterone (200 mg daily) for short cervix without dilation.

Monitor with ultrasound every 1–2 weeks; restrict activity if high risk.

ii. Cervical polyps: Observation if asymptomatic; polypectomy for persistent bleeding (safe in pregnancy).

iii. Cervical cancer

Early stage (IA–IB1): Cone biopsy or trachelectomy in second trimester; delay definitive treatment (hysterectomy) to postpartum.

Advanced stage (IB2–IV): Chemotherapy (e.g., cisplatin) after first trimester; radiation avoided (fetal harm).

Delivery: Cesarean preferred to avoid tumor bleeding; timing based on stage and gestational age.

Fetal monitoring: Ultrasound for preterm labor (cervical incompetence) or growth restriction (cancer).

Complications

Maternal: Preterm labor, bleeding, or cancer progression.

Fetal: Preterm birth, IUGR, or stillbirth (cancer or severe preterm labor).

Prognosis: Good for incompetence with cerclage/progesterone; polyps benign; cervical cancer outcomes depend on stage and treatment timing.

4. Endometriosis

Definition: Presence of endometrial tissue outside the uterus, affecting 0.5–5% of pregnant women with pre-existing disease, often improved by pregnancy.

Etiology

Pre-existing endometriosis; pregnancy hormones (progesterone) typically suppress disease activity.

Risk factors: Nulliparity, infertility, or prior endometriosis diagnosis.

Pathophysiology

Progesterone inhibits endometrial proliferation, reducing symptoms; however, endometriomas or adhesions may persist or cause complications.

Rarely, endometriomas rupture or cause pain due to mass effect.

Clinical Features

Asymptomatic in most pregnant women; persistent pelvic pain, dyspareunia, or mass effect (endometrioma).

Rare complications: Rupture, infection, or obstruction.

Diagnosis

Ultrasound: Identifies endometriomas (cystic masses with ground-glass appearance).

MRI: For complex masses or suspected adhesions (avoid gadolinium).

History: Prior endometriosis diagnosis or infertility.

Management

Asymptomatic: Observation; monitor endometrioma size with ultrasound.

Symptomatic: Analgesics (acetaminophen); surgery (laparoscopy) rarely needed for rupture or torsion.

Delivery: Vaginal delivery unless adhesions or masses obstruct pelvis.

Fetal monitoring: Ultrasound for growth or preterm labor risk.

Complications

Maternal: Pain, endometrioma rupture, or infertility recurrence postpartum.

Fetal: Preterm birth or IUGR (rare, with severe disease).

Prognosis: Symptoms often improve in pregnancy; recurrence common postpartum.

5. Bacterial Vaginosis (BV)

Definition: A polymicrobial vaginal dysbiosis, not a true infection but associated with adverse pregnancy outcomes, affecting 10–30% of pregnant women.

Etiology

Overgrowth of anaerobic bacteria (Gardnerella vaginalis, Mobiluncus, Bacteroides) with reduced Lactobacillus.

Risk factors: Multiple sexual partners, douching, smoking, or African descent.

Pathophysiology

Altered vaginal flora increases pH (>4.5), promoting inflammation and cytokine release, which may trigger preterm labor or PROM.

Clinical Features

Thin, grayish-white vaginal discharge with fishy odor (after KOH whiff test).

Often asymptomatic; detected via screening in high-risk women (e.g., prior preterm birth).

Diagnosis

Amsel criteria (≥3/4): Homogeneous discharge, pH >4.5, positive whiff test, clue cells on wet mount.

Gram stain: Nugent score ≥7 confirms BV.

Culture: Not routinely needed.

Management

Symptomatic or high-risk (prior preterm birth)

Metronidazole (500 mg orally twice daily or 250 mg three times daily for 7 days) or clindamycin (300 mg orally twice daily for 7 days).

Avoid vaginal metronidazole gel in first trimester.

Asymptomatic low-risk: Treatment controversial; consider if prior preterm birth.

Follow-up: Repeat testing if symptoms persist.

Delivery: Vaginal delivery unless obstetric indications.

Complications

Maternal: Chorioamnionitis, postpartum endometritis, or preterm labor.

Fetal: Preterm birth, low birth weight, or PROM.

Prognosis: Good with treatment; reduces preterm birth risk in high-risk women.

6. Gestational Trophoblastic Disease (GTD)

Definition: A spectrum of disorders from abnormal trophoblastic proliferation, including hydatidiform mole (complete/partial), invasive mole, choriocarcinoma, or placental-site trophoblastic tumor, rare in pregnancy.

Etiology

Abnormal fertilization leading to excess paternal chromosomes (complete mole: 46,XX, paternal origin; partial mole: triploidy).

Risk factors: Extremes of maternal age (<20 or >35), prior GTD, or Asian descent.

Pathophysiology

Abnormal trophoblast growth forms cystic placental tissue (mole) or invasive tumors, producing high hCG levels.

Can metastasize (choriocarcinoma) or persist post-evacuation (invasive mole).

Clinical Features

Vaginal bleeding (first trimester), hyperemesis, uterine size larger than gestational age, or theca lutein cysts.

Choriocarcinoma: Irregular bleeding, respiratory symptoms (lung metastases), or neurological signs (brain metastases).

Diagnosis

Ultrasound: Snowstorm appearance (complete mole), cystic spaces (partial mole), or invasive mass.

Labs: Elevated hCG (>100,000 mIU/mL in mole), anemia, or thyroid function abnormalities (hCG mimics TSH).

Histopathology: Post-evacuation to confirm GTD type.

Metastatic workup: Chest X-ray, CT/MRI (if choriocarcinoma suspected).

Management

i. Hydatidiform mole

Suction curettage (first-line); hysterectomy for women not desiring fertility.

Monitor hCG weekly until undetectable for 6 months to rule out persistent GTD.

ii. Invasive mole/choriocarcinoma

Chemotherapy (methotrexate or dactinomycin) for non-metastatic disease; multi-agent (EMA-CO regimen) for metastatic disease.

Safe after first trimester if pregnancy continuation desired (rare); usually managed postpartum.

Delivery: Cesarean if invasive disease or obstetric indications.

Fetal monitoring: Ultrasound for anomalies or growth restriction (partial mole).

Complications

Maternal: Hemorrhage, preeclampsia (before 24 weeks), thyrotoxicosis, or metastatic disease.

Fetal: Miscarriage, preterm birth, or fetal anomalies (partial mole).

Prognosis: Excellent for hydatidiform mole with curettage; choriocarcinoma curable with chemotherapy (>90% survival).

Diagnosis of Gynecological Disorders

History: Assess for vaginal bleeding, pelvic pain, pressure, discharge, or history of gynecological conditions (e.g., fibroids, endometriosis).

Physical Examination: Speculum exam for cervical lesions or discharge; bimanual exam for uterine/ adnexal masses or tenderness.

Investigations

Ultrasound: First-line for fibroids, ovarian cysts, cervical incompetence, or GTD; transvaginal for cervical length or adnexal masses.

MRI: For complex masses or suspected malignancy (avoid gadolinium).

Labs: hCG (GTD), hemoglobin (bleeding), or tumor markers (CA-125, limited use in pregnancy).

Cervical screening: Pap smear, colposcopy, or biopsy for suspected cervical cancer.

Microscopy: Wet mount or Gram stain for BV.

Differential Diagnosis

Obstetric: Ectopic pregnancy, miscarriage, or placental abruption.

Non-gynecological: Appendicitis, nephrolithiasis, or gastroenteritis.

Complications

Maternal

Preterm labor, PROM, or PPH (fibroids, cervical incompetence, BV).

Hemorrhage or infection (ovarian cysts, polyps, GTD).

Malignancy progression (cervical cancer, GTD).

Fetal

Preterm birth, IUGR, or stillbirth (fibroids, BV, GTD).

Congenital anomalies (partial mole, cervical cancer treatment).

Fetal distress from maternal instability (e.g., hemorrhage, malignancy). Prognosis

Fibroids: Most asymptomatic; complications rare with monitoring;

regression postpartum.

Ovarian cysts: Functional cysts resolve spontaneously; benign tumors manageable; malignancy rare but serious.

Cervical cancer: Early-stage treatable with good outcomes; advanced stages challenging.

Endometriosis: Symptoms improve in pregnancy; recurrence common postpartum.

BV: Treatment reduces preterm birth risk; low-risk cases often resolve.

GTD: Hydatidiform mole curable; choriocarcinoma highly treatable with chemotherapy.

Prevention

Antenatal

Routine cervical length screening (transvaginal ultrasound) at 18–24 weeks for high-risk women (prior preterm birth).

Pap smear at first prenatal visit to detect cervical abnormalities.

Screen for BV in high-risk women (prior preterm birth).

Monitor pre-existing fibroids or endometriosis with ultrasound.

Preconception

Optimize gynecological conditions: Myomectomy for large fibroids, endometriosis treatment, or cervical dysplasia management.

HPV vaccination (pre-pregnancy) to reduce cervical cancer risk.

Counsel on pregnancy risks in women with known gynecological disorders.

Lifestyle

Avoid douching or multiple sexual partners to reduce BV risk.

Maintain healthy weight to minimize fibroid growth.

Public Health

Access to prenatal screening and HPV vaccination programs.

Education on BV prevention and early reporting of abnormal bleeding or pain.

Key Points

Gynecological disorders in pregnancy include uterine fibroids, ovarian cysts, cervical disorders, endometriosis, BV, and GTD, influenced by hormonal and anatomical changes.

Fibroids: Often asymptomatic; degeneration causes pain; monitor with ultrasound, rarely need surgery.

Ovarian cysts: Functional cysts resolve; surgery for torsion or malignancy; malignancy rare.

Cervical incompetence: Short cervix (<25 mm); cerclage or progesterone prevents preterm birth.

Cervical cancer: Rare; early-stage managed conservatively, advanced requires chemotherapy or postpartum surgery.

Endometriosis: Symptoms improve in pregnancy; endometriomas may cause pain or rupture.

BV: Associated with preterm birth; treat high-risk or symptomatic cases with metronidazole.

GTD: Hydatidiform mole treated with curettage; choriocarcinoma requires chemotherapy.

Diagnosis: Relies on ultrasound, MRI, Pap smear, or hCG; avoid teratogenic interventions.

Complications: Preterm birth, IUGR, hemorrhage, or malignancy progression; timely management improves outcomes.

Prevention: Screening (cervical length, Pap smear, BV), preconception optimization, and lifestyle measures reduce risks

Long Answer Questions (LAQs)

1. Describe emesis gravidarum and hyperemesis gravidarum with causes, complications, and management.
2. Discuss diabetes mellitus in pregnancy including GDM, its diagnosis, complications, and management.
3. Explain hypertensive disorders in pregnancy and their effects on mother and fetus.
4. Describe anemia in pregnancy with types, causes, clinical features, and management.
5. Discuss infections in pregnancy and their maternal and fetal consequences.

Short Answer Questions (SAQs)

1. Define hyperemesis gravidarum.
2. What is gestational diabetes mellitus?
3. Mention causes of anemia in pregnancy.
4. List common infections during pregnancy.
5. What is Rh isoimmunization?

Multiple Choice Questions (1 Mark Each)

1. Hyperemesis gravidarum most commonly occurs in:

A. Second trimester B. Third trimester

C. First trimester D. Postpartum period

Answer: C

2. Hormone mainly responsible for hyperemesis gravidarum is:

A. Progesterone B. Estrogen

C. hCG D. Oxytocin

Answer: C

3. Most common anemia in pregnancy is:

A. Megaloblastic anemia B. Aplastic anemia

C. Iron deficiency anemia D. Hemolytic anemia

Answer: C

4. Gestational diabetes mellitus is diagnosed usually by:

A. Fasting blood sugar B. Random blood sugar

C. Oral glucose tolerance test (OGTT) D. HbA1c

Answer: C

5. Most common complication of diabetes in pregnancy is:

A. IUGR B. Preterm labor

C. Macrosomia D. Congenital infection

Answer: C

6. Rh isoimmunization occurs when:

A. Rh positive mother, Rh negative fetus B. Rh positive mother, Rh positive fetus

C. Rh negative mother, Rh positive fetus D. Rh negative mother, Rh negative fetus

Answer: C

7. Most common thyroid disorder in pregnancy is:

A. Hypothyroidism B. Hyperthyroidism

C. Thyroiditis D. Subclinical hypothyroidism

Answer: D

8. Most common urinary tract infection organism in pregnancy is:

A. Staphylococcus B. Klebsiella

C. Proteus D. Escherichia coli

Answer: D

9. Viral infection most commonly causing congenital anomalies is:

A. HIV B. Hepatitis B

C. Rubella D. Influenza

Answer: C

10. Severe vomiting in pregnancy may lead to deficiency of:

A. Vitamin A B. Vitamin D

C. Vitamin B1 (Thiamine) D. Vitamin K

Answer:

09

Obstetrical Hemorrhage

(Nazf-al-Tauliid)

9.1 *Isqat* (Abortion)
9.2 *Qwaneen -i-isqat-i-Tibbi* (MTP Act)
9.3 *Haml Kharij-al-Rahin* (Ectopic Pregnancy)
9.4 *Daul-aroma ghaziyah Hamli* (Gestational Trophoblastic Disease)
9.5 *Jiryan-al-Dam qabl-i-Wiladat* (Ante partum Hemorrhage)
9.6 *Jiryan-al-Dam bad-i-Wiladat* (Post partum hemorrhage)

Learning Objective (At the end of the session, the students should be able to)

Define *Isqat* (Abortion) & describe its causes, diagnosis, management, and complications and enlist the methods of Induction of abortion and causes of Recurrent Abortion
Explain the MTP Act
Observe and describe MTP procedure
Review the sample Abortion consent.
Describe *Hamal Kharij Ur Reham* (Ectopic Pregnancy) and its classification, etiology, diagnosis & complications
Identify Gestational Trophoblastic Diseases & briefly explain its pathophysiology, diagnosis & complications
Define *Jiryan-Ud-Dam Qabl Wiladat* (Ante Partum Hemorrhage) and discuss the etiology, diagnosis & complications of Placenta Previa and Abruptio placentae
Elaborate the types, causes, and complications of *Jiryan-Ud- Dam Bad Azwiladat* (Post Partum Hemorrhage)

9.1 Abortion

(*Isqat*)

Definition

Abortion is the termination of a pregnancy before the fetus reaches viability, typically defined as before 24–28 weeks of gestation or a fetal weight less than 500 grams, depending on regional guidelines. It may occur spontaneously (miscarriage) or be induced for medical, therapeutic, or elective reasons. The World Health Organization (WHO) defines abortion as the expulsion or extraction of a fetus or embryo from the uterus before it can survive independently.

Classification of Abortion

Abortions are classified based on etiology, timing and method:

1. Spontaneous Abortion (Miscarriage):

Occurs naturally without medical or surgical intervention.

Incidence: Approximately 10–20% of confirmed pregnancies end in spontaneous abortion, with most occurring in the first trimester.

Risk factors: Chromosomal abnormalities (50–60% of cases), maternal age (>35 years), endocrine disorders (e.g., diabetes, hypothyroidism), infections, uterine anomalies, and lifestyle factors (e.g., smoking, alcohol).

2. Induced Abortion:

Deliberate termination of pregnancy via medical or surgical intervention.

Subcategories:

Therapeutic Abortion: Performed to preserve maternal health or in cases of severe fetal abnormalities.

Elective Abortion: Performed at the request of the pregnant individual, often for personal, social, or economic reasons.

3. Timing:

First Trimester: Up to 12–14 weeks gestation.

Second Trimester: 14–24 weeks gestation.

Third Trimester: After 24 weeks (rare, typically for severe maternal or fetal indications, subject to legal restrictions).

Indications for Induced Abortion

1. Maternal Indications:

Life-threatening conditions (e.g., severe preeclampsia, heart disease, cancer requiring immediate treatment). Mental health risks (e.g., severe psychiatric conditions exacerbated by pregnancy).

2. Fetal Indications:

Lethal fetal anomalies (e.g., anencephaly, trisomy 13 or 18).

Severe congenital malformations incompatible with life.

3. Elective Indications:

Personal choice, socioeconomic factors, unintended pregnancy, or contraceptive failure.

4. Other Indications:

Pregnancy resulting from rape or incest.

Legal and cultural factors vary by region, influencing access and indications.

Methods of Induced Abortion

The choice of method depends on gestational age, patient health, provider expertise, and local regulations.

1. Medical Abortion

Medical abortion involves the use of pharmacological agents to terminate a pregnancy. It is most effective in the first trimester and increasingly used in the second trimester.

First Trimester (Up to 10–12 Weeks):

Regimen:

Mifepristone (antiprogestin): 200 mg orally, blocks progesterone, leading to decidual breakdown and uterine contractions.

Misoprostol (prostaglandin E1 analog): 800 µg vaginally, buccally, or sublingually 24–48 hours later to induce uterine contractions and expel pregnancy tissue.

Efficacy: 95–98% when used in combination; misoprostol alone has lower efficacy (85–90%).

Follow-Up: Ultrasound or serum β-hCG levels to confirm complete abortion (1–2 weeks post-procedure).

Second Trimester:

Regimen: Mifepristone followed by repeated doses of misoprostol (400–800 µg every 3–6 hours, up to 5 doses).

Efficacy: 90–95% within 24 hours.

Considerations: Higher doses of misoprostol may be required; hospitalization is often recommended for pain management and monitoring.

Contraindications

Ectopic pregnancy, chronic adrenal failure, severe anemia, or allergy to medications.

Caution in patients with bleeding disorders or on anticoagulants.

Advantages

Non-invasive, avoids surgical risks, suitable for outpatient settings.

Preferred by patients seeking privacy or avoiding anesthesia.

Disadvantages

Prolonged process (hours to days), heavy bleeding, cramping.

Incomplete abortion requiring surgical intervention in 2–5% of cases.

2. Surgical Abortion

Surgical methods involve mechanical removal of pregnancy tissue and are highly effective across gestational ages.

First Trimester

Vacuum Aspiration (Manual or Electric):

Procedure: Cervical dilation followed by suction of uterine contents using a manual vacuum aspirator (MVA) or electric vacuum aspiration (EVA).

Anesthesia: Local (paracervical block) or conscious sedation.

Efficacy: >99% when performed by trained providers.

Duration: 5–10 minutes.

Advantages: Quick, highly effective, performed in a single visit.

Disadvantages: Requires skilled provider, minor risk of uterine perforation or infection.

Second Trimester

Dilation and Evacuation (D&E):

Procedure: Cervical preparation (e.g., misoprostol or osmotic dilators like laminaria) followed by evacuation using suction and forceps under ultrasound guidance.

Anesthesia: General anesthesia or deep sedation often required.

Efficacy: >99%.

Indications: Preferred for second-trimester terminations due to safety and efficacy.

Dilation and Curettage (D&C):

Less common, involves scraping the uterine lining with a curette.

Used in cases of incomplete abortion or when vacuum aspiration is unavailable.

Third Trimester (Rare)

Induction of Labor: Using high-dose misoprostol or oxytocin, often with feticide (e.g., intracardiac potassium chloride) to ensure fetal demise prior to delivery.

Performed in specialized centers under strict legal and medical indications.

Contraindications

Unstable hemodynamics, severe infections (e.g., chorioamnionitis), or anatomical barriers (e.g., large uterine fibroids).

Complications

While abortion is generally safe when performed by trained providers in appropriate settings, complications can occur:

1. Immediate Complications

Hemorrhage: Excessive bleeding (1–2% of cases), more common in second-trimester procedures.

Uterine Perforation: Rare (<0.5%), associated with surgical methods.

Infection: Endometritis or pelvic inflammatory disease (<1%), preventable with prophylactic antibiotics.

Incomplete Abortion: Retained products of conception (2–5% in medical abortion, <1% in surgical abortion), requiring further intervention.

2. Delayed Complications

Asherman Syndrome: Intrauterine adhesions leading to infertility or abnormal menstruation (rare).

Psychological Impact: Most patients experience relief post-abortion, but some may report transient feelings of guilt or sadness. Long-term mental health risks are not significantly increased compared to continuing pregnancy, per studies like the Turnaway Study (2018).

3. Mortality

Legal abortion in developed settings: <1 per 100,000 procedures.

Unsafe abortion (common in restrictive settings): 30–220 per 100,000, per WHO estimates.

Post-Abortion Care

Monitoring: Vital signs, bleeding, and pain management post-procedure.

Contraception Counseling: Immediate initiation of contraception (e.g., IUD, implants) to prevent unintended pregnancies.

Follow-Up: Assess for complications and confirm complete abortion (ultrasound or β-hCG).

Psychosocial Support: Offer counseling for emotional or ethical concerns, particularly in cases of therapeutic abortion.

9.2 MTP Act

(*Qwaneen -i-isqat-i-Tibbi*)

Introduction

The Medical Termination of Pregnancy (MTP) Act, 1971 is a landmark legislation in India that legalized abortion under specific conditions to reduce maternal mortality and morbidity associated with unsafe abortions. Enacted on August 10, 1971, it provides a legal framework for safe and regulated termination of pregnancy by registered medical practitioners (RMPs). The Act was amended in 2002 and significantly updated in 2021 to expand access, address reproductive justice, and adapt to advancements in medical science.

Historical Background

Pre-MTP Act Era: Prior to 1971, abortion was illegal under Section 312 of the IPC, leading to widespread unsafe abortions, which contributed to high maternal mortality (estimated 8–11% of global maternal deaths due to unsafe abortions).(https://pmc.ncbi.nlm.nih.gov/articles/PMC8575235/)

Shantilal Shah Committee (1964): Formed by the Ministry of Health and Family Welfare to address the rising incidence of unsafe abortions, this committee recommended legalizing abortion under specific conditions, leading to the MTP Act in 1971.

Objective: The Act aims to provide safe, legal, and accessible abortion services to reduce maternal morbidity and mortality, empower women's reproductive autonomy, and address public health concerns related to unsafe abortions.(https://chahalacademy.com/mtp-act)

The MTP Act, 1971, establishes a legal framework for abortion, specifying who can perform abortions, under what conditions, where, and with whose consent. Below are its core provisions:

Medical Termination of Pregnancy (MTP) refers to the deliberate termination of a pregnancy before fetal viability, typically defined as before 24–28 weeks of gestation or a fetal weight less than 500 grams, using medical or surgical methods. In India, MTP is regulated by the Medical Termination of Pregnancy Act, 1971, and its amendments, which provide a legal framework for safe and accessible abortion services. MTP encompasses both therapeutic (medically indicated) and elective (patient choice) abortions, performed by registered medical practitioners (RMPs) in approved facilities.

Indications for MTP

MTP is performed under specific conditions as outlined in the MTP Act, 1971 (amended 2021). These include:

1. Maternal Indications

Risk to the woman's life or grave injury to her physical or mental health (e.g., severe preeclampsia, cardiac disease, cancer requiring immediate treatment).

Mental health risks, including psychological distress from rape or incest (presumed to cause grave mental injury).

Contraceptive failure (extended to unmarried women in 2021 amendment).

2. Fetal Indications

Substantial risk of serious physical or mental abnormalities in the fetus (e.g., anencephaly, trisomy 13 or 18, severe congenital malformations).

3. Social and Special Categories (2021 Amendment)

Pregnancies resulting from rape or incest.

Minors (under 18 years).

Women with physical or mental disabilities (per Rights of Persons with Disabilities Act, 2016).

Mentally ill women.

Women in humanitarian crises or emergencies (e.g., natural disasters).

4. Emergency Indications

Immediate termination to save the woman's life (per Section 5, MTP Act), bypassing standard gestational limits and dual RMP opinions.

MTP (Amendment) Act, 2021

Effective from September 24, 2021, this amendment expanded access and addressed gaps in the 1971 Act.

1. Extended Gestational Limits

Up to 20 weeks: Requires one RMP's opinion (simplified from two for 12–20 weeks)

20–24 weeks: Requires two RMPs' opinions for special categories of women, including:

Survivors of rape or incest.

Minors.

Women with physical or mental disabilities (per the Rights of Persons with Disabilities Act, 2016).

Mentally ill women.

Women in humanitarian crises or emergencies (e.g., disasters).

Beyond 24 weeks: Permitted only for substantial fetal abnormalities, as diagnosed by a state-level Medical Board.

2. Contraceptive Failure

Extended to unmarried women, recognizing changing social norms and destigmatizing pregnancies outside marriage. Previously limited to married women.

3. Medical Boards

Each state or union territory must establish a Medical Board with multi-specialty expertise (gynecology, pediatrics, radiology, etc.) to evaluate terminations beyond 24 weeks for fetal anomalies

Criticism: No time-bound decision-making process, potentially delaying care.

4. Transgender Inclusion

While the Act uses “woman,” the Transgender Persons (Protection of Rights) Act, 2019, recognizes transgender individuals who may become pregnant. However, clarity on their inclusion under the MTP Act remains ambiguous.

5. Confidentiality

Strengthened provisions to protect the privacy of women undergoing abortion.

Methods of MTP

The choice of MTP method depends on gestational age, patient health, provider expertise, and facility resources. Methods are broadly categorized as medical or surgical, with protocols aligned with WHO guidelines and Indian standards.

1. Medical Abortion

Medical abortion uses pharmacological agents to terminate pregnancy and is primarily used in the first trimester, with increasing application in the second trimester.

First Trimester (Up to 9–12 Weeks)

Regimen

Mifepristone: 200 mg orally, an antiprogestin that blocks progesterone, causing decidual breakdown and cervical softening.

Misoprostol: 800 μg vaginally, buccally, or sublingually 24–48 hours later to induce uterine contractions and expel pregnancy tissue.

Efficacy: 95–98% when used in combination; misoprostol alone has lower efficacy (85–90%).

Setting: Outpatient clinics with access to approved facilities (per MTP Rules, 2003). Hospitalization is rarely required unless complications arise.

Follow-Up: Ultrasound or serum β-hCG levels 1–2 weeks post-procedure to confirm complete abortion.

Contraindications: Ectopic pregnancy, chronic adrenal failure, severe anemia, bleeding disorders, or allergy to medications.

Second Trimester (13–24 Weeks)

Regimen

Mifepristone (200 mg orally) followed by misoprostol (400–800 µg every 3–6 hours, u to 5 doses) vaginally or orally.

Alternative: Misoprostol alone in settings where mifepristone is unavailable.

Efficacy: 90–95% within 24 hours.

Setting: Hospitalization recommended for pain management, monitoring, and management of potential complications.

Considerations: Higher doses of misoprostol increase the risk of side effects (e.g., nausea, fever, diarrhea).

Advantages

Non-invasive, avoids surgical risks.

Suitable for early pregnancies and outpatient settings.

Preferred by patients seeking privacy or avoiding anesthesia.

Disadvantages

Prolonged process (hours to days).

Heavy bleeding and cramping.

Risk of incomplete abortion (2–5%), requiring surgical intervention.

2. Surgical Abortion

Surgical methods involve mechanical removal of pregnancy tissue and are highly effective across gestational ages. They require trained providers and approved facilities.

First Trimester (Up to 12 Weeks)

Vacuum Aspiration (Manual or Electric)

Procedure: Cervical dilation (using misoprostol or mechanical dilators) followed by suction of uterine contents using a manual vacuum aspirator (MVA) or electric vacuum aspiration (EVA).

Anesthesia: Local (paracervical block) or conscious sedation.

Duration: 5–10 minutes.

Efficacy: >99%.

Advantages: Quick, single-visit procedure with minimal complications.

Disadvantages: Requires skilled provider; rare risks include uterine perforation or infection.

Second Trimester (13–24 Weeks)

Dilation and Evacuation (D&E)

Procedure: Cervical preparation with osmotic dilators (e.g., laminaria) or misoprostol, followed by evacuation using suction and forceps under ultrasound guidance.

Anesthesia: General anesthesia or deep sedation.

Efficacy: >99%.

Indications: Preferred for second-trimester MTP due to safety and efficacy.

Considerations: Requires advanced training and specialized equipment.

Dilation and Curettage (D&C)

Less common, involves scraping the uterine lining with a curette.

Used for incomplete abortions or in settings without vacuum aspiration.

Beyond 24 Weeks (Rare)

Induction of Labor

Procedure: High-dose misoprostol or oxytocin to induce uterine contractions, often preceded by feticide (e.g., intracardiac potassium chloride) to ensure fetal demise, as required by Medical Boards for fetal anomaly cases.

Setting: Specialized centers with intensive care capabilities.

Indications: Severe fetal abnormalities or life-threatening maternal conditions.

Contraindications: Unstable hemodynamics, severe infections (e.g., chorioamnionitis), or anatomical barriers (e.g., large uterine fibroids).

Complications of MTP

While MTP is generally safe when performed by trained providers in approved facilities, complications can occur. These are categorized as immediate or delayed.

1. Immediate Complications

Hemorrhage: Excessive bleeding (1–2%), more common in second-trimester procedures or medical abortions.

Uterine Perforation: Rare (<0.5%), associated with surgical methods, particularly D&E.

Infection: Endometritis or pelvic inflammatory disease (<1%), preventable with prophylactic antibiotics (e.g., doxycycline or azithromycin).

Incomplete Abortion: Retained products of conception (2–5% in medical abortion, <1% in surgical abortion), requiring further intervention (e.g., repeat aspiration or curettage).

Post-Abortal Triad: Pain, bleeding, and low-grade fever, indicating possible retained tissue or infection.

2. Delayed Complications

Asherman Syndrome: Intrauterine adhesions leading to infertility or abnormal menstruation (rare, <1%).

Menstrual Disturbances: Irregular cycles post-procedure, typically resolving within 1–2 cycles.

Chronic Pelvic Inflammation: Rare, associated with untreated infections.

Future Obstetric Risks: Minimal evidence of increased risk of ectopic pregnancy, preterm labor, or perinatal loss, though poorly performed procedures may contribute.

3. Mortality

Legal MTP in India: <1 per 100,000 procedures in approved settings.

Unsafe abortions (outside MTP Act): 30–220 per 100,000 (WHO estimates), contributing to 8–11% of maternal mortality in India.

Post-Abortion Care

Comprehensive post-abortion care is critical to ensure patient safety and recovery:

Monitoring: Assess vital signs, bleeding, and pain post-procedure. Monitor for signs of infection or hemorrhage.

Pain Management: Nonsteroidal anti-inflammatory drugs (NSAIDs) like ibuprofen for cramping; stronger analgesics for second-trimester procedures.

Contraception Counseling: Immediate initiation of contraception (e.g., intrauterine devices, implants, oral contraceptives) to prevent unintended pregnancies. Post-abortion is an ideal time for IUD insertion due to cervical dilation.

Follow-Up

Medical abortion: Ultrasound or β-hCG levels 1–2 weeks post-procedure to confirm completion.

Surgical abortion: Follow-up within 1–2 weeks to assess for complications.

Antibiotic Prophylaxis: Recommended for surgical abortions to reduce infection risk (e.g., doxycycline 100 mg twice daily for 7 days).

Special Cases in MTP

1. Adolescent Patients

Minors require guardian consent, posing challenges in cases of family conflict or lack of support.

High risk of unsafe abortions due to stigma and lack of awareness.

2. Rural and Underserved Areas

Shortage of RMPs (75% deficit in rural India) and approved facilities limits access.

Telemedicine and self-managed medical abortion (e.g., via mifepristone/misoprostol kits) are emerging solutions but require regulatory oversight.

3. Fetal Anomalies

Diagnosis via ultrasound, amniocentesis, or chorionic villus sampling (CVS) is critical for terminations beyond 20 weeks.

Medical Boards evaluate cases beyond 24 weeks, ensuring multi-specialty input (gynecology, radiology, pediatrics).

4. Ethical Dilemmas

Balancing patient autonomy with provider conscientious objection (providers must refer patients if refusing non-emergency MTP). Ethical debates over late-term abortions, particularly for fetal anomalies or social reasons.

9.3 Ectopic Pregnancy

(*Haml Kharij-al-Rahim*)

Definition

An ectopic pregnancy is a pregnancy in which the fertilized ovum implants and develops outside the endometrial cavity of the uterus. The most common site is the fallopian tube (95–98% of cases), but ectopic pregnancies can also occur in the ovary, cervix, abdominal cavity, or cesarean scar. Ectopic pregnancy is a life-threatening condition due to the risk of rupture and hemorrhage, requiring prompt diagnosis and management.

Epidemiology

Incidence: Approximately 1–2% of all pregnancies globally, with higher rates in populations with risk factors (e.g., 2–5% in assisted reproductive technology [ART] pregnancies).

India: Estimated incidence is 1 in 100–200 pregnancies, with higher rates in urban centers due to increased use of ART and delayed childbearing.

Maternal Mortality: Ectopic pregnancy accounts for 3–4% of pregnancy-related deaths in developed countries and up to 10% in low-resource settings, including parts of India, due to delayed diagnosis and limited access to care.

Etiology and Risk Factors

Ectopic pregnancy results from impaired embryo transport or implantation, often due to tubal damage or dysfunction. Key risk factors include:

1. Tubal Factors

Previous tubal surgery (e.g., tubal ligation, reversal).

History of pelvic inflammatory disease (PID), often caused by Chlamydia trachomatis or Neisseria gonorrhoeae, leading to tubal scarring.

Prior ectopic pregnancy (10–15% recurrence risk).

2. Reproductive Factors

Use of ART, particularly in vitro fertilization (IVF), due to altered tubal transport.

Intrauterine contraceptive devices (IUCDs), especially progesterone-releasing devices, which increase ectopic risk if pregnancy occurs.

History of infertility or ovulation induction.

3. Maternal Factors

Maternal age >35 years (increased risk due to tubal dysfunction).

Smoking (impairs ciliary function in fallopian tubes).

Endometriosis or uterine anomalies (e.g., fibroids obstructing tubal ostia).

4. Other Factors

Previous abdominal or pelvic surgery (e.g., appendectomy, cesarean section).

Congenital tubal abnormalities (e.g., diverticula).

Rarely, hormonal imbalances or medications (e.g., progestin-only contraceptives).

Pathophysiology

Implantation Sites

Fallopian Tube (95–98%): Ampulla (70%), isthmus (12%), fimbria (11%), interstitial/cornual (2–3%).

Non-Tubal Sites (2–5%): Ovary (0.5%), cervix (0.1%), abdominal cavity (1%), cesarean scar (<1%).

Mechanism: Impaired tubal motility or structural damage prevents the embryo from reaching the uterus, leading to extrauterine implantation. The trophoblast invades the implantation site, potentially causing rupture (e.g., tubal rupture in 20–30% of untreated cases) and life-threatening hemorrhage.

Outcomes: Without intervention, ectopic pregnancies may result in spontaneous resolution (rare), tubal abortion (expulsion into the peritoneal cavity), or rupture with hemoperitoneum.

Clinical Presentation

Ectopic pregnancy typically presents in the first trimester (6–8 weeks gestation). Symptoms and signs vary based on whether the ectopic pregnancy is unruptured or ruptured.

1. Unruptured Ectopic Pregnancy

Symptoms

Amenorrhea or irregular vaginal bleeding (spotting or light bleeding in 50–80% of cases).

Unilateral pelvic or lower abdominal pain (mild to moderate, often cramp-like).

Referred shoulder pain (due to diaphragmatic irritation from hemoperitoneum, rare in unruptured cases).

Signs

Mild tenderness on pelvic examination.

Adnexal mass (palpable in 10–20% of cases).

Normal or slightly enlarged uterus.

2. Ruptured Ectopic Pregnancy

Symptoms

Severe, sudden-onset abdominal or pelvic pain.

Syncope, dizziness, or collapse due to hypovolemic shock.

Heavy vaginal bleeding (less common than in miscarriage).

Signs

Signs of shock (tachycardia, hypotension, pallor).

Peritoneal signs (rebound tenderness, guarding).

Cervical motion tenderness on bimanual examination.

Hemoperitoneum on culdocentesis (if performed).

Diagnosis

Prompt and accurate diagnosis is critical to prevent rupture and complications. The diagnostic approach integrates clinical evaluation, laboratory tests, and imaging.

1. History and Physical Examination

Assess for risk factors, amenorrhea, pain, and bleeding.

Perform pelvic examination to detect adnexal tenderness, mass, or cervical motion tenderness.

2. Laboratory Tests

Serum β-hCG

Levels are typically lower than in normal intrauterine pregnancies (IUPs) for the same gestational age.

Discriminatory zone: β-hCG >1,500–2,000 IU/L without an IUP on transvaginal ultrasound suggests ectopic pregnancy.

Serial β-hCG: In IUPs, β-hCG doubles every 48–72 hours; in ectopic pregnancy, it rises suboptimally (<66% increase) or plateaus.

Progesterone: Levels <5 ng/mL suggest non-viable pregnancy (ectopic or miscarriage); >20 ng/mL suggests IUP.

Complete Blood Count: Assess for anemia or leukocytosis in suspected rupture.

Blood Group and Rh Status: Essential for transfusion planning and Rh immunoglobulin administration in Rh-negative women.

3. Imaging

Transvaginal Ultrasound (TVUS)

Gold standard for diagnosis.

Findings suggestive of ectopic pregnancy:

Empty uterine cavity (no gestational sac) with β-hCG above discriminatory zone.

Adnexal mass (e.g., echogenic ring or “tubal ring” sign in 60–70% of cases).

Extrauterine gestational sac with yolk sac or fetal pole (diagnostic but rare, <10%).

Free fluid in the cul-de-sac (suggests hemoperitoneum, especially if echogenic).

Differential diagnosis: Corpus luteum cyst, early IUP, or miscarriage.

Transabdominal Ultrasound: Used if TVUS is unavailable or for assessing free intraperitoneal fluid.

MRI/CT: Rarely used, reserved for atypical cases (e.g., abdominal or cesarean scar ectopic).

4. Diagnostic Algorithm

Step 1: Confirm pregnancy with urine or serum β-hCG.

Step 2: Perform TVUS to locate the pregnancy.

Step 3: If no IUP is seen and β-hCG is above the discriminatory zone, presume ectopic pregnancy until proven otherwise.

Step 4: Serial β-hCG and repeat ultrasound if initial findings are inconclusive (e.g., pregnancy of unknown location [PUL]).

Differential Diagnosis

Early intrauterine pregnancy.

Spontaneous miscarriage.

Corpus luteum cyst.

Appendicitis, ovarian torsion, or ruptured ovarian cyst.

Pelvic inflammatory disease or tubo-ovarian abscess.

Gastrointestinal disorders (e.g., gastroenteritis, bowel obstruction).

Management

Management depends on the patient's clinical stability, β-hCG levels, ectopic size, and patient preferences. Options include medical, surgical, and expectant management.

1. Medical Management

Indications

Hemodynamically stable patient.

Unruptured ectopic pregnancy.

β-hCG <5,000 IU/L (ideally <3,000 IU/L).

Ectopic mass <3.5 cm on ultrasound.

No fetal cardiac activity.

Patient compliance with follow-up.

Regimen

Methotrexate: A folate antagonist that inhibits trophoblast proliferation.

Single-Dose Protocol: 50 mg/m^2 intramuscularly (IM), followed by serial β-hCG on days 4 and 7. Success if β-hCG drops >15% between days 4 and 7, with weekly monitoring until β-hCG <5 IU/L.

Two-Dose or Multi-Dose Protocols: Used for higher β-hCG levels or larger ectopic masses, with additional doses if β-hCG decline is inadequate.

Success Rate: 85–95% for single-dose protocol; higher with multi-dose.

Contraindications

Ruptured ectopic pregnancy.

Hemodynamic instability.

Renal or hepatic dysfunction.

Active peptic ulcer disease or immunodeficiency.

Breastfeeding.

Side Effects: Abdominal pain (common, 2–3 days post-injection), nausea, stomatitis, bone marrow suppression (rare).

Follow-Up: Weekly β-hCG until undetectable; counsel patients to avoid alcohol, NSAIDs, and pregnancy for 3 months due to teratogenic risks.

2. Surgical Management

Indications

Hemodynamic instability or suspected rupture.

β-hCG >5,000 IU/L or ectopic mass >3.5 cm.

Fetal cardiac activity.

Patient preference or inability to comply with medical follow-up.

Failed medical management.

Procedures

Laparoscopy (preferred)

Salpingectomy: Removal of the affected fallopian tube, indicated for rupture, extensive tubal damage, or completed family planning.

Salpingostomy: Removal of the ectopic pregnancy with preservation of the tube, indicated for unruptured ectopic and desire for future fertility.

Success rate: >95%.

Laparotomy: Reserved for severe hemorrhage, unstable patients, or lack of laparoscopic expertise.

Anesthesia: General anesthesia for laparoscopy/laparotomy; local anesthesia for salpingostomy in select cases.

Advantages: Definitive treatment, rapid resolution.

Disadvantages: Surgical risks (e.g., bleeding, infection), potential impact on future fertility (salpingectomy).

3. Expectant Management

Indications

Asymptomatic patients with low β-hCG (<1,000 IU/L and declining).

Small ectopic mass (<2 cm) without cardiac activity.

High likelihood of spontaneous resolution.

Protocol: Serial β-hCG and ultrasound monitoring every 2–7 days until β-hCG is undetectable.

Success Rate: 50–70%, higher with lower initial β-hCG.

Risks: Requires strict compliance; 10–20% progress to rupture or require intervention.

4. Management of Non-Tubal Ectopic Pregnancies

Cervical Ectopic: Methotrexate (systemic or local injection), uterine artery embolization, or surgical evacuation (e.g., curettage with tamponade).

Ovarian Ectopic: Laparoscopic resection or oophorectomy (rare).

Cesarean Scar Ectopic: Methotrexate, surgical excision, or hysterectomy in severe cases.

Abdominal Ectopic: Laparotomy or laparoscopy, with high risk of maternal morbidity.

Complications

1. Immediate

Hemorrhage: Most common cause of morbidity/mortality, especially with tubal rupture.

Hypovolemic Shock: Due to massive hemoperitoneum.

Infection: Post-surgical sepsis or pelvic abscess (rare, <1%).

2. Delayed

Persistent Trophoblastic Tissue: After salpingostomy or medical management (5–10%), requiring additional methotrexate or surgery.

Reduced Fertility: Salpingectomy reduces fertility by 15–20%; salpingostomy carries a 10–15% risk of recurrent ectopic pregnancy.

Chronic Pelvic Pain: Due to adhesions or residual tubal damage.

3. Rare Complications

Asherman syndrome (post-surgical intrauterine adhesions).

Psychological distress, particularly in patients with desired pregnancies.

Post-Management Care

Monitoring

Medical management: Weekly β-hCG until <5 IU/L.

Surgical management: Assess for postoperative complications (e.g., infection, hematoma).

Rh Immunoglobulin: Administer 50–300 µg anti-D immunoglobulin to Rh-negative women within 72 hours to prevent isoimmunization.

Contraception Counseling: Advise contraception for 3–6 months post-methotrexate or surgical management to optimize tubal healing and reduce recurrence risk.

Psychosocial Support: Offer counseling for emotional impact, especially in cases of desired pregnancy or recurrent ectopic pregnancies.

Future Pregnancy Planning: Discuss recurrence risk (10–15%) and early ultrasound in subsequent pregnancies to confirm intrauterine location.

Special Cases

1. Pregnancy of Unknown Location (PUL)

Defined as positive β-hCG without visible IUP or ectopic on ultrasound.

Management: Serial β-hCG and repeat ultrasound; methotrexate or surgery if ectopic is confirmed.

2. Heterotopic Pregnancy

Rare (1 in 10,000–30,000 spontaneous pregnancies, higher with ART).

Coexistence of IUP and ectopic pregnancy; requires selective management of ectopic while preserving IUP.

Key points

Ectopic pregnancy is a medical emergency requiring high clinical suspicion, especially in women with risk factors presenting with pain and bleeding.

Diagnosis relies on a combination of β-hCG, transvaginal ultrasound, and clinical assessment.

Management options (medical, surgical, expectant) are tailored to clinical stability, β-hCG levels, and patient preferences, with laparoscopy as the preferred surgical approach.

Post-management care includes β-hCG monitoring, Rh immunoglobulin, contraception counseling, and psychosocial support.

9.4 Gestational Trophoblastic Disease

(Daul-aroma ghaziyah Hamli)

Definition

Gestational trophoblastic disease (GTD) comprises a spectrum of disorders originating from the trophoblastic tissue of the placenta, characterized by abnormal proliferation of trophoblasts. It includes both benign and malignant entities, the malignant forms being collectively termed gestational trophoblastic neoplasia (GTN). The disease arises following abnormal fertilization and is associated with excessive secretion of human chorionic gonadotropin (hCG).

Classification

Gestational trophoblastic disease includes the following entities:

1. Hydatidiform mole

Complete mole

Partial mole

2. Invasive mole

3. Choriocarcinoma

4. Placental site trophoblastic tumor (PSTT)

5. Epithelioid trophoblastic tumor (ETT)

The first two are benign or pre-malignant, while the remaining forms constitute malignant varieties of GTD.

Incidence

The incidence varies widely with geographic region and socioeconomic status. It is more common in Asian countries compared to Western nations. The estimated incidence is approximately 1 in 1000 pregnancies in developed countries and 1 in 200–400 pregnancies in some parts of Asia.

Etiology and Risk Factors

The exact etiology is unknown, but several risk factors are associated:

1. Extremes of maternal age: More common in women below 20 years and above 40 years.
2. Previous molar pregnancy: Recurrence risk increases after a prior mole.

3. Nutritional deficiency: Particularly of carotene and animal fat (Vitamin A deficiency).
4. Genetic factors: Abnormal fertilization resulting in paternal disomy or triploidy.
5. Socioeconomic factors: More common in low-income groups.

Pathogenesis and Genetic Basis

Normal Conception

In a normal pregnancy, a haploid ovum (23,X) is fertilized by a haploid sperm (23,X or Y) to form a diploid zygote (46,XX or XY), with equal contribution from both parents. The trophoblast develops normally to form the placenta.

Complete Mole

An empty ovum (lacking maternal chromosomes) is fertilized by:

A single sperm that duplicates its chromosomes (monospermic), or two sperms (dispermic).

The resulting karyotype is 46,XX or 46,XY, entirely paternal in origin. There is no fetal tissue, and all villi become hydropic with diffuse trophoblastic hyperplasia.

Partial Mole

A normal ovum is fertilized by two sperms, producing a triploid karyotype (69,XXY; 69,XXX; or 69,XYY). Some fetal parts or membranes may develop, and only a proportion of villi are edematous with focal trophoblastic proliferation.

Invasive Mole

Represents a locally invasive form of complete mole in which molar villi and trophoblasts invade the myometrium and sometimes penetrate into venous channels, leading to embolic spread.

Choriocarcinoma

A highly malignant neoplasm composed of proliferating cytotrophoblasts and syncytiotrophoblasts without villous formation. It is characterized by hemorrhage, necrosis, and early hematogenous metastasis.

Placental Site and Epithelioid Trophoblastic Tumors

These arise from the intermediate trophoblast at the implantation site. They are rare, produce low levels of hCG, and are less responsive to chemotherapy.

Pathology

1. Complete Mole

Gross: The uterus is enlarged and filled with numerous translucent vesicles resembling a cluster of grapes. No fetus or amniotic sac is present.

Microscopy: Diffuse hydropic degeneration of all villi with circumferential proliferation of trophoblasts. Fetal vessels are absent.

2. Partial Mole

Gross: Some normal placental tissue is present along with cystic degeneration. A malformed fetus or fetal parts may be seen.

Microscopy: Focal villous edema with irregular shapes and focal trophoblastic hyperplasia. Fetal vessels and nucleated RBCs may be present.

3. Invasive Mole

Hydropic villi and trophoblastic tissue invade the myometrium and may reach the serosa or parametrium. Villi can be seen within blood vessels.

4. Choriocarcinoma

Soft, hemorrhagic, and necrotic mass, often replacing the uterine wall. Microscopically composed of proliferating cytotrophoblasts and syncytiotrophoblasts, with no chorionic villi.

5. PSTT and ETT

Solid tumors infiltrating the myometrium, composed predominantly of intermediate trophoblasts, showing less mitotic activity and absence of villi.

Clinical Features

Hydatidiform Mole

Vaginal bleeding in early pregnancy is the most common symptom.

Excessive uterine enlargement disproportionate to gestational age.

Passage of vesicles per vaginam.

Severe nausea and vomiting (hyperemesis gravidarum).

Early-onset preeclampsia before 20 weeks of gestation.

Bilateral theca lutein ovarian cysts.

Features of hyperthyroidism due to elevated hCG.

Invasive Mole

Persistent or irregular uterine bleeding following evacuation of a mole.

Subinvolution of uterus.

Elevated or plateauing hCG titers.

Pelvic pain due to uterine invasion.

Choriocarcinoma

Irregular or heavy bleeding weeks to months after any pregnancy—molar, abortion, or even normal delivery.

Uterine enlargement without pregnancy.

Symptoms of metastasis, such as cough, hemoptysis (lungs), headache or seizures (brain), or vaginal nodules.

Investigations

1. Laboratory Tests

Serum β-hCG: Markedly elevated (>100,000 mIU/mL) in complete mole; used for diagnosis and follow-up.

Thyroid function tests: May show hyperthyroidism.

CBC, liver and renal function tests: Baseline before evacuation or chemotherapy.

Blood group and Rh typing: For Rh prophylaxis.

2. Imaging

Ultrasonography:

Complete mole: “Snowstorm” or “cluster of grapes” appearance; absence of fetus and amniotic sac.

Partial mole: Gestational sac with fetal parts and cystic changes in placenta.

Chest X-ray: To detect lung metastases.

CT/MRI: For evaluation of metastatic spread to liver, brain, or pelvis.

3. Histopathology

Confirms the diagnosis and differentiates between complete and partial mole.

p57 immunostaining is absent in complete mole and present in partial mole.

Management

1. Molar Pregnancy

Pre-evacuation: Preparation

Stabilize patient and correct anemia or preeclampsia.

Baseline hCG estimation and imaging.

Blood cross-matching and availability of oxytocics.

Evacuation

Suction evacuation and curettage is the preferred method.

Oxytocics are administered after evacuation to minimize bleeding.

Prophylactic antibiotics are given.

Anti-D immunoglobulin to Rh-negative women.

Post-evacuation: Follow-up

Serum β-hCG monitoring:

Weekly until three consecutive normal readings.

Monthly thereafter for at least six months.

Contraception: Pregnancy should be avoided during the surveillance period.

Criteria for Postmolar GTN (FIGO):

Plateau of hCG in four values over three weeks.

Rising hCG in three consecutive weekly values.

Persistence of detectable hCG >6 months post-evacuation.

Histological diagnosis of choriocarcinoma.

2. Management of GTN

FIGO Staging

Stage Description

I. Disease confined to uterus
II. Extension to genital structures
III. Lung metastasis (with/without genital tract involvement)
IV. Other distant metastasis (brain, liver, etc.)

WHO Risk Scoring System

A prognostic score is calculated based on factors such as maternal age, antecedent pregnancy, interval since pregnancy, pre-treatment hCG level, tumor size, site and number of metastases, and prior chemotherapy.

Score 0–6: Low-risk GTN

Score ≥7: High-risk GTN

3. Chemotherapy

Low-risk GTN (Score 0–6)

Single-agent chemotherapy with Methotrexate (with folinic acid rescue) or Actinomycin D.

Continued until hCG is normal for three weeks, followed by 1–2 consolidation cycles.

High-risk GTN (Score ≥7)

Combination chemotherapy with EMA-CO regimen:

Etoposide, Methotrexate, Actinomycin D, Cyclophosphamide, Vincristine (Oncovin).

Continued until hCG normalization, followed by 2–3 consolidation cycles.

Resistant Disease

Alternative multi-agent regimens or surgical excision of localized lesions.

Surgery

Hysterectomy may be considered in women who have completed childbearing or have localized uterine disease.

Excision of isolated metastases in resistant cases.

Radiotherapy

Reserved for brain metastases, used along with chemotherapy.

4. PSTT and ETT

These tumors are less sensitive to chemotherapy.

Primary treatment is hysterectomy.

Chemotherapy is reserved for metastatic or recurrent cases.

Prognosis

The prognosis of GTD is excellent with appropriate therapy.

Hydatidiform mole: Nearly 100% cure after evacuation and follow-up.

Invasive mole: >95% cure rate.

Choriocarcinoma: Cure rate exceeds 90% for low-risk and about 70–80% for high-risk cases.

PSTT/ETT: Prognosis depends on extent; poor in metastatic disease.

Follow-up and Subsequent Pregnancy

Regular hCG monitoring for at least 6–12 months.

Effective contraception during the follow-up period.

Recurrence risk after one mole is about 1%.

Early ultrasound and hCG testing are advised in subsequent pregnancies.

Complications

Hemorrhage

Infection

Uterine perforation during evacuation

Trophoblastic embolism

Persistent GTN or metastatic choriocarcinoma

Summary

GTD represents a spectrum from benign hydatidiform mole to malignant choriocarcinoma.

The disease results from abnormal fertilization and proliferation of trophoblastic tissue.

Serum hCG estimation is the cornerstone of diagnosis and follow-up.

Early evacuation, close monitoring, and chemotherapy based on risk classification ensure nearly complete cure in most cases.

Fertility is usually preserved, and most women achieve normal future pregnancies.

9.5 Ante partum Hemorrhage)

(*Jiryan-al-Dam qabl-i-Wiladat*)

Definition

Antepartum hemorrhage (APH) is defined as bleeding from or into the genital tract, occurring after the period of viability (usually after 28 weeks of gestation) and before the birth of the baby.

It is a major obstetric emergency associated with significant maternal and perinatal morbidity and mortality.

Incidence

The incidence of APH ranges from 2–5% of all pregnancies. It remains an important cause of maternal death in developing countries.

Classification

Antepartum hemorrhage is broadly classified into:

1. Placental Causes

Placenta Previa

Placental Abruption (Abruptio Placentae)

2. Extra-placental or Local Causes

Local lesions of the cervix or vagina (cervicitis, erosion, carcinoma cervix, vaginal varices, lacerations).

Trauma to genital tract (coitus, examination).

3. Unexplained or Indeterminate Causes

In some cases, no cause is detected even after delivery.

Importance

APH is an obstetric emergency because:

It endangers both mother and fetus by causing hemorrhage and shock.

It may lead to fetal hypoxia, prematurity, or death.

The underlying cause (especially abruption) may involve coagulopathy or uteroplacental insufficiency.

Causes and Pathophysiology

1. Placenta Previa

Placenta previa refers to placental implantation in the lower uterine segment, partially or completely covering the internal os.

Types

Type I (Low-lying): Placenta in lower segment but not reaching the os.

Type II (Marginal): Placenta reaches the margin of the os.

Type III (Partial): Placenta partially covers the os.

Type IV (Complete): Placenta completely covers the os.

Etiopathogenesis

The cause is low implantation of the blastocyst. Associated risk factors include:

Multiparity

Previous cesarean section or uterine surgery

Multiple pregnancy

Advanced maternal age

Smoking

Previous placenta previa

Pathology

The lower uterine segment forms late and stretches during pregnancy and labor. This causes partial separation of the placenta and painless vaginal bleeding. The amount of bleeding is often disproportionate to visible loss because the uterus remains relaxed and non-tender.

2. Abruptio Placentae (Placental Abruption)

Definition

Premature separation of a normally implanted placenta after 20 weeks of gestation and before the birth of the baby.

Types

Revealed type: Blood escapes through the cervix and appears externally.

Concealed type: Blood collects behind the placenta and does not escape externally.

Mixed type: Both concealed and revealed bleeding present.

Etiopathogenesis

The basic event is rupture of decidual spiral arteries leading to bleeding into the decidua basalis.

A hematoma forms, separating the placenta from the uterine wall, causing uteroplacental insufficiency.

The cause is multifactorial:

Hypertensive disorders (most common)

Abdominal trauma

Sudden uterine decompression (as in rupture of membranes of polyhydramnios)

Short umbilical cord

Smoking, cocaine use

Multiparity and maternal age >35 years

Pathology

Revealed abruption: Blood tracks down between membranes and decidua, escaping externally.

Concealed abruption: Blood is retained behind the placenta, may infiltrate the myometrium, and cause Couvelaire uterus (uteroplacental apoplexy) — where the uterine wall becomes bluish and ecchymosed due to extravasation of blood.

Clotting factors get consumed, leading to consumptive coagulopathy (DIC).

3. Local Causes

Cervical erosion, polyps, carcinoma cervix

Vaginal varices

Trauma from coitus or examination

Infection (cervicitis, vaginitis)

Clinical Features

General Presentation

Vaginal bleeding after 28 weeks of gestation

Pallor, anxiety, and tachycardia depending on blood loss

Uterine size and tone vary depending on cause

Placenta Previa

Bleeding: Bright red, painless, and recurrent.

Uterus: Soft, relaxed, non-tender.

Fetal parts: Easily felt; presenting part high and may be malpresented.

Fetal heart sounds: Usually present.

General condition: Often better than apparent blood loss.

No signs of preeclampsia.

Abruptio Placentae

Bleeding: Dark, may be revealed or concealed, often associated with pain.

Pain: Constant abdominal pain with uterine tenderness.

Uterus: Hard, tender, "woody" in consistency.

Fetal parts: Difficult to feel.

Fetal heart sounds: Often absent (intrauterine death common).

Associated features: Shock, preeclampsia, DIC, and Couvelaire uterus.

Local Causes

Bleeding usually slight, following examination or coitus.

No uterine tenderness or alteration in fetal condition.

Diagnosis

History

Onset, amount, and nature of bleeding

Associated pain or trauma

Obstetric history, especially previous cesarean section, placenta previa, or hypertension

Physical Examination

General Examination: Assess severity of blood loss, pulse, blood pressure, pallor, and shock.

Abdominal Examination

Uterine size and tone:

Soft and relaxed → Placenta previa

Hard and tender → Abruption

Fetal parts:

Easily felt → Placenta previa

Difficult to feel → Abruption

Fetal heart sounds:

Present → Placenta previa

Absent → Abruption

Vaginal Examination

Never perform a digital vaginal examination until placenta previa is excluded by ultrasound.

Speculum examination may be done to rule out local lesions.

If placenta previa is excluded: Gentle vaginal examination may be done to assess cervical status and confirm diagnosis.

Investigations

Ultrasound scan: Diagnostic for placenta previa. May detect retroplacental clot in abruption (though less sensitive).

Blood grouping and cross-matching

Hemoglobin and hematocrit.

Coagulation profile (fibrinogen, PT, aPTT, D-dimer).

Liver and renal function tests in hypertensive or severe cases.

Kleihauer-Betke test (for fetomaternal hemorrhage, Rh prophylaxis).

Differential Diagnosis

Placenta previa

Abruptio placentae

Vasa previa (fetal vessel rupture)

Local genital lesions

Management

General Principles

Hospitalization of all cases.

Immediate assessment of maternal and fetal condition.

IV access, blood grouping, cross-matching.

Resuscitation: IV fluids, blood transfusion as needed.

Monitor: Pulse, BP, urine output, fetal heart rate.

Avoid vaginal examination until placenta previa is ruled out.

Management of Placenta Previa

Expectant Management (Conservative)

Indicated when:

Bleeding is mild and stops spontaneously.

Fetus is alive and preterm (<37 weeks).

Maternal condition is stable.

Measures:

Admit to hospital ("watchful expectancy").

Bed rest, sedation, and avoidance of vaginal examination.

Blood reserved for transfusion if required.

Corticosteroids for fetal lung maturity (<34 weeks).

Monitor maternal and fetal status regularly.

Active Management

Indicated when:

Bleeding is severe or recurrent.

Maternal or fetal condition deteriorates.

Fetus mature or term gestation.

Delivery:

Cesarean section is the preferred mode for major placenta previa (Type III and IV).

Vaginal delivery may be attempted in minor cases (Type I and II posterior) if bleeding is mild and membranes rupture spontaneously.

Management of Abruptio Placentae

Initial Management

Stabilize the patient: airway, breathing, circulation.

Replace blood loss with crystalloids and blood transfusion.

Monitor urine output.

Correct coagulopathy if present.

Definitive Management

If fetus alive and no contraindication: Expedite delivery — usually cesarean section.

If fetus dead: Aim for vaginal delivery unless there is obstetric contraindication.

Artificial rupture of membranes helps relieve uterine distension and reduce bleeding.

Oxytocics may be used cautiously to aid delivery once cervix is favorable.

Monitor for DIC and renal failure.

Management of Local Causes

Treat underlying cervical or vaginal lesions (cauterization, excision).

Avoid trauma and coitus until cause is treated.

Complications

Maternal

Hemorrhagic shock

Anemia

Postpartum hemorrhage

DIC (especially in abruption)

Renal failure

Infection

Maternal death

Fetal

Hypoxia and asphyxia

Preterm birth

Intrauterine growth restriction (IUGR)

Intrauterine death

Prognosis

Maternal prognosis: Generally good with prompt management, though mortality remains significant in severe abruption.

Fetal prognosis: Poorer, especially in abruption placentae and severe placenta previa.

Prevention

Early detection and management of risk factors such as anemia, hypertension, and smoking.

Routine antenatal care and ultrasound for placental localization.

Avoid unnecessary uterine curettage or trauma.

Institutional delivery with blood and surgical backup.

Summary

Antepartum hemorrhage is bleeding after 28 weeks of pregnancy but before delivery.

The two main causes are placenta previa and placental abruption.

Placenta previa causes painless, bright red bleeding; abruption causes painful, dark bleeding with uterine tenderness.

Ultrasound confirms the diagnosis of placenta previa.

Never perform vaginal examination until previa is ruled out.

Management aims to stabilize the mother and deliver the fetus safely.

Prompt diagnosis, resuscitation, and appropriate delivery route can significantly reduce maternal and fetal mortality.

9.6 Postpartum hemorrhage (PPH)

(*Jiryan-al-Dam bad-i-Wiladat*)

Definition

Postpartum hemorrhage (PPH) is defined as excessive bleeding from the genital tract following the birth of the baby, which adversely affects the maternal condition.

According to Time of Onset

1. Primary (Early) PPH:

Bleeding occurring within 24 hours of delivery.

2. Secondary (Late) PPH:

Bleeding occurring after 24 hours and up to 12 weeks postpartum.

According to Quantity

Traditionally defined as blood loss exceeding:

500 mL after vaginal delivery, or

1000 mL after cesarean section. However, any blood loss causing hemodynamic instability should be regarded as PPH, regardless of estimated amount.

Incidence

Occurs in 4–6% of all deliveries.

Remains one of the leading causes of maternal mortality worldwide, particularly in developing countries, accounting for about 25–30% of maternal deaths.

Importance

PPH is an obstetric emergency that can lead to hypovolemic shock, disseminated intravascular coagulation (DIC), renal failure, and death if not treated promptly.

It is largely preventable by active management of the third stage of labor and timely intervention.

Physiological Basis of Hemostasis after Delivery

Normally, after separation of the placenta:

1. The myometrial fibers around the placental bed contract and compress the uterine sinuses — this acts as a “living ligature.”

2. Thrombosis and clot formation further occlude open vessels.

3. The uterus remains firmly contracted (known as a “retracted uterus”).

Failure of these mechanisms results in postpartum hemorrhage.

Etiological Classification (The Four Ts)

1. Tone (Uterine Atony) — 70–80% cases
2. Tissue (Retained Products of Conception)
3. Trauma (Genital Tract Lacerations, Hematomas, Rupture)
4. Thrombin (Coagulopathy)

1. Atonic Postpartum Hemorrhage

Definition

Failure of the uterus to contract and retract effectively after delivery leads to continuous bleeding from open sinuses of the placental site.

Predisposing Factors

Uterine Overdistension: Multiple pregnancy, Polyhydramnios, Macrosomic baby

Uterine Exhaustion: Prolonged labor, Precipitate labor, Induction or augmentation with oxytocin, Grand multiparity

Uterine Inertia: Chorioamnionitis, Deep anesthesia (halothane, magnesium sulfate), Full bladder

Other Causes: Retained placenta or membranes, Placenta accreta spectrum, Previous history of PPH

Pathophysiology

Lack of uterine contraction leaves the large venous sinuses at the placental bed open.

Continuous bleeding occurs, often leading to massive hemorrhage.

As blood loss continues, the myometrium becomes flabby, and shock develops rapidly.

Clinical Features

Sudden profuse vaginal bleeding soon after delivery.

Uterus is soft, boggy and enlarged on palpation.

Placenta may or may not have been delivered.

Signs of shock appear early and are often disproportionate to visible blood loss due to concealed bleeding.

2. Traumatic Postpartum Hemorrhage

Causes

Cervical, vaginal or perineal lacerations

Extension of episiotomy

Rupture of the uterus or vaginal vault

Broad ligament or vulvovaginal hematoma

Clinical Features

Uterus is well contracted.

Persistent bleeding despite firm uterine tone.

May have signs of hematoma — pain, swelling, or pelvic pressure.

3. Tissue (Retained Placental Tissue)

Causes

Retained cotyledon or succenturiate lobe

Incomplete separation of placenta

Abnormal adherence (placenta accreta, increta, percreta)

Retained membranes or clots interfering with uterine contraction.

Clinical Features

Uterus fails to contract adequately.

Irregular uterine contour and persistent bleeding.

Inspection of delivered placenta reveals missing cotyledons or torn membranes.

4. Thrombin (Coagulopathy)

Causes

Disseminated intravascular coagulation (DIC) secondary to:

Abruption placentae

Amniotic fluid embolism

Severe preeclampsia or eclampsia

Intrauterine fetal death

Sepsis

Preexisting coagulation disorders (hemophilia carrier, thrombocytopenia).

Clinical Features

Oozing from puncture sites, gums, and wounds.

No clot formation after blood collection.

Prolonged clotting time and low fibrinogen.

Diagnosis

Clinical Diagnosis

Excessive vaginal bleeding after delivery.

Uterine tone and height assessed by abdominal palpation.

Inspection of genital tract and placenta.

Assessment of maternal vital signs and shock.

Investigations

Hemoglobin, hematocrit, blood grouping and cross-match.

Coagulation profile (PT, aPTT, fibrinogen).

Platelet count.

Bedside clotting test (no clot after 7–10 minutes suggests coagulopathy).

Management of PPH

Management of PPH must be prompt, organized and simultaneous.

The goals are to arrest bleeding, restore blood volume, and treat the cause.

Step 1: Immediate Resuscitation

1. Call for help.

Senior obstetrician, anesthetist, pediatrician, and nursing staff.

2. Assess airway, breathing, circulation (ABC).

3. IV Access: Two wide-bore (14G) cannulas.

4. Blood sampling: For Hb, group, cross-match, coagulation screen.

5. Resuscitation:

Rapid infusion of crystalloids (Ringer's lactate or normal saline, up to 2 L).

Blood transfusion if loss >1000 mL or patient in shock.

6. Oxygen 10–15 L/min by mask.

7. Monitor vital signs — pulse, BP, urine output (>30 mL/hour), oxygen saturation.

Step 2: Identify and Treat the Cause (4 Ts)

(A) Tone – Uterine Atony

Uterotonic Drugs

1. Oxytocin: 10 IU IV slow bolus followed by infusion (20–40 IU in 1 L fluid at 60 drops/min).
2. Ergometrine: 0.2 mg IM/IV (contraindicated in hypertension, preeclampsia).
3. Carboprost (15-methyl $PGF_2\alpha$): 250 µg IM every 15–20 min (max 8 doses) — avoid in asthma.
4. Misoprostol: 800–1000 µg rectally if others unavailable.

Bimanual Uterine Compression

One hand in the vagina compresses the anterior fornix against the posterior wall while the other hand compresses the fundus abdominally.

Uterine Massage

Stimulates contraction if the uterus is flabby.

If bleeding persists despite medical therapy:

Mechanical Measures

Uterine balloon tamponade: Bakri balloon, condom catheter, or Sengstaken tube filled with 300–500 mL saline.

Compression sutures: B-Lynch, Hayman, or Cho sutures applied during laparotomy.

Uterine artery ligation or internal iliac artery ligation to reduce blood flow.

Hysterectomy: Definitive life-saving measure when conservative methods fail.

(B) Tissue – Retained Products

Explore uterus manually under anesthesia to remove retained placental tissue or membranes.

Send removed tissue for examination.

Administer uterotonics after evacuation.

(C) Trauma – Genital Tract Injuries

Inspect cervix, vagina, and perineum thoroughly.

Repair lacerations under good light.

Drain hematomas if large.

Surgical repair for rupture uterus.

(D) Thrombin – Coagulopathy

Replace clotting factors:

Fresh frozen plasma (15–20 mL/kg)

Platelet concentrates if <50,000/mm^3

Cryoprecipitate if fibrinogen <1 g/L

Treat underlying cause (abruption, sepsis, etc.).

Step 3: Post-Control Care

Continue IV fluids and blood as required.

Monitor vitals, urine output, and uterine tone.

Correct anemia and coagulation abnormalities.

Administer antibiotics.

Document blood loss and interventions.

Surgical Options (Stepwise Approach)

Step	Procedure	Remarks
1.	Uterine tamponade	Balloon/condom catheter; simple and fertility-sparing
2.	Compression sutures	B-Lynch, Hayman; useful in atony
3.	Uterine artery ligation	Reduces uterine perfusion by 40–50%
4.	Internal iliac artery ligation	Decreases pelvic blood flow; technically demanding
5.	Hysterectomy	Last resort; life-saving when conservative measures fail

Secondary Postpartum Hemorrhage

Definition: Bleeding occurring after 24 hours up to 12 weeks postpartum.

Causes

Retained placental bits or membranes

Subinvolution of placental site

Endometritis or infection

Trophoblastic disease (rare)

Secondary uterine atony

Clinical Features

Irregular, sometimes profuse bleeding days or weeks after delivery.

Uterus larger and softer than expected.

Often associated with offensive lochia and fever (if infection present).

Management

Resuscitation as required.

Antibiotics for infection.

Uterotonics to aid involution.

Evacuation of retained tissue under antibiotic cover.

Investigate for coagulation defect if recurrent.

Complications of PPH

Maternal

Hypovolemic shock

Acute renal failure (from tubular necrosis)

Sheehan's syndrome (postpartum pituitary necrosis)

DIC

Infection

Death

Fetal/Neonatal (Indirect)

Preterm delivery in high-risk mothers

Maternal anemia impacting neonatal outcome

Prevention

A. Antenatal

Correction of anemia

Identification of high-risk cases (multiple pregnancy, polyhydramnios, placenta previa, etc.)

Good nutrition and antenatal care

B. Intrapartum

Skilled birth attendants

Avoid prolonged or obstructed labor

Judicious use of oxytocics

C. Active Management of Third Stage of Labor (AMTSL)

1. Prophylactic oxytocin 10 IU IM after delivery of the anterior shoulder or within 1 minute of birth.
2. Controlled cord traction (CCT) for placental delivery (Brandt–Andrews method).
3. Uterine massage immediately after placental delivery.

This reduces incidence of PPH by 60–70%.

Prognosis

With prompt recognition and treatment, prognosis is excellent.

Delay in diagnosis and resuscitation is the main cause of mortality.

Future pregnancies: Slightly increased risk of recurrence (5–10%).

Summary

Postpartum hemorrhage is defined as blood loss >500 mL after vaginal delivery or any loss causing hemodynamic instability.

It is classified into primary (within 24 hours) and secondary (after 24 hours) types.

Atony is the commonest cause.

Management includes resuscitation, identification of cause (4 Ts), uterotonics, mechanical and surgical measures.

Active management of the third stage is the most effective preventive strategy.

Timely intervention saves lives — "Every minute counts in PPH management."

Long Answer Questions (LAQs)

Describe abortion (Isqat) with types, causes, clinical features, and management.

Discuss ectopic pregnancy including risk factors, diagnosis, and management.

Explain gestational trophoblastic disease with types and complications.

Describe antepartum hemorrhage with causes, diagnosis, and management.

Discuss postpartum hemorrhage with causes, prevention, and treatment.

Short Answer Questions (SAQs)

Define abortion.

What is ectopic pregnancy?

List causes of antepartum hemorrhage.

Define postpartum hemorrhage.

What is gestational trophoblastic disease?

Multiple Choice Questions (1 Mark Each)

1. Abortion is defined as termination of pregnancy before:

A. 20 weeks B. 28 weeks

C. 32 weeks D. 36 weeks

Answer: B

2. Most common site of ectopic pregnancy is:

A. Ovary B. Cervix

C. Fallopian tube D. Abdominal cavity

Answer: C

3. Classical triad of ectopic pregnancy includes:

A. Bleeding, fever, pain B. Amenorrhea, pain abdomen, vaginal bleeding

C. Vomiting, pain, fever D. Bleeding, shock, anemia

Answer: B

4. Most common cause of antepartum hemorrhage is:

A. Placental abruption B. Placenta previa

C. Uterine rupture D. Cervical polyp

Answer: B

5. Painless vaginal bleeding in late pregnancy suggests:

A. Abruptio placentae B. Uterine rupture

C. Placenta previa D. Vasa previa

Answer: C

6. Most common cause of postpartum hemorrhage is:

A. Trauma B. Tissue retention

C. Thrombin disorder D. Uterine atony

Answer: D

7. Primary postpartum hemorrhage occurs within:

A. 12 hours B. 24 hours

C. 48 hours D. 7 days

Answer: B

8. Gestational trophoblastic disease is best diagnosed by:

A. Ultrasound only B. X-ray

C. Serum β-hCG levels D. CT scan

Answer: C

9. Grape-like vesicles are seen in:

A. Ectopic pregnancy B. Placenta accreta

C. Hydatidiform mole D. Placental abruption

Answer: C

10. Most important preventive measure for PPH is:

A. Antibiotics B. Blood transfusion

C. Active management of third stage of labor D. Early induction

Answer: C

10

Obstetrical Complications

(Awaredat -i-Wiladat)

10.1 *Dauran-i-haml irtefay-i-Daght-al-Dam ke awaredat (*Hypertensive disorders in pregnancy)
10.2 *Qillat-i-Ma' Amniosi* (Oligohydramnios) & *Kasrat-i-an' amniosi* (Polyhydramnios)
10.3 *Haml-i-adeed aur haml-i-tawam* (Multifetal & Twins pregnancy)
10.4 *Takhal-luf-i-nam-we-dakhillur-rahim* (Intra Uterine Growth Retardation)
10.5 *Tamzzuk-i-aghshiyahya-i-janeen mubtasir* (Preterm Rupture of membrane)
10.6 *Wiladat-i-Mubakkerah* (Preterm labor)
10.7 *Wiladat-i-mutajawejah linnuzj* (Post Maturity)
10.8 *Maut-i-janeen Dakhil-al-Rahim* (Intra Uterine Fetal Death)

Learning Objective (At the end of the session, the students should be able to)

Discuss the etiopathogenesis, classification diagnosis & complications of Hypertensive Disorders in Pregnancy

Describe the etiopathogenesis, types, diagnosis & complications of *Qilatt-i-Mae Amniosi* (Oligohydramnios) & *Kasrat-i-Mae Amniosi* (Polyhydramnios)

Discuss the etiopathogenesis, types, diagnosis & complications of Multifetal & Twins Pregnancy

Discuss the etiopathogenesis, types, diagnosis & complications of Intra Uterine Growth Retardation (IUGR)

Discuss the etiology, diagnosis & complications of Preterm Labor

Discuss the causes, diagnosis & complications of Pre-term Rupture of Membrane

Describe the etiology, diagnosis & complications of Post Maturity

Discuss the etiopathogenesis, diagnosis & complications of *Faut e Janeeni* (Intra Uterine Fetal Death)

10.1 Hypertensive disorders in pregnancy

(Dauran-i-haml irtefay-i-Daght-al-Dam ke awaredat)

Hypertensive Disorders in Pregnancy

Definition

Hypertensive disorders of pregnancy (HDP) include a spectrum of conditions associated with raised blood pressure during pregnancy, labor or puerperium.

They are among the leading causes of maternal and perinatal morbidity and mortality worldwide.

Classification (As per ACOG and Dutta)

1. Gestational Hypertension
2. Preeclampsia–Eclampsia Syndrome
3. Chronic (Pre-existing) Hypertension
4. Chronic Hypertension with Superimposed Preeclampsia

Normal Blood Pressure in Pregnancy

Normal: <140/90 mmHg

Blood pressure is slightly reduced during mid-pregnancy due to decreased peripheral resistance and increases near term.

Definition of Hypertension in Pregnancy

Systolic BP ≥140 mmHg and/or Diastolic BP ≥90 mmHg on two occasions, 4 hours apart, after 20 weeks of gestation.

Severe hypertension: ≥160/110 mmHg.

I. Gestational Hypertension

Definition

New-onset hypertension (≥140/90 mmHg) after 20 weeks of gestation without proteinuria or end-organ dysfunction.

Blood pressure normalizes within 12 weeks postpartum.

Features

Transient condition, may progress to preeclampsia in 20–25% cases.

No proteinuria.

No evidence of hemolysis, liver dysfunction, or thrombocytopenia.

Management

Monitoring: BP, urine albumin and fetal growth every 1–2 weeks.

Lifestyle: Rest, reduced salt intake.

Antihypertensives: Labetalol, Methyldopa, or Nifedipine (oral).

Termination of pregnancy if BP uncontrolled or maternal/fetal compromise.

II. Preeclampsia

Definition

A multisystem disorder of pregnancy characterized by:

Hypertension (≥140/90 mmHg)

Proteinuria (≥300 mg/24 h or ≥+1 on dipstick)

Occurring after 20 weeks of gestation in a previously normotensive woman.

Incidence

Occurs in about 5–8% of pregnancies.

Etiopathogenesis

Exact cause unknown; multifactorial.

The central pathology is abnormal placentation and endothelial dysfunction.

Mechanisms

1. Abnormal trophoblastic invasion → failure of spiral arteries to remodel → placental ischemia.
2. Placental ischemia → release of antiangiogenic factors (sFlt-1, endoglin) → endothelial injury.
3. Endothelial dysfunction → vasospasm, increased vascular permeability, platelet activation, and coagulation abnormalities.
4. Result: Hypertension, proteinuria, edema and multiorgan involvement.

Risk Factors

Maternal	**Medical**	**Obstetric**
Nulliparity	Chronic hypertension	Multiple pregnancy
Family history	Diabetes mellitus	Hydatidiform mole
Obesity	Renal disease	Placental abnormalities
Age <20 or >35 years	Antiphospholipid syndrome	Previous preeclampsia

Clinical Features

Symptoms

Headache

Visual disturbances (blurred vision, scotoma)

Epigastric or right upper quadrant pain

Swelling of face, hands

Decreased urine output

Signs

BP ≥140/90 mmHg

Proteinuria on urine test

Pedal and facial edema

Hyperreflexia and clonus (signs of CNS irritability)

Investigations

Maternal Evaluation

1. Urine analysis – albumin, 24-hour protein.

2. Blood tests

CBC, Platelet count

Liver function tests (AST, ALT, LDH)

Renal function (Urea, Creatinine, Uric acid)

Coagulation profile (PT, aPTT, Fibrinogen)

3. Fundus examination – Hypertensive retinopathy.

Fetal Evaluation

Ultrasound – fetal growth, amniotic fluid volume.

Doppler velocimetry – uterine and umbilical artery resistance.

Non-stress test (NST) and biophysical profile (BPP).

Severity Criteria

Parameter	Mild Preeclampsia	Severe Preeclampsia
BP	≥140/90 to <160/110 mmHg	≥160/110 mmHg
Proteinuria	≥300 mg/24 h	≥5 g/24 h
Symptoms	None or mild	Headache, visual changes, epigastric pain
Platelets	Normal	<100,000/mm^3
Liver enzymes	Normal	Elevated
Serum Creatinine	Normal	>1.1 mg/dL
Fetus	Normal growth	IUGR, oligohydramnios, abnormal Doppler

Complications

Maternal

Eclampsia (seizures)

HELLP syndrome

Acute renal failure

Pulmonary edema

DIC

Abruptio placentae

Cerebral hemorrhage

Maternal death

Fetal

IUGR

Prematurity

Hypoxia, acidosis

Stillbirth

Neonatal death

Management of Preeclampsia

A. General Principles

Control blood pressure.

Prevent seizures.

Monitor maternal and fetal condition.

Plan delivery at optimal time.

B. Mild Preeclampsia

Rest and observation (preferably hospital admission).

BP monitoring every 4–6 hours.

Antihypertensives:

Labetalol (oral, 100–400 mg twice daily)

Methyldopa (250–500 mg 3 times daily)

Nifedipine (10–20 mg orally).

Monitor fetal well-being by NST, ultrasound, and Doppler.

Delivery: At 37 weeks or earlier if condition worsens.

C. Severe Preeclampsia

Hospitalize in intensive care setting.

Antihypertensive therapy:

Labetalol IV (20–80 mg bolus)

Hydralazine IV (5–10 mg)

Nifedipine oral.

Seizure prophylaxis: Magnesium sulfate ($MgSO_4$) regimen.

Pritchard's Regimen:

4 g IV + 10 g IM (5 g in each buttock),

Maintenance: 5 g IM every 4 hours × 24 h after last seizure.

Monitor: Knee jerk, respiratory rate (>16/min), urine output (>30 mL/hr).

Fluid balance: Avoid overload.

Corticosteroids: For fetal lung maturity if <34 weeks.

Delivery: Definitive cure is delivery of fetus and placenta.

Induction if cervix favorable; otherwise cesarean section if maternal/fetal distress.

III. Eclampsia

Definition

Occurrence of generalized tonic–clonic convulsions and/or coma in a woman with preeclampsia, not due to epilepsy or other causes.

Timing

Antepartum: 50%

Intrapartum: 30%

Postpartum: 20% (usually within 48 hours)

Clinical Features

Prodromal symptoms: Headache, visual disturbance, epigastric pain.

Convulsions: Tonic–clonic seizures lasting 1 minute, followed by coma.

May have repeated fits, cyanosis, tongue bite or pulmonary edema.

Management of Eclampsia

1. Control of Convulsions

Magnesium sulfate – drug of choice.

Pritchard or Zuspan regimen.

If seizures persist, diazepam 10 mg IV slowly.

2. Control of Blood Pressure

Labetalol or Hydralazine IV to maintain BP <150/100 mmHg.

3. Supportive Therapy

Oxygen, maintain airway.

Catheterize bladder; strict input-output charting.

Fluid: 80 mL/hour (avoid overload).

Treat complications (e.g., pulmonary edema, DIC).

4. Delivery

After maternal stabilization. Induce labor if cervix favorable; cesarean if urgent delivery needed. Continue $MgSO_4$ for 24 hours after last fit.

IV. Chronic Hypertension

Definition

Hypertension (≥140/90 mmHg) present before pregnancy or detected before 20 weeks, or persists beyond 12 weeks postpartum.

Complications

Superimposed preeclampsia

Abruptio placentae

IUGR

Preterm delivery

Management

Continue safe antihypertensives (Labetalol, Methyldopa).

Monitor for superimposed preeclampsia.

Low-dose aspirin (75–150 mg/day) prophylaxis from 12 weeks.

Fetal surveillance by growth scans and Doppler.

V. Chronic Hypertension with Superimposed Preeclampsia

Definition

Development of new-onset proteinuria or sudden rise in BP in a woman with pre-existing hypertension.

Management

Similar to severe preeclampsia.

Delivery often required once fetal maturity is reasonable or if maternal condition deteriorates.

HELLP Syndrome

Definition: A severe form of preeclampsia characterized by:

Hemolysis

Elevated Liver enzymes

Low Platelets

Clinical Features

Epigastric pain, nausea, vomiting

Jaundice, malaise.

Laboratory

LDH >600 IU/L, AST/ALT elevated.

Platelets <100,000/mm^3.

Peripheral smear: Schistocytes.

Complications

DIC, hepatic rupture, renal failure, maternal death.

Management

Stabilize and deliver immediately.

Blood and platelet transfusion as needed.

Magnesium sulfate prophylaxis.

Intensive monitoring.

Prevention of Preeclampsia

1. Low-dose aspirin (75–150 mg daily from 12–16 weeks) for high-risk women.
2. Calcium supplementation (1–1.5 g/day).
3. Early antenatal registration and regular BP monitoring.
4. Rest and avoidance of stress.
5. Treatment of underlying disorders like hypertension, renal or autoimmune disease.

Summary Table

Disorder	Onset	Proteinuria	Time of Resolution
Gestational HTN	After 20 wks	Absent	<12 wks postpartum
Preeclampsia	After 20 wks	Present	<12 wks postpartum
Eclampsia	After 20 wks	Present	<12 wks postpartum
Chronic HTN	Before 20 wks	Variable	>12 wks postpartum

Key Points

Hypertensive disorders account for nearly 15% of maternal deaths in developing countries.

Preeclampsia is a disease of theories, with endothelial dysfunction at its core.

Magnesium sulfate is the drug of choice for seizure prophylaxis and control.

Delivery of the placenta is the only definitive cure.

Early recognition and careful monitoring are vital to prevent maternal and fetal complications.

10.2 Oligohydramnios (*Qillat-i-Ma' Amniosi*)

& Polyhydramnios (*Kasrat-i-an' amniosi*)

Oligohydramnios (*Qillat-i-Ma' Amniosi*)

Definition

Oligohydramnios is a condition characterized by deficient amniotic fluid volume for gestational age.

Diagnostic Criteria

1. Amniotic Fluid Index (AFI):

< 5 cm → Oligohydramnios

(Measured as the sum of vertical fluid pockets in 4 quadrants of uterus using ultrasound)

2. Single Deepest Pocket (SDP):

< 2 cm → Oligohydramnios

Normal AFI by Gestational Age

16–20 weeks: ~12–14 cm

28–32 weeks: peaks at 14–18 cm

Term (≥ 37 weeks): declines to 8–10 cm

Etiology (Causes)

1. Fetal Causes

Renal anomalies:

Bilateral renal agenesis (Potter syndrome)

Polycystic kidneys

Multicystic dysplastic kidneys

Obstructive uropathy (posterior urethral valves)

Chromosomal abnormalities

2. Placental Causes

Uteroplacental insufficiency (e.g., preeclampsia, IUGR, chronic hypertension)

Placental infarction

Post-term pregnancy (placental senescence)

3. Maternal Causes

Dehydration

Hypovolemia

Use of ACE inhibitors, prostaglandin synthetase inhibitors (NSAIDs)

4. Membrane Causes

Premature rupture of membranes (PROM)

Leakage of amniotic fluid

Pathophysiology

The majority of amniotic fluid in the second half of pregnancy is derived from fetal urine.

Any condition reducing fetal urine output (renal anomalies, hypoxia) or fluid loss (ruptured membranes) leads to low AF volume.

Prolonged oligohydramnios causes fetal compression deformities and pulmonary hypoplasia.

Clinical Features

Maternal

Decreased abdominal girth or fundal height less than gestational age

Difficulty in palpating fetal parts due to close apposition

Fetal movements felt more intensely

Fetal

Restricted movements

Abnormal presentation (e.g., breech)

Growth restriction (IUGR)

Complications

Maternal

Prolonged or obstructed labor (due to poor lubrication)

Increased rate of cesarean delivery

Fetal

Pulmonary hypoplasia (especially if early onset)

Skeletal deformities (Potter facies, club foot)

Umbilical cord compression → fetal distress

Meconium aspiration

IUGR

Increased perinatal morbidity and mortality

Diagnosis

1. Ultrasound Findings

AFI < 5 cm or SDP < 2 cm

Fetal anomalies (especially renal)

IUGR

Cord compression signs

2. Additional Tests

Doppler studies of umbilical artery

Non-stress test (NST) or biophysical profile (BPP)

Fetal well-being monitoring

Screening for PROM (if suspected)

Management

1. Evaluation of Cause

Exclude rupture of membranes (speculum exam, Amnisure test)

Screen for fetal anomalies (detailed anomaly scan)

Assess placental function (Doppler)

2. Conservative Management (if preterm and stable)

Adequate maternal hydration (oral/IV)

Bed rest (left lateral position)

Serial ultrasound for AFI and fetal growth

NST / BPP for fetal well-being

Stop causative drugs (e.g., ACE inhibitors, NSAIDs)

3. Interventions

Amnioinfusion (during labor):

Infusion of warm saline into amniotic cavity via intrauterine catheter to relieve cord compression.

Amniocentesis / Amnioinfusion (antenatal):

Sometimes done in severe cases to improve visualization or relieve compression.

4. Delivery

If term or fetal distress → Induce labor or perform cesarean section

Continuous fetal heart rate monitoring during labor

Polyhydramnios (*Kasrat-i-an' amniosi*)

Definition

Polyhydramnios (hydramnios) is the excess accumulation of amniotic fluid beyond normal limits for gestational age.

Diagnostic Criteria

1. Amniotic Fluid Index (AFI):

> 24 cm → Polyhydramnios

2. Single Deepest Pocket (SDP):

> 8 cm

Types

1. Acute Polyhydramnios:

Rapid accumulation (usually in 2nd trimester)

Sudden abdominal distension, respiratory distress

Commonly associated with twin-to-twin transfusion syndrome (TTTS)

2. Chronic Polyhydramnios:

Gradual accumulation (usually in 3rd trimester)

More common, less symptomatic

Etiology (Causes)

1. Fetal Causes

Congenital anomalies:

Esophageal or duodenal atresia (impaired swallowing)

Anencephaly (absent swallowing reflex)

Cleft lip/palate

Neural tube defects

Chromosomal abnormalities:

Trisomy 21, 18, 13

Fetal anemia:

Rh isoimmunization, parvovirus infection

Twin-to-twin transfusion syndrome (recipient twin)

2. Maternal Causes

Diabetes mellitus (maternal hyperglycemia → fetal polyuria)

Multiple pregnancy

Infections (TORCH, syphilis)

3. Idiopathic

~50–60% cases (no identifiable cause)

Pathophysiology

Amniotic fluid balance depends on fetal swallowing and urination.

Excess production (fetal polyuria) or decreased absorption (impaired swallowing) → accumulation.

Clinical Features

Maternal

Rapid increase in abdominal size

Respiratory distress or orthopnea (due to diaphragmatic pressure)

Abdominal discomfort, tightness, stretch marks

Difficulty in palpating fetal parts or hearing FHR

Uterine overdistension → preterm labor

Fetal

Malpresentation (transverse lie, breech)

Increased risk of cord prolapse after rupture of membranes

Complications

Maternal

Preterm labor

Premature rupture of membranes (PROM)

Malpresentation

Placental abruption (due to sudden decompression)

Postpartum hemorrhage (uterine atony)

Respiratory distress due to uterine distension

Fetal

Cord prolapse

Prematurity

Malformations

Intrauterine death

Growth abnormalities (macrosomia or IUGR depending on cause)

Diagnosis

1. Clinical

Fundal height much more than gestational age

Difficulty in palpating fetal parts

Fluid thrill on abdominal examination

2. Ultrasound

AFI > 24 cm or SDP > 8 cm

Look for fetal anomalies, twins, placental lesions

Assess fetal growth and presentation

3. Additional Investigations

Oral glucose tolerance test (OGTT) for diabetes

TORCH screening

Rh typing and antibody screen

Detailed anomaly scan

Karyotyping (if structural anomalies present)

Management

1. Mild / Idiopathic Polyhydramnios

Close monitoring with serial ultrasounds

Maternal rest and symptom relief

Control maternal blood sugar if diabetic

Fetal surveillance with NST / BPP

2. Moderate to Severe Cases

Amnioreduction:

Therapeutic removal of excess fluid via amniocentesis (under USG guidance)

Indomethacin (NSAID):

Reduces fetal urine output

Dose: 25–50 mg orally every 6 hours

Used before 32 weeks only (monitor ductus arteriosus by Doppler)

Treat underlying cause:

(e.g., control diabetes, manage Rh isoimmunization)

3. Delivery

At term: Induction of labor under controlled conditions

During labor: Artificial rupture of membranes under controlled setting to prevent cord prolapse

Monitor for: PPH and fetal distress

Summary

Oligohydramnios → Deficient fluid, often due to renal or placental problems → compression & distress.

Polyhydramnios → Excess fluid, often due to diabetes or swallowing defects → overdistension & preterm risk.

Both conditions require fetal surveillance, cause evaluation and timely delivery to reduce perinatal morbidity and mortality.

10.3 Multifetal & Twins pregnancy

(Haml-i-adeed aur haml-i-tawam)

Introduction

Multi-fetal pregnancy refers to the development of more than one fetus in the uterus.

Twin pregnancy is the most common type (~1 in 80 pregnancies).

Increasing incidence due to advanced maternal age and assisted reproductive technologies (ART).

High-risk pregnancy due to increased maternal and fetal complications.

Definition

When more than one fetus simultaneously develops in the uterus, it is called multiple pregnancy. Simultaneous development of two fetuses (twins) is most common ; other types like development of three fetuses (triplets), four fetuses (quadruplets), five fetuses (quintuplets) or six fetuses (sextuplets) may also occur. (*Dutta)*

Embryology and Zygosity

Zygosity

1. Monozygotic (Identical) twins: 20%, Single ovum, divides after fertilization

Genetically identical

Division timing determines chorionicity and amnionicity:

Timing	Placenta	Amnion	Clinical Significance
0–4 days	Dichorionic, diamniotic	2	Lowest risk
4–8 days	Monochorionic, diamniotic	2	Risk of TTTS
8–12 days	Monochorionic, monoamniotic	1	Cord entanglement
>13 days	Conjoined	1	Rare, high mortality

2. Dizygotic (Fraternal/binovular) twins: 80%, Two separate ova fertilized by two sperm.

Always dichorionic diamniotic

Influenced by maternal age, genetics, parity

Chorionicity & Amnionicity

Chorionicity: Number of placentas

Amnionicity: Number of amniotic sacs

Clinically more important than zygosity; determines risk and management

Types: DCDA, MCDA, MCMA, conjoined

Epidemiology

Twin births: 1–2% of live births

Monozygotic: ~0.3–0.4%

Dizygotic: Variable (higher with fertility treatment)

Maternal age 30–35 years increases dizygotic twin incidence

ART increases multi-fetal pregnancies significantly

Etiology / Risk Factors

1. Genetic: Family history of twins (maternal side for dizygotic)
2. Maternal age: Peak incidence at 30–35 years
3. Parity: Increased parity → higher dizygotic twin rate
4. Race: African > Caucasian > Asian
5. Fertility treatment: IVF, ovulation induction
6. Short interpregnancy interval
7. High BMI

Pathophysiology

Implantation and Placental Development

Monozygotic division affects the placentation: mono vs. dichorionic

Shared placenta in monochorionic twins → vascular anastomoses → risk of TTTS

Hemodynamic Changes

Maternal blood volume expands more (~40–50% increase vs. 30–40% in singleton)

Cardiac output rises more → predisposition to heart failure in high-risk mothers

Increased renal load → higher risk of hydronephrosis, proteinuria

Fetal Interactions

Monozygotic monochorionic twins: Risk of unequal blood flow → Donor-recipient syndrome

Risk of growth restriction, anemia, polycythemia

Clinical Features

Maternal Signs

Rapid uterine growth

Multiple fetal heart sounds (>12 weeks)

Palpable multiple parts after 20 weeks

Excessive nausea and vomiting

Diagnosis

1. Clinical suspicion: Large uterus for gestational age. Excessive fundal height.
2. Ultrasonography (Gold Standard):

First trimester: Number of gestational sacs, yolk sacs, heartbeats

Chorionicity determination:

Lambda sign: dichorionic

T-sign: monochorionic

Second trimester: Growth monitoring, anomalies

3. Other investigations:

Serial hemoglobin and hematocrit

Blood pressure, urine protein

Early referral to high-risk obstetrics

Maternal Complications

1. Early Pregnancy:

Miscarriage, hyperemesis, molar pregnancy risk higher.

2. Second & Third Trimester:

Preeclampsia / gestational hypertension

Gestational diabetes

Anemia

Polyhydramnios (especially in MC twins)

Preterm labor (50–60% in twins)

Placental complications: previa, abruption

Increased cesarean section rate

Fetal / Neonatal Complications

1. Prematurity: Leading cause of morbidity/mortality
2. Growth restriction: More in monochorionic twins
3. Twin-to-Twin Transfusion Syndrome (TTTS):

Only in monochorionic twins

Donor twin: growth restriction, oligohydramnios

Recipient twin: polycythemia, heart failure, polyhydramnios

4. Congenital anomalies: More common in monozygotic twins
5. Cord complications: Particularly in monoamniotic twins
6. Stillbirth: Higher in monochorionic twins
7. Neonatal complications: Respiratory distress, intraventricular hemorrhage, NICU admission

Antenatal Management

Maternal Care

Frequent antenatal visits: Every 2–4 weeks initially, weekly in late pregnancy for high-risk twins

Nutrition: Extra 300–600 kcal/day, iron, folic acid, calcium

Monitoring: BP, proteinuria, hematocrit, thyroid if indicated

Fetal Surveillance

Ultrasound:

11–14 weeks → Confirm number, chorionicity

18–22 weeks → Anomaly scan

Every 4 weeks → Growth scan (2–3 weeks for monochorionic)

Doppler studies: Umbilical artery, MCA, ductus venosus in growth-restricted twins

Fetal echocardiography: If monochorionic twins or anomalies

Prevention of Preterm Labor

Progesterone supplementation (if indicated)

Cervical length assessment

Bed rest: Only if complications or preterm contractions

Delivery

Timing

Type	Recommended Gestation
Dichorionic twins	38 weeks
Monochorionic twins	36–37 weeks
Monoamniotic twins	32–34 weeks

Mode of Delivery

Vaginal: If first twin cephalic, no complications

Cesarean: Non-cephalic presentation of first twin, placental issues, cord entanglement

Continuous fetal monitoring during labor

Peripartum preparation

Availability of NICU

Preparedness for postpartum hemorrhage

Multi-disciplinary team: Obstetrician, anesthesiologist, neonatologist

Postpartum Care

High risk of hemorrhage → careful monitoring

Early ambulation, iron and fluid supplementation

Lactation support: Multiple infants requires guidance

Psychological support: Anxiety and stress higher in multiple births

Prognosis

Maternal outcomes: Generally good if managed in high-risk settings

Fetal outcomes: Depend on chorionicity, prematurity, growth discordance, TTTS

Long-term: Monochorionic twins have higher perinatal morbidity

Summary

Multi-fetal pregnancies are high-risk; early detection and chorionicity determination are key.

Monozygotic vs dizygotic helps predict complications; chorionicity guides management.

Major complications: Preterm labor, TTTS, growth restriction, preeclampsia.

Requires frequent monitoring, nutrition, timely delivery planning and neonatal care.

Multidisciplinary approach significantly improves maternal and fetal outcomes.

Multi-Fetal Pregnancy

```
├── Types
│   ├── Twins (Most common)
│   │   ├── Zygosity
│   │   │   ├── Monozygotic (Identical)
│   │   │   │   ├── 0–4 days → DCDA (Dichorionic, Diamniotic)
│   │   │   │   ├── 4–8 days → MCDA (Monochorionic, Diamniotic)
│   │   │   │   ├── 8–12 days → MCMA (Monochorionic, Monoamniotic)
│   │   │   │   └── >13 days → Conjoined Twins
│   │   │   └── Dizygotic (Fraternal) → Always DCDA
│   │   └── Chorionicity & Amnionicity
│   │   ├── DCDA → 2 placentas, 2 sacs, lowest risk
│   │   ├── MCDA → 1 placenta, 2 sacs, risk of TTTS
│   │   ├── MCMA → 1 placenta, 1 sac, cord entanglement
│   │   └── Conjoined → 1 placenta, 1 sac, fused bodies
│   └── Triplets / Quadruplets → Rare, high-risk
├── Maternal Complications
│   ├── Early Pregnancy → Miscarriage, Hyperemesis, GTD risk ↑
```

│ ├─ Second/Third Trimester → Preeclampsia, Gestational diabetes, Polyhydramnios, Preterm labor, Placental complications, Anemia
│ └─ Peripartum/Postpartum → PPH, High C-section rate, Psychological stress
├─ Fetal / Neonatal Complications
│ ├─ Prematurity → NICU, RDS
│ ├─ Growth restriction / IUGR
│ ├─ TTTS (MC only)
│ │ ├─ Donor → Oligohydramnios, anemia
│ │ └─ Recipient → Polyhydramnios, polycythemia, heart failure
│ ├─ Congenital anomalies ↑ (Monozygotic)
│ ├─ Cord complications → Entanglement (MCMA)
│ └─ Stillbirth → Monochorionic twins > Dichorionic twins
├─ Antenatal Monitoring
│ ├─ Ultrasound
│ │ ├─ 11–14 weeks → Number, chorionicity, viability
│ │ ├─ 18–22 weeks → Anomaly scan
│ │ └─ Every 2–4 weeks → Growth, AFI, Doppler (MC twins every 2–3 weeks)
│ ├─ Maternal
│ │ ├─ BP & proteinuria → Preeclampsia
│ │ ├─ Hb & iron supplementation
│ │ ├─ Weight gain & nutrition
│ │ └─ Blood sugar → Gestational diabetes
│ └─ Preterm labor prevention
│ ├─ Cervical length monitoring
│ ├─ Progesterone if indicated
│ └─ Bed rest only if complications
├─ Delivery Planning
│ ├─ Timing
│ │ ├─ Dichorionic → 38 weeks
│ │ ├─ Monochorionic → 36–37 weeks
│ │ └─ Monoamniotic → 32–34 weeks
│ ├─ Mode
│ │ ├─ Vaginal → First twin cephalic, no contraindication
│ │ └─ Cesarean → First twin non-cephalic, cord entanglement, previa, MCMA
│ └─ Peripartum Care
│ ├─ NICU availability
│ ├─ Uterotonics → Prevent PPH
│ └─ Multidisciplinary team → Obstetrician + Anesthesiologist + Neonatologist
└─ High-Yield Summary
├─ Chorionicity > Zygosity for management
├─ TTTS only in monochorionic twins
├─ MCMA → Highest risk of cord accidents & stillbirth

├─ Maternal complications ↑ (preeclampsia, PPH, diabetes)
├─ Fetal complications ↑ (prematurity, IUGR, anomalies)
└─ Early detection + frequent monitoring = Improved outcomes

10.4 Intrauterine Growth Retardation (IUGR)

(*Takhal-luf-i-nam-we-dakhillur-rahim*)

Definition

A condition in which a fetus fails to achieve its genetically determined growth potential.

Alternative terms: Fetal growth restriction (FGR), small-for-gestational-age (SGA).

Clinical definition: Fetal weight < 10th percentile for gestational age on standard growth charts.

Severe IUGR: Weight < 3rd percentile or < 5th percentile (depending on reference).

Epidemiology

Incidence: 5–10% of all pregnancies.

Higher in developing countries, low socioeconomic status, maternal malnutrition, multiple pregnancies.

Maternal/fetal factors contribute equally.

Associated with perinatal morbidity and mortality.

Etiology / Risk Factors

IUGR causes are broadly divided into maternal, placental, fetal and environmental factors.

Maternal Factors

Chronic diseases: Hypertension, preeclampsia, diabetes mellitus, renal disease, autoimmune disorders

Malnutrition: Low BMI, anemia, vitamin deficiencies

Infections: TORCH infections (Toxoplasmosis, Rubella, CMV, HSV), malaria, syphilis

Substance use: Smoking, alcohol, cocaine, drugs

Multiple pregnancies: Twins/triplets

Advanced maternal age (<18 or >35 years)

Placental Factors

Abnormal placentation → poor perfusion

Placental insufficiency

Placental infarcts or thrombosis

Placenta previa or abruption

Fetal Factors

Chromosomal abnormalities: Trisomy 13, 18, 21

Congenital anomalies: Cardiac, renal, CNS defects

Infections: Congenital TORCH infections

Environmental Factors

High altitude → chronic hypoxia

Exposure to toxins or radiation

Classification of IUGR

Symmetric (Proportional) IUGR

Early onset (<28 weeks)

Head, body and organs proportionally small

Usually caused by chromosomal abnormalities or early maternal disease

Asymmetric (Disproportional) IUGR

Late onset (>28 weeks)

Head sparing: Brain size preserved, body thin

Commonly due to placental insufficiency or maternal hypertension/preeclampsia

Clinical Classification (Based on Risk)

1. Mild: 5th–10th percentile
2. Moderate: 3rd–5th percentile
3. Severe: $<3^{rd}$ percentile

Pathophysiology

Maternal Hypoperfusion

Chronic hypertension or preeclampsia → decreased uteroplacental blood flow → fetal hypoxia → nutrient restriction

Placental Dysfunction

Infarcts, thrombosis, or abnormal villi → impaired exchange of oxygen and nutrients → growth restriction

Fetal Adaptations

Brain-sparing effect: preferential blood flow to brain, heart and adrenals

Reduced liver perfusion: decreased glycogen and fat storage

Altered metabolism: catabolism of muscle → thin extremities

Clinical Feature

Maternal Signs

Small-for-gestational-age uterus

Fundal height lag (>3 cm below expected)

Reduced fetal movements

Fetal Signs

Ultrasound: estimated fetal weight <10th percentile

Abnormal Doppler studies:

Umbilical artery: increased resistance

Middle cerebral artery: decreased resistance (brain-sparing)

Ductus venosus: abnormal flow in severe cases

Diagnosis

Clinical Diagnosis: Symphyseal-fundal height (SFH) measurement

Fetal movement assessment: Ultrasound

Biometry:

Biparietal diameter (BPD)

Head circumference (HC)

Abdominal circumference (AC) → most sensitive for IUGR

Femur length (FL)

Estimated fetal weight (EFW) using Hadlock formula

Amniotic fluid index (AFI): Oligohydramnios common

Doppler Studies

Umbilical artery: high resistance → placental insufficiency

Middle cerebral artery: low resistance → brain-sparing

Ductus venosus: absent or reversed a-wave → fetal compromise

Biophysical Profile (BPP)

Fetal tone, movement, breathing, amniotic fluid, NST

Score <6/10 → fetal distress

Complications

Perinatal

Preterm birth

Birth asphyxia

Meconium aspiration

Hypoglycemia

Hypothermia

Polycythemia

Long-term

Neurodevelopmental delay

Learning disabilities

Cardiovascular disease in adulthood (Barker hypothesis)

Maternal

Higher cesarean section rate

Preeclampsia

Anxiety and stress

Management

Maternal Optimization

Treat underlying maternal disease (hypertension, diabetes)

Improve nutrition

Avoid smoking, alcohol, and drugs

Monitor weight gain

Fetal Surveillance

Serial ultrasound every 2–4 weeks (biometry, Doppler, AFI)

Non-stress test (NST) weekly

Biophysical profile (BPP) weekly

Timing of Delivery

Mild IUGR with normal Doppler: continue pregnancy to term

Severe IUGR with abnormal Doppler: consider early delivery

Delivery route: Vaginal if fetal status favorable; cesarean if compromise present

Intrauterine Interventions

Corticosteroids for fetal lung maturity if preterm delivery anticipated

Magnesium sulfate for neuroprotection in <32 weeks

Prognosis

Depends on severity, gestational age at onset, cause, and fetal surveillance

Symmetric IUGR (early onset) → poor prognosis

Asymmetric IUGR (late onset) → better prognosis if managed timely

Prevention

Early prenatal care

Optimize maternal nutrition

Treat maternal diseases promptly

Avoid teratogens (smoking, alcohol, drugs)

Aspirin prophylaxis in high-risk mothers (prevention of preeclampsia

Important Points

IUGR: Estimated fetal weight <10th percentile

Symmetric vs Asymmetric: Early vs late onset; proportional vs brain-sparing

Most sensitive ultrasound parameter: Abdominal circumference (AC)

Doppler abnormality: Umbilical artery high resistance → worst prognosis

Management: Maternal optimization, close fetal surveillance, timely delivery

Complications: Perinatal asphyxia, hypoglycemia, neurodevelopmental delay

Symmetric vs Asymmetric IUGR

Feature	Symmetric IUGR	Asymmetric IUGR
Onset	Early (<28 weeks)	Late (>28 weeks)
Fetal Proportions	Proportionally small (head, body, organs all reduced)	Disproportionate; head normal ("brain-sparing"), body thin
Cause	Chromosomal abnormalities, congenital infections (TORCH), early maternal chronic disease	Placental insufficiency, maternal hypertension/preeclampsia, late malnutrition
Most Affected Organ	Entire body equally	Liver and fat stores more affected; brain spared
Ultrasound Findings	All biometry parameters <10th percentile	Abdominal circumference <10th percentile; head circumference preserved
Doppler Findings	Usually normal early; may show chronic hypoxia later	Umbilical artery: ↑ resistance; MCA: ↓ resistance (brain sparing); Ductus venosus: abnormal in severe cases
Amniotic Fluid	Often normal	Oligohydramnios common
Growth Pattern	Slow from early gestation	Normal early growth, slows in third trimester
Delivery Considerations	Early delivery may be needed if severe or fetal compromise	Monitor with Doppler; deliver based on fetal status and gestational age
Prognosis	Poorer, higher risk of perinatal morbidity	Better if detected and managed timely
Associated Complications	Congenital anomalies, neurodevelopmental delay	Preterm birth, hypoglycemia, perinatal asphyxia, polycythemia

Intrauterine Growth Retardation (IUGR)

```
│
├── Definition
│   ├── Fetal weight <10th percentile for gestational age
│   ├── Severe: <3rd percentile
│   └── AKA: Fetal Growth Restriction (FGR), Small-for-Gestational-Age (SGA)
│
├── Classification
│   ├── Symmetric (Proportional)
```

```
│   │   ├── Early onset (<28 weeks)
│   │   ├── Head, body, organs all proportionally small
│   │   └── Causes: Chromosomal anomalies, congenital infections, maternal chronic disease
│   └── Asymmetric (Disproportional)
│   ├── Late onset (>28 weeks)
│   ├── Brain sparing: Head normal, body thin
│   └── Causes: Placental insufficiency, maternal hypertension, preeclampsia
│
├── Etiology / Risk Factors
│   ├── Maternal
│   │   ├── Hypertension / Preeclampsia
│   │   ├── Diabetes (poorly controlled)
│   │   ├── Malnutrition / Anemia
│   │   ├── Infections: TORCH, malaria
│   │   └── Smoking, alcohol, drugs
│   ├── Placental
│   │   ├── Placental insufficiency
│   │   ├── Infarcts / Thrombosis
│   │   └── Previa or abruption
│   ├── Fetal
│   │   ├── Chromosomal anomalies (Trisomy 13, 18, 21)
│   │   ├── Congenital anomalies (cardiac, renal, CNS)
│   │   └── Intrauterine infections
│   └── Environmental
│   ├── High altitude
│   └── Toxins / radiation
│
├── Pathophysiology
│   ├── Maternal hypoperfusion → ↓ uteroplacental blood flow → fetal hypoxia
│   ├── Placental dysfunction → impaired nutrient & oxygen delivery
│   └── Fetal adaptations
│   ├── Brain sparing (↑ cerebral perfusion)
│   ├── ↓ liver perfusion → ↓ glycogen & fat
│   └── Muscle catabolism → thin extremities
│
├── Clinical Features
│   ├── Maternal: Small uterus, lag in fundal height, reduced fetal movements
│   └── Fetal: Estimated weight <10th percentile, Doppler abnormalities
│
├── Diagnosis
│   ├── Clinical: Symphyseal-fundal height, fetal movements
│   ├── Ultrasound: BPD, HC, AC (most sensitive), FL, EFW, AFI
```

```
│  ├── Doppler: Umbilical artery ↑ resistance, MCA ↓ resistance, Ductus venosus a-wave reversal
│  └── Biophysical profile (BPP): score <6/10 → fetal compromise
│
├── Complications
│  ├── Perinatal: Preterm birth, asphyxia, RDS, hypoglycemia, hypothermia, polycythemia
│  ├── Long-term: Neurodevelopmental delay, learning disabilities, adult cardiovascular disease
│  └── Maternal: Preeclampsia, cesarean section, anxiety/stress
│
├── Management
│  ├── Maternal optimization: Treat chronic disease, nutrition, lifestyle modifications
│  ├── Fetal surveillance
│  │  ├── Serial ultrasound (biometry, Doppler, AFI)
│  │  ├── NST weekly
│  │  └── BPP weekly
│  ├── Timing of delivery
│  │  ├── Mild IUGR, normal Doppler → continue to term
│  │  └── Severe IUGR, abnormal Doppler → early delivery
│  ├── Delivery route: Vaginal if fetal status favorable, C-section if compromise
│  └── Intrauterine interventions: Corticosteroids for lung maturity, magnesium sulfate (<32 weeks)
│
└── Prognosis
├── Depends on severity, gestational age, cause, fetal surveillance
├── Symmetric IUGR → poorer prognosis
└── Asymmetric IUGR → better prognosis if managed timely
```

10.5 Preterm Rupture of membrane

(*Tamzzuk-i-aghshiyahya-i-janeen mubtasir*)

Definition

Rupture of membranes (ROM): Spontaneous rupture/tearing of the amniotic sac before the onset of labor.

Term PROM: Rupture of membranes ≥37 weeks of gestation before labor onset.

Preterm PROM (PPROM): Rupture of membranes <37 weeks gestation.

Latency period: Time between rupture and onset of labor.

Key distinction:

Type	Gestational Age	Timing
Term PROM	≥37 weeks	Before labor
PPROM	<37 weeks	Before labor

Epidemiology

PPROM complicates 2–3% of all pregnancies.

Responsible for 30–40% of preterm births.

Associated with significant perinatal morbidity and mortality.

Incidence higher in: multiple pregnancies, low socioeconomic status, prior PROM, infections.

Etiology / Risk Factors

PPROM is multifactorial; causes are maternal, fetal or environmental.

Maternal Factors

Infections: Genital tract infections (bacterial vaginosis, UTI, chorioamnionitis, STIs)

History of PROM: 30% recurrence risk

Low socioeconomic status / Malnutrition

Smoking, alcohol, drug use

Multiple pregnancy → overdistension of uterus

Cervical incompetence or short cervix

Fetal Factors

Polyhydramnios → overdistension

Multiple gestation → mechanical stress on membranes

Placental / Amniotic Factors

Placental abruption

Structural weakness of membranes (collagen defect)

Prior invasive procedures (amniocentesis, cervical cerclage)

Pathophysiology

1. Mechanical Stress: Overdistension of uterus → rupture of membranes.
2. Infection: Bacterial enzymes (collagenases) weaken membranes → rupture.
3. Inflammatory Mediators: Cytokines and prostaglandins → membrane weakening and uterine contractions.
4. Membrane Structural Defects: Deficient collagen crosslinking, abnormal extracellular matrix.

Classification of PROM

Type	Gestational Age	Notes
Term PROM	≥37 weeks	Usually labor ensues within 24 hrs
Preterm PROM (PPROM)	<37 weeks	Preterm labor risk ↑; requires specialized management
Prolonged ROM	≥24 hours before delivery	↑ risk of infection for mother & fetus
Recurrent PROM	Multiple pregnancies affected	High recurrence risk

Clinical Features

Maternal:

Sudden gush of fluid per vagina or continuous trickle

Often painless

May be associated with uterine contractions (if labor begins)

Fever, foul-smelling discharge → suggest infection

Fetal:

Variable fetal heart rate (FHR) changes if infection or cord prolapse present

Reduced fetal movements if severe oligohydramnios

Signs of chorioamnionitis: fetal tachycardia

Diagnosis

Clinical + Investigative

History & Examination

History of fluid leakage, color, amount, odor

Sterile speculum exam: pooling of fluid in the posterior fornix

Avoid digital exam unless labor is imminent (↑ infection risk)

Tests

Nitrazine test: pH of amniotic fluid ~7.0–7.5 → turns paper blue

Fern test: Amniotic fluid dries → "ferning" pattern under microscope

Amnisure / IGFBP-1 test: Commercial rapid immunoassay for PROM

Ultrasound: Assess amniotic fluid index (AFI) → oligohydramnios common. Evaluate fetal growth and well-being

Complications

Maternal

Infection: Chorioamnionitis, endometritis

Sepsis (rare, severe cases)

Increased cesarean delivery

Postpartum hemorrhage

Fetal / Neonatal

Prematurity → RDS, IVH, NEC, sepsis

Umbilical cord compression / prolapse

Fetal growth restriction

Oligohydramnios → pulmonary hypoplasia if <26 weeks

Neonatal sepsis

Management

Depends on gestational age, fetal status, and presence of infection.

General Principles

Hospitalization for observation. Monitor for infection: Maternal temp, WBC count, CRP

Avoid digital vaginal examination unless labor or delivery imminent

Gestational Age-Specific Management

<34 Weeks (Conservative / Expectant Management)

Goal: Prolong pregnancy safely for fetal maturity

Fetal surveillance: Daily NST / BPP every 24–48h

Ultrasound for growth and AFI

Maternal prophylaxis:

Antibiotics (e.g., Ampicillin → Erythromycin) → reduces infection & latency

Corticosteroids (e.g., Betamethasone) → fetal lung maturity

Tocolysis (if contractions present, short-term) → delay labor 48h for steroids

34–36+6 Weeks

Individualized approach:

If no infection or labor → consider delivery

Antibiotics may be continued

Corticosteroids usually not needed

≥37 Weeks

Delivery indicated

Vaginal route preferred if no contraindication

Indications for Immediate Delivery

Chorioamnionitis

Non-reassuring fetal status

Significant placental abruption

Severe oligohydramnios compromising fetus

Monitoring

Maternal: Vital signs, uterine tenderness, WBC, CRP

Fetal: FHR monitoring, daily NST, AFI, growth scans

Infection signs: Fever, uterine tenderness, fetal tachycardia

Prognosis

Depends on gestational age at rupture and latency period

PPROM <28 weeks: High perinatal morbidity/mortality

Term PROM: Usually good outcome if labor managed promptly

With infection: Increased maternal and neonatal complications

Prevention

Treat maternal infections early

Avoid smoking, alcohol, drugs

Cervical cerclage in selected women with cervical incompetence

Adequate prenatal care

High-Yield Points

PPROM: ROM <37 weeks

Complications: Prematurity, chorioamnionitis, oligohydramnios, cord prolapse

Diagnosis: History, sterile speculum, Nitrazine, Fern test, AFI

Management: Expectant <34 weeks with steroids + antibiotics; delivery ≥37 weeks

Avoid digital exam unless labor imminent

Latent infection: Early recognition reduces maternal & fetal morbidity

Rupture of Membranes (ROM)

```
│
├─ Definition
│  ├─ PROM: ≥37 weeks before labor
│  └─ PPROM: <37 weeks before labor
├─ Risk Factors / Etiology
│  ├─ Maternal
│  │  ├─ Genital tract infections (bacterial vaginosis, chorioamnionitis)
│  │  ├─ Urinary tract infection
│  │  ├─ History of PROM
│  │  ├─ Multiple gestation
│  │  ├─ Short cervix / cervical incompetence
│  │  └─ Smoking, alcohol, drugs, malnutrition
│  ├─ Fetal
│  │  ├─ Polyhydramnios → overdistension
│  │  └─ Multiple gestation → mechanical stress
│  └─ Placental / Membrane Factors
│  ├─ Placental abruption
│  ├─ Structural weakness of membranes (collagen defect)
│  └─ Prior invasive procedures (amniocentesis, cerclage)
├─ Pathophysiology
```

```
│ ├─ Mechanical stress → membrane rupture
│ ├─ Infection → collagenase activity → membrane weakening
│ └─ Inflammatory mediators (cytokines, prostaglandins) → labor onset
├─ Classification
│ ├─ Term PROM ≥37 weeks
│ ├─ Preterm PROM (PPROM) <37 weeks
│ ├─ Prolonged ROM ≥24 hours before delivery
│ └─ Recurrent PROM → multiple pregnancies affected
├─ Clinical Features
│ ├─ Maternal: Sudden gush / continuous leakage of fluid, usually painless
│ ├─ Fetal: Reduced movements, non-reassuring FHR if infection or cord prolapse
│ └─ Infection signs: Fever, uterine tenderness, foul discharge
├─ Diagnosis
│ ├─ History: Leakage of fluid, color, amount, odor
│ ├─ Speculum exam: Pooling of fluid in posterior fornix
│ ├─ Bedside tests:
│ │ ├─ Nitrazine (pH paper turns blue)
│ │ ├─ Fern test (ferning pattern)
│ │ └─ IGFBP-1 test (Amnisure)
│ └─ Ultrasound: AFI → oligohydramnios, fetal growth, presentation
├─ Complications
│ ├─ Maternal: Chorioamnionitis, sepsis, endometritis, postpartum hemorrhage
│ └─ Fetal / Neonatal:
│ ├─ Prematurity → RDS, IVH, NEC, sepsis
│ ├─ Cord prolapse / compression
│ ├─ Oligohydramnios → pulmonary hypoplasia (<26 weeks)
│ └─ Fetal growth restriction
├─ Management
│ ├─ General Principles
│ │ ├─ Hospitalization
│ │ ├─ Monitor maternal vitals, labs
│ │ └─ Avoid digital vaginal exam unless labor imminent
│ ├─ Gestational Age-Specific
│ │ ├─ <34 weeks: Expectant management
│ │ │ ├─ Fetal monitoring: NST, BPP, growth scans
│ │ │ ├─ Antibiotics (Ampicillin + Erythromycin)
│ │ │ ├─ Corticosteroids for lung maturity
│ │ │ └─ Tocolysis if contractions present
│ │ ├─ 34–36+6 weeks: Individualized approach
│ │ │ ├─ Consider delivery if risk factors present
│ │ │ └─ Continue antibiotics if needed
│ │ └─ ≥37 weeks: Delivery indicated (usually vaginal)
```

```
│  └─ Immediate Delivery Indications
│  ├─ Chorioamnionitis
│  ├─ Non-reassuring fetal status
│  ├─ Placental abruption
│  └─ Severe oligohydramnios compromising fetus
└─ Prognosis
├─ Depends on gestational age and latency period
├─ PPROM <28 weeks → high perinatal morbidity/mortality
└─ Term PROM → usually good outcome with timely delivery
```

10.6 Preterm labor

(Wiladat-i-Mubakkerah)

Definition

Preterm labor (PTL): Onset of regular uterine contractions causing cervical changes before 37 completed weeks of gestation.

Preterm birth: Delivery occurring before 37 weeks, regardless of onset of labor.

Late preterm: 34–36+6 weeks

Early preterm: <34 weeks

Very preterm: <32 weeks

PTL is labor before 37 weeks; preterm birth is the outcome.

Epidemiology

PTL complicates 5–12% of all pregnancies globally.

Leading cause of neonatal morbidity and mortality.

High-risk groups: Multiple pregnancy, prior PTL, low socioeconomic status.

Etiology / Risk Factors

Maternal Factors

History of preterm birth (strongest predictor)

Short cervical length / cervical incompetence

Uterine anomalies (bicornuate, septate uterus)

Maternal infections:

Genital tract infections (bacterial vaginosis, STIs)

Urinary tract infections

Multiple pregnancies → uterine overdistension

Polyhydramnios

Environmental

Smoking, alcohol, drug abuse

Heavy physical work or stress

Low socioeconomic status / malnutrition

Obstetric Factors

PPROM or PROM

Antepartum bleeding (placenta previa, abruption)

Short interpregnancy interval (<6 months)

Hydramnios or polyhydramnios

Fetal Factors

Multiple gestation

Congenital anomalies

Pathophysiology

PTL is multi-factorial; involves uterine activation, cervical remodeling, and fetal signals.

Uterine Activation: Increased oxytocin receptors in myometrium. Increased prostaglandin synthesis → contractions

Cervical Changes: Cervical ripening: Collagen breakdown → softening and shortening

Inflammation: Cytokines → prostaglandins → cervical remodeling

Triggering Factors

Infection / inflammation: ↑ cytokines, prostaglandins

Mechanical stretch: Uterine overdistension (twins, polyhydramnios)

Maternal-fetal endocrine signals: Corticotropin-releasing hormone (CRH), fetal adrenal cortisol

Classification

Type - Description

Spontaneous preterm labor - Labor before 37 weeks without obvious cause (~70%)

Medically indicated / iatrogenic - Preterm delivery due to maternal or fetal indications (preeclampsia, IUGR, fetal compromise)

Threatened preterm labor - Uterine contractions without cervical changes

Established preterm labor - Contractions + cervical changes (dilatation ≥1 cm or effacement ≥80%)

Clinical Features

Maternal

Regular uterine contractions (>4 per 20 min or >8 per hour)

Lower abdominal pain or cramps

Backache (dull, intermittent)

Vaginal discharge: Blood-tinged or watery (if associated with PROM)

Cervical changes: shortening (<25 mm) or dilatation

Fetal

Increased fetal heart rate variability if fetal compromise

Reduced fetal movements (if severe hypoxia or distress)

Diagnosis

Clinical Assessment

History: contractions, pain, leakage of fluid

Abdominal exam: uterine tone, contraction frequency

Speculum: check for ROM, bleeding

Digital exam: assess cervical dilatation & effacement (if ROM present)

Investigations

Ultrasound: Cervical length measurement (<25 mm predictive)

Fetal fibronectin test (fFN): Predicts risk of delivery within 7–14 days

Amniotic fluid assessment if ROM suspected

Maternal labs: CBC, urinalysis, infection markers (if indicated)

Complications

Maternal

Increased risk of cesarean delivery

Infection: chorioamnionitis

Anxiety and stress

Fetal / Neonatal

Prematurity → RDS, IVH, NEC, hypothermia, hypoglycemia

Low birth weight

Long-term: neurodevelopmental delay, cerebral palsy, learning disabilities

Management

Goals: Delay delivery to allow fetal maturation, prevent infection, and reduce maternal/fetal complications.

General Measures

Hospitalization

Bed rest (though evidence limited, may reduce contractions in selected cases)

Hydration (IV fluids if contractions)

Identify and treat underlying infection

Tocolysis (Uterine Contraction Suppression)

Indicated: <34 weeks with viable fetus, no infection, no fetal compromise

Drugs:

Beta-agonists: Ritodrine, Terbutaline (rarely used now)

Calcium channel blockers: Nifedipine (first-line)

NSAIDs: Indomethacin (<32 weeks, short-term)

Magnesium sulfate: For neuroprotection and tocolysis

Corticosteroids

Accelerate fetal lung maturity

Indicated: 24–34 weeks gestation

Regimens: Betamethasone 12 mg IM q24h × 2 doses or Dexamethasone 6 mg IM q12h × 4 doses

Antibiotic Prophylaxis

If associated with PROM or infection risk

Reduces risk of chorioamnionitis and neonatal sepsis

Magnesium Sulfate for Neuroprotection

Indicated for <32 weeks gestation

Reduces risk of cerebral palsy in preterm infants

Delivery Mode

If contractions cannot be stopped, fetal compromise, or maternal indications → proceed to delivery

Mode of delivery: Usually vaginal unless obstetric indications

Prognosis

Dependent on gestational age at birth and fetal maturity

>34 weeks: Usually favorable outcome

<32 weeks: High neonatal morbidity and mortality

Prevention

Progesterone supplementation (17-OH progesterone) in high-risk women (prior PTL)

Cervical cerclage in cervical insufficiency

Treat infections early

Adequate prenatal care, nutrition, avoid smoking/alcohol

High-Yield Points

PTL: Regular contractions + cervical changes before 37 weeks

Most common cause of preterm birth

Risk factors: prior PTL, multiple pregnancy, infection, cervical incompetence

Diagnosis: Clinical + ultrasound cervical length + fFN

Management <34 weeks: Tocolysis + corticosteroids + infection prophylaxis

Magnesium sulfate: neuroprotection <32 weeks

Early recognition and intervention improve neonatal outcomes

Preterm Labor (PTL)

- Definition
  - Regular uterine contractions causing cervical changes
  - Occurs before 37 completed weeks of gestation
- Classification
  - Threatened PTL → contractions without cervical changes
  - Established PTL → contractions + cervical changes (dilatation ≥1 cm or effacement ≥80%)
  - Spontaneous PTL → idiopathic, ~70% cases
  - Medically indicated PTL → maternal/fetal compromise (e.g., preeclampsia, IUGR)
- Risk Factors / Etiology
  - Maternal
    - Prior PTL
    - Short cervical length / incompetence
    - Uterine anomalies
    - Infection: genital tract, UTI, chorioamnionitis
    - Multiple pregnancy, polyhydramnios
  - Lifestyle / Environmental
    - Smoking, alcohol, drugs
    - Heavy physical work / stress
    - Malnutrition, low socioeconomic status
  - Obstetric / Fetal
  - PPROM / PROM
  - Antepartum bleeding (placenta previa/abruption)
  - Fetal anomalies or multiples
- Pathophysiology
  - Uterine activation → ↑oxytocin receptors, ↑prostaglandins → contractions
  - Cervical changes → collagen breakdown, cervical ripening
  - Triggers: Infection/inflammation, mechanical stretch, fetal-maternal endocrine signals (CRH, cortisol)
- Clinical Features
  - Maternal: Regular contractions (>4/20 min), abdominal cramps, backache, vaginal discharge
  - Fetal: Possible distress, reduced movements if severe

```
├── Diagnosis
│   ├── Clinical: Contraction frequency, cervical exam, ROM assessment
│   ├── Ultrasound: Cervical length <25 mm predictive
│   ├── Fetal fibronectin (fFN) test: Predicts delivery risk within 7–14 days
│   └── Labs: CBC, urinalysis, infection markers (if indicated)
│
├── Complications
│   ├── Maternal: Increased cesarean delivery, chorioamnionitis, stress/anxiety
│   └── Fetal / Neonatal: Prematurity → RDS, IVH, NEC, hypothermia, hypoglycemia, low birth weight, long-term neurodevelopmental issues
│
├── Management
│   ├── General Measures
│   │   ├── Hospitalization, monitoring
│   │   ├── Bed rest / hydration
│   │   └── Treat underlying infection
│   ├── Tocolysis (<34 weeks, viable fetus, no infection)
│   │   ├── Nifedipine (first-line)
│   │   ├── Indomethacin (<32 weeks)
│   │   ├── Magnesium sulfate (neuroprotection <32 weeks)
│   │   └── Beta-agonists (rarely used)
│   ├── Corticosteroids (24–34 weeks) → accelerate fetal lung maturity
│   ├── Antibiotics if PROM / infection risk
│   └── Delivery Indications
│   ├── Failed tocolysis
│   ├── Maternal/fetal compromise
│   └── Obstetric indications
└── Prognosis
├── Dependent on gestational age, fetal maturity, severity
├── >34 weeks → usually favorable
└── <32 weeks → high neonatal morbidity/mortality
```

10.7 Post Maturity

(*Wiladat-i-mutajawejah linnuzj*)

Post-term pregnancy: Pregnancy that extends beyond 42 completed weeks (294 days) of gestation from the first day of the last menstrual period (LMP).

Prolonged pregnancy: Pregnancy >40 weeks but <42 weeks.

Postmaturity syndrome: Clinical features seen in infants of post-term pregnancies (skin, body fat, and meconium changes).

Epidemiology

Incidence: 3–12% of all pregnancies (varies by population).

More common in primigravidas than multigravidas.

Risk of post-term pregnancy is increased with prior post-term pregnancies.

Less common in women with accurate early dating (first trimester US).

Etiology / Risk Factors

Maternal Factors

Nulliparity (primigravida)

Previous post-term pregnancy (strongest predictor)

Obesity

Male fetus

Fetal Factors

Anencephaly → impaired labor initiation

Other fetal anomalies causing decreased fetal cortisol production

Placental / Hormonal Factors

Defective placental aging / insufficiency

Delayed fetal hypothalamic-pituitary-adrenal (HPA) axis maturation → ↓ cortisol → ↓ labor onset

Genetic Factors

Familial tendency for post-term pregnancy

Pathophysiology

Labor initiation is triggered by fetal HPA axis → cortisol → placental prostaglandin synthesis → myometrial contractions.

Post-term pregnancy occurs due to failure of fetal signals or altered maternal responsiveness, leading to continued uterine quiescence.

Placental aging → decreased nutrient and oxygen transfer → risk of fetal compromise.

Clinical Features

Maternal

Usually asymptomatic

May report reduced fetal movements if placental insufficiency develops

Fetal / Neonatal (Postmaturity Syndrome)

Physical appearance: Dry, cracked skin; peeling; long nails; reduced subcutaneous fat

Hair and nails: Long, abundant hair; meconium-stained skin

Meconium staining: Common in amniotic fluid

Body habitus: Thin, “wasted” appearance due to fat loss

Placenta: Small, old, and calcified

Diagnosis

Clinical

Gestational age >42 weeks based on LMP or first trimester US

Fundal height may lag due to reduced amniotic fluid

Ultrasound

Confirm gestational age (crown-rump length early in pregnancy is gold standard)

Assess amniotic fluid index (AFI) → oligohydramnios common

Fetal well-being: Biophysical profile (BPP)

Fetal Monitoring

Non-stress test (NST)

Doppler studies if fetal compromise suspected

Complications

Maternal

Prolonged labor

Increased risk of cesarean section

Perineal trauma

Postpartum hemorrhage

Fetal / Neonatal

Macrosomia → birth injury (shoulder dystocia, brachial plexus injury)

Oligohydramnios → cord compression → variable decelerations

Meconium aspiration syndrome

Stillbirth / neonatal death

Hypoglycemia, polycythemia

Fetal distress due to placental insufficiency

Management

Antepartum

Fetal surveillance: NST twice weekly. Biophysical profile. Amniotic fluid assessment (AFI)

Induction of labor: Considered at 41–42 weeks

Methods:

Prostaglandins (Cervidil, Misoprostol)

Oxytocin infusion if cervix favorable

Balloon catheter for cervical ripening

Intrapartum

Continuous fetal monitoring due to risk of fetal compromise

Prepare for operative delivery if labor not progressing or signs of fetal distress

Postpartum

Evaluate neonate for postmaturity syndrome, hypoglycemia, polycythemia

Monitor mother for PPH and infection

Prognosis

Maternal prognosis: Usually good with proper monitoring and timely delivery

Fetal prognosis:

Increased risk if gestation extends beyond 42 weeks

Early intervention and close fetal surveillance improve outcomes

Prevention

Accurate early dating using first trimester ultrasound

Consider induction at 41–42 weeks to prevent post-term complications

Manage maternal conditions (obesity, diabetes) to reduce risk

High-Yield Points

Post-term pregnancy: >42 weeks gestation

Risk factors: Primigravida, prior post-term, male fetus, obesity

Complications: Macrosomia, oligohydramnios, meconium aspiration, stillbirth

Management: Fetal surveillance + induction at 41–42 weeks

Neonatal care: Watch for postmaturity syndrome, hypoglycemia, polycythemia

Post-term Pregnancy (Postmaturity)

```
├── Definition
│   ├── Gestation >42 completed weeks
│   ├── Prolonged pregnancy: 40–42 weeks
│   └── Postmaturity syndrome: Clinical features in neonates (skin, fat, meconium)
├── Risk Factors / Etiology
│   ├── Maternal
│   │   ├── Primigravida (nulliparity)
│   │   ├── Previous post-term pregnancy
│   │   ├── Obesity
│   │   └── Male fetus
│   ├── Fetal
│   │   ├── Anencephaly → impaired labor initiation
│   │   └── Congenital anomalies → ↓ fetal cortisol
│   ├── Placental / Hormonal
│   │   ├── Defective placental aging / insufficiency
```

```
│  │  └─ Delayed fetal HPA axis maturation → ↓ cortisol → ↓ prostaglandins
│  └─ Genetic Factors: Familial tendency
├─ Pathophysiology
│  ├─ Failure of fetal HPA axis → delayed cortisol production
│  ├─ ↓ placental prostaglandin synthesis → delayed myometrial contractions
│  └─ Placental aging → decreased nutrient & oxygen supply → fetal compromise
├─ Clinical Features
│  ├─ Maternal: Usually asymptomatic; may report reduced fetal movements
│  └─ Fetal / Neonatal (Postmaturity Syndrome)
│  ├─ Dry, cracked, peeling skin
│  ├─ Thin, "wasted" appearance
│  ├─ Long hair & nails
│  ├─ Meconium-stained skin or fluid
│  └─ Small, calcified placenta
├─ Diagnosis
│  ├─ Gestational age >42 weeks (LMP / first trimester US)
│  ├─ Ultrasound: Confirm age, AFI (oligohydramnios common)
│  └─ Fetal monitoring: NST, biophysical profile
├─ Complications
│  ├─ Maternal
│  │  ├─ Prolonged labor
│  │  ├─ Increased cesarean section
│  │  ├─ Perineal trauma
│  │  └─ Postpartum hemorrhage
│  └─ Fetal / Neonatal
│  ├─ Macrosomia → shoulder dystocia, birth injury
│  ├─ Oligohydramnios → cord compression → variable decelerations
│  ├─ Meconium aspiration syndrome
│  ├─ Stillbirth / neonatal death
│  └─ Hypoglycemia, polycythemia
├─ Management
│  ├─ Antepartum
│  │  ├─ Fetal surveillance: NST twice weekly, BPP, AFI
│  │  └─ Consider induction at 41–42 weeks
│  ├─ Induction Methods
│  │  ├─ Prostaglandins (Cervidil, Misoprostol)
│  │  ├─ Oxytocin infusion (if cervix favorable)
│  │  └─ Balloon catheter for cervical ripening
│  ├─ Intrapartum
│  │  ├─ Continuous fetal monitoring
│  │  └─ Prepare for operative delivery if labor abnormal
│  └─ Postpartum
```

```
│ ├─ Evaluate neonate for postmaturity syndrome
│ └─ Monitor mother for PPH & infection
└─ Prognosis
├─ Maternal: Usually good with timely delivery
└─ Fetal: Increased risk if gestation extends beyond 42 weeks; close surveillance improves outcome
```

10.8 Intra Uterine Fetal Death

(*Maut-i-janeen Dakhil-al-Rahim*)

Definition

Intrauterine Fetal Death (IUFD): Death of the fetus after 20 weeks of gestation but before delivery, irrespective of fetal weight. Also called stillbirth.

Some sources use:

Early stillbirth: 20–28 weeks

Late stillbirth: >28 weeks

Key distinction: IUFD occurs in utero, stillbirth includes death at birth.

Epidemiology

Incidence: ~2–6 per 1000 births in developed countries; higher in developing countries.

Major contributors: Maternal health, antenatal care quality, fetal anomalies, infections.

High-risk groups: Advanced maternal age, hypertension, diabetes, previous IUFD.

Etiology / Risk Factors

IUFD is multifactorial, broadly classified into maternal, fetal, and placental causes.

Maternal Factors

Hypertensive disorders: Preeclampsia, eclampsia

Diabetes mellitus: Poorly controlled

Maternal infections: TORCH (Toxoplasma, Rubella, CMV, Herpes), malaria, syphilis, bacterial infections

Trauma

Autoimmune disorders: SLE, antiphospholipid antibody syndrome

Advanced maternal age (>35 years)

Substance abuse: Smoking, alcohol, drugs

Fetal Factors

Chromosomal anomalies: Trisomy 13, 18, 21

Structural malformations (cardiac, renal, CNS)

Multiple gestations → higher IUFD risk in one twin

Placental Factors

Placental insufficiency

Placental abruption

Placenta previa with bleeding

Umbilical cord accidents: Prolapse, true knot, velamentous insertion

Infarcts or thrombosis

Unexplained IUFD

20–50% of cases remain idiopathic after investigation

Pathophysiology

Maternal, fetal, or placental insult → hypoxia → fetal death

Timing of fetal death may vary:

Acute events: Cord accident, abruption → sudden death

Chronic events: Placental insufficiency, infection → gradual demise

Postmortem changes in uterus:

Cessation of fetal movements

Loss of heart sounds

Intrauterine maceration of fetal tissues if death occurs >24–48 hours before delivery

Clinical Features

Maternal

Cessation of perceived fetal movements

Sometimes associated with abdominal pain or vaginal bleeding depending on cause

Signs of labor may develop spontaneously if death occurred weeks earlier

Fetal

No heart sounds on auscultation / Doppler

Ultrasound confirms absence of cardiac activity

Fetal maceration may be visible if death occurred >24–48 hours

Diagnosis

Clinical

History of absent fetal movements

Abdominal exam: No fetal movements, soft fetal parts

Auscultation: No fetal heart sounds with Doppler or fetoscope

Investigations

Ultrasound: Confirms absence of fetal cardiac activity; evaluates placenta and amniotic fluid

Maternal labs: CBC, coagulation profile if DIC suspected

Infection screen: TORCH, syphilis, malaria (if indicated)

Fetal karyotyping: For recurrent IUFD or suspected anomalies

Complications

Maternal

Disseminated Intravascular Coagulation (DIC): Especially if IUFD >4 weeks

Infection: Chorioamnionitis, endometritis

Psychological trauma: Grief, depression, PTSD

Prolonged labor or difficult delivery

Fetal

Already deceased; postmortem changes if retained in utero

Maceration: Skin peeling, discoloration, soft tissues breakdown

Management

Goals: Safe delivery of the fetus, prevention of maternal complications, and psychological support.

Maternal Stabilization

Assess maternal vitals

Check for infection or coagulopathy (DIC)

Emotional support and counseling

Timing and Mode of Delivery

Spontaneous labor: Often occurs within 1–2 weeks

Induction of labor: Indicated if fetal demise diagnosed

Methods:

Misoprostol / prostaglandins

Oxytocin infusion if cervix favorable

Mechanical methods: Balloon catheter for cervical ripening

Cesarean section: Rare; reserved for maternal indications (placenta previa, obstruction)

Supportive Care

Psychological counseling

Discuss autopsy or karyotyping if indicated

Family support for grief

Prognosis

Maternal: Usually excellent if managed promptly

Fetal: Intrauterine death is irreversible; prognosis depends on underlying cause

Prevention

Early identification and management of maternal risk factors (hypertension, diabetes, infections)

Routine antenatal care and fetal surveillance

Ultrasound dating early in pregnancy

Counseling women with previous IUFD for preconception care and close monitoring

High-Yield Points

IUFD: Fetal death after 20 weeks gestation before delivery

Common causes: Maternal hypertension, diabetes, infections, placental insufficiency, cord accidents

Diagnosis: Absent fetal movements + absent heart sounds + ultrasound confirmation

Management: Induce labor, prevent maternal complications, provide emotional support

Complications: DIC if prolonged retention, infection, maternal psychological trauma

Recurrent IUFD → investigate fetal karyotype, maternal thrombophilia, autoimmune disorders

Intrauterine Fetal Death (IUFD)

```
│
├─ Definition
│ ├─ Death of fetus after 20 weeks gestation but before delivery
│ ├─ Also called stillbirth
│ └─ Early stillbirth: 20–28 weeks; Late stillbirth: >28 weeks
├─ Risk Factors / Etiology
│ ├─ Maternal
│ │ ├─ Hypertension / preeclampsia / eclampsia
│ │ ├─ Diabetes mellitus (poorly controlled)
│ │ ├─ Infections: TORCH, malaria, syphilis, bacterial infections
│ │ ├─ Trauma
│ │ ├─ Autoimmune: SLE, antiphospholipid syndrome
│ │ └─ Advanced maternal age, smoking, alcohol, drugs
│ ├─ Fetal
│ │ ├─ Chromosomal anomalies: Trisomy 13, 18, 21
│ │ ├─ Structural malformations (cardiac, renal, CNS)
│ │ └─ Multiple gestation (higher risk in one twin)
│ └─ Placental
│ ├─ Placental insufficiency / infarction
```

```
│ ├─ Placental abruption
│ ├─ Placenta previa with bleeding
│ └─ Umbilical cord accidents: prolapse, true knot, velamentous insertion
│
├─ Pathophysiology
│ ├─ Maternal, fetal, or placental insult → hypoxia → fetal death
│ ├─ Acute events: cord accident, abruption → sudden death
│ └─ Chronic events: placental insufficiency, infection → gradual demise
│
├─ Clinical Features
│ ├─ Maternal: Cessation of fetal movements, sometimes abdominal pain or bleeding
│ └─ Fetal: No heart sounds, confirmed on Doppler/ultrasound; maceration if death >24–48 hrs
│
├─ Diagnosis
│ ├─ Clinical: Absent fetal movements, soft fetal parts, absent heart sounds
│ ├─ Ultrasound: No cardiac activity, assess placenta & amniotic fluid
│ ├─ Maternal labs: CBC, coagulation profile if DIC suspected
│ ├─ Infection screen: TORCH, syphilis, malaria if indicated
│ └─ Fetal karyotyping: For recurrent IUFD or suspected anomalies
│
├─ Complications
│ ├─ Maternal
│ │ ├─ DIC (especially if IUFD >4 weeks)
│ │ ├─ Infection: chorioamnionitis, endometritis
│ │ ├─ Psychological trauma: grief, depression, PTSD
│ │ └─ Prolonged/difficult labor
│ └─ Fetal
│ └─ Maceration: skin peeling, tissue breakdown if retained in utero
│
├─ Management
│ ├─ Maternal stabilization: Vitals, infection/coagulopathy assessment, counseling
│ ├─ Timing/mode of delivery
│ │ ├─ Spontaneous labor: usually within 1–2 weeks
```

│ │ ├─ Induction: Misoprostol/prostaglandins, oxytocin infusion, balloon catheter
│ │ └─ Cesarean: Rare, only for maternal indications
│ └─ Supportive care: Psychological counseling, autopsy/karyotyping if indicated, family support
│
└─ Prognosis
├─ Maternal: Usually excellent if managed promptly
└─ Fetal: Already deceased; prognosis depends on underlying cause

Long Answer Questions (LAQs)

Describe hypertensive disorders of pregnancy with classification, complications, and management.

Discuss oligohydramnios and polyhydramnios with causes, diagnosis, and management.

Explain preterm labor with risk factors, diagnosis, and prevention.

Describe post-maturity and its maternal and fetal complications.

Discuss intrauterine fetal death with causes, diagnosis, and management.

Short Answer Questions (SAQs)

Define preterm labor.

What is oligohydramnios?

Define polyhydramnios.

What is intrauterine growth restriction (IUGR)?

Define post-maturity.

Multiple Choice Questions (1 Mark Each)

1. Preeclampsia is characterized by hypertension after:

A. 12 weeks B. 16 weeks

C. 20 weeks D. 28 weeks

Answer: C

2. Oligohydramnios is defined when AFI is less than:

A. 10 cm B. 8 cm

C. 5 cm D. 2 cm

Answer: C

3. Most common cause of polyhydramnios is:

A. Renal agenesis B. Rh incompatibility

C. Diabetes mellitus D. PROM

Answer: C

4. Preterm labor occurs before:

A. 34 weeks B. 37 weeks

C. 38 weeks D. 40 weeks

Answer: B

5. Most common cause of intrauterine growth restriction is:

A. Multiple pregnancy B. Fetal anomaly

C. Placental insufficiency D. Polyhydramnios

Answer: C

6. Post-maturity is pregnancy continuing beyond:

A. 40 weeks B. 41 weeks

C. 42 weeks D. 44 weeks

Answer: C

7. Most common complication of post-maturity is:

A. Polyhydramnios B. Meconium aspiration

C. Macrosomia D. Placenta previa

Answer: B

8. Premature rupture of membranes refers to rupture before:

A. Onset of labor B. Cervical dilatation

C. Onset of labor pains D. Full term

Answer: C

9. Most common cause of intrauterine fetal death is:

A. Congenital anomaly B. Infection

C. Placental abruption D. Diabetes

Answer: C

10. Best method to monitor fetal growth in high-risk pregnancy is:

A. Abdominal girth B. Fundal height

C. Ultrasonography D. CTG

Answer: C

11

Normal & Abnormal Puerperium

(Zamana -i-Nafas Taba I wa Ghaiyr Taba'i)

11.1 *Umumu Manafi' ul-A'da'I Tabdiliyan* (General Physiological Changes)
11.2 *Sael-e-Nafasi/ Hulabah* (Lochia)
11.3 *Rada'at* (Lactation)
11.4 *Taba'I Zamana-i-Nifas ka Mu'alajah* (Management of normal puerperium)
11.5 *Nighdast bad Wilada* (Post Natal Care)
11.6 *Humma Nefasiyah* (Puerperal Pyrexia)
11.7 *Enten-e-nafasi* (Puerperal Sepsis)
11.8 *Aubur-Rahim Juz'i* (Sub Involution)
11.9 *Awaridat-e-Majra Bawl* (Urinary Tract Complications)
11.10 *Aridat-e-Thad I* (Breast Complications)
11.11 *Khusar-e-Waridi Nefasi aur insed-e-Ri'wi* (Puerperal venous Thrombosis & Pulmonary embolism)
11.12 *Nafsiyati khlal* (Psychiatric Disorders)

Learning Objective (At the end of the session, the students should be able to)

Explain General physiological changes during puerperium (Normal & Abnormal) and describe Lochia
Elaborate physiology of Lactation
Demonstrate the procedure of Post-Natal Care (PNC)
Present & describe the management of normal puerperium & its minor ailments
Distinguish Puerperal Pyrexia & Puerperal Sepsis
Define Sub Involution & explain its causes, diagnosis & management
Explain the causes, diagnosis & management of UTI, Retention of urine & Incontinence of urine in puerperium
Elaborate causes, diagnosis & management of Breast Engorgement, Cracked and Retracted Nipple, Acute Mastitis & Lactation failure in puerperium
Summarize the Puerperal Venous Thrombosis & Pulmonary Embolism in puerperium
Describe in brief Puerperal Blues, Postpartum Depression & Postpartum Psychosis during puerperium

11.1 General Physiological Changes

(*Umumu Manafi' ul-A'da'l Tabdiliyan*)

General physiological changes of puerperium

Puerperium (also called postpartum period) is the period following childbirth during which the maternal organs, particularly the uterus and genital tract, return to their pre-pregnant state — both anatomically and physiologically.

Duration: Approximately 6 weeks (42 days).

The changes involve involution, restoration of normal functions and initiation of lactation.

1. Uterine changes

a. Involution of the Uterus

Involution means the process by which the uterus returns to its pre-pregnant size, shape, and condition.

Immediately after delivery: Uterus is firm, globular, and reaches midway between the pubic symphysis and umbilicus.

Weight: ~1000 g.

After 24 hours: Fundus at the level of umbilicus.

By the end of 1 week: Fundus midway between umbilicus and symphysis pubis; weight: ~500 g.

By 2 weeks: Fundus not palpable abdominally; weight: ~300 g.

By 6 weeks: Uterus returns to non-pregnant size (~100 g).

Mechanisms of Involution:

1. Autolysis: Degeneration of hypertrophied muscle fibers through enzymatic digestion.
2. Phagocytosis: Removal of cellular debris by macrophages.
3. Regeneration: Endometrium regenerates from basal layer.

b. Endometrial Regeneration

Superficial layer (decidua) is shed off as lochia.

Basal layer remains to regenerate new endometrium.

Complete regeneration:

Except at placental site → within 10 days.

At placental site → within 6 weeks.

c. Placental Site Involution

After placental separation, the site (~7–8 cm in diameter) appears as an irregular elevated area.

Gradually shrinks due to thrombosis and fibrosis of blood vessels.

Healing complete by 6 weeks.

2. Lochia (postpartum vaginal discharge)

Definition: Lochia is the vaginal discharge from the uterus, cervix, and vagina following childbirth, consisting of blood, mucus and tissue debris.

Type	Duration	Composition	Color
Lochia rubra	1–4 days	Blood, decidual tissue, fetal membranes	Red
Lochia serosa	5–10 days	Serous fluid, leukocytes, mucus	Pinkish-brown
Lochia alba	11–21 days (up to 4–6 weeks)	Leukocytes, epithelial cells, mucus	Whitish or yellowish-white

Normal characteristics: Faint musty odor.

Not offensive (foul smell indicates infection).

Gradually decreases in amount and changes color from red → brown → white.

3. Cervix, vagina and perineum

a. Cervix

Immediately after delivery: soft, edematous, and patulous.

External os admits 2 fingers initially, then 1 finger by end of 1 week.

By 6 weeks, the cervix becomes firm and well-formed but external os becomes slit-like (not circular as in nulliparous women).

b. Vagina

Greatly distended at delivery, edematous, and smooth.

Gradually regains tone over 3 weeks due to restoration of muscular and connective tissue elasticity.

Rugae reappear by 3rd week.

c. Perineum

Stretched and possibly lacerated during delivery.

Gradually regains tone by 6 weeks if properly supported (pelvic floor exercises help).

Healing of episiotomy/lacerations occurs within 7–10 days.

4. Ovarian and hormonal changes

After placental delivery, estrogen and progesterone levels fall abruptly.

Prolactin level rises (from anterior pituitary) due to loss of negative feedback.

Stimulates lactogenesis (milk secretion).

FSH and LH remain suppressed in lactating women due to prolactin inhibition → lactational amenorrhea.

In non-lactating women, FSH and LH rise → ovulation may resume within 6–8 weeks.

5. Menstruation and ovulation

Lactating women: Amenorrhea persists for 3–6 months (or longer) due to high prolactin levels.

Non-lactating women: Ovulation may occur by 4–6 weeks postpartum. Menstruation resumes by 6–8 weeks.

Note: Ovulation can occur before first menstruation → possible conception during lactational amenorrhea.

6. Breast changes and lactation

Phases

1. Mammogenesis: Development during pregnancy under estrogen & progesterone.

2. Lactogenesis: Initiation of milk secretion after delivery (due to fall in estrogen/progesterone, rise in prolactin).

3. Galactokinesis: Ejection of milk via oxytocin reflex (posterior pituitary).

4. Galactopoiesis: Maintenance of milk secretion due to suckling stimulus and continued prolactin secretion.

Composition of milk:

Colostrum: Thick yellowish secretion for first 3–5 days → rich in proteins, antibodies (IgA), and vitamin A.

Mature milk: Established by 5–10 days.

7. Cardiovascular system

Blood volume: Falls to normal within 1–2 weeks due to diuresis and decreased plasma volume.

Cardiac output: Elevated immediately after delivery → returns to normal by 2 weeks.

Pulse rate: Slight bradycardia for first few days (50–60 bpm).

Blood pressure: Usually stable; transient fall may occur from blood loss.

Hemoglobin and hematocrit: May transiently fall but rise as diuresis occurs.

8. Hematological changes

Leukocytosis: Common in early puerperium (WBC up to 20,000–25,000/mm^3).

Coagulation: Hypercoagulable state persists → risk of deep vein thrombosis (DVT).

ESR: Remains elevated for few days.

9. Urinary system

Bladder: Atonic and edematous immediately after delivery → risk of urinary retention.

Diuresis: Begins within 24–48 hours; helps remove excess fluid from pregnancy.

Urine output: Increases to 2–3 L/day initially.

Risk: Infection due to trauma, catheterization, or stasis.

10. Gastrointestinal system

Appetite: Usually returns within 1–2 days.

Constipation: Common due to dehydration, decreased tone, and pain.

Hemorrhoids: May worsen due to straining.

11. Endocrine changes

Estrogen & Progesterone: Sharp fall after placenta expulsion.

Prolactin: Rises and maintained in lactating women.

Cortisol: Gradually returns to normal.

Thyroid activity: May fluctuate; transient postpartum thyroiditis possible.

12. Body temperature and weight

Temperature: Slight rise (≤38°C) in first 24 hours is physiological due to dehydration and breast engorgement.

Persistent fever → infection (puerperal sepsis, UTI, mastitis).

Weight: Immediate loss of 5–6 kg (fetus, placenta, amniotic fluid) + gradual loss of 2–3 kg over next few weeks.

13. Psychological changes

Emotional instability ("postpartum blues") common due to hormonal shifts, fatigue, and role change.

Usually resolves in 1–2 weeks.

Severe or persistent symptoms → postpartum depression.

11.2 Lochia

(*Sael-e-Nafasi/ Hulabah*)

Definition

Lochia is the vaginal discharge that occurs during the puerperium, resulting from the shedding and regeneration of the uterine lining after childbirth.

It consists of blood, mucus, decidual tissue, bacterial debris and represents the healing process of the endometrium and placental site.

Origin of Lochia

The lochial discharge comes from three main sources:

1. Decidua (Endometrium)

Superficial necrotic layer of decidua is shed after delivery.

Basal layer remains intact and regenerates the new endometrium.

2. Placental Site

Blood and debris from thrombosed vessels and necrotic tissue.

Contributes to the blood-stained component of early lochia.

3. Cervical and Vaginal Secretions

Mucus, epithelial cells and normal flora.

Add to the later serous and mucoid components of lochia.

Composition of Lochia

Lochia is a mixture of the following components:

Component	Source/Explanation
Blood	From open uterine vessels at placental site
Serum	From uterine surface exudation
Decidual tissue	Shredded necrotic decidual cells
Leukocytes	Due to inflammatory response and defense
Epithelial cells	From uterine and vaginal lining
Mucus	From cervix and vagina
Bacteria	Mostly saprophytic; non-pathogenic if asepsis maintained

Types and Duration of Lochia

After delivery, the lochia changes in color, composition, and amount over time. These changes occur gradually and are classified into three distinct types:

Type of Lochia	Duration	Color & Appearance	Composition	Normal Odor
Lochia Rubra	Day 1–4	Bright red, bloody discharge	Blood, shreds of decidua, fetal membranes, vernix caseosa, lanugo, and meconium (occasionally)	Fresh, non-foul odor
Lochia Serosa	Day 5–10	Brownish-pink or serous discharge	Serum, leukocytes, mucus, and less blood	Faint, musty odor
Lochia Alba	Day 11–21 (may persist up to 4–6 weeks)	Whitish or yellowish-white	Mucus, leukocytes, epithelial cells, cholesterol crystals, and bacteria	No foul smell

Quantity of Lochia

Total amount: Approximately 250–500 mL over the entire puerperium.

Daily average: First 2 days: ~200 mL/day. Gradually decreases thereafter

Normal course: Decrease in amount and change in color from red → brown → white.

Physiological Characteristics

Odor: Musty or fleshy, but not foul.

Consistency: Non-coagulated, though small clots may appear early.

Flow: May increase during breastfeeding due to oxytocin-induced uterine contractions (milk let-down reflex also triggers uterine contractions).

Amount varies with:

Parity (more in multiparae)

Type of delivery (more after cesarean)

Uterine tone and involution speed

Microscopic Features

Lochia rubra: Predominantly RBCs, decidual fragments and bacteria.

Lochia serosa: Mainly leukocytes, necrotic decidual cells and some RBCs.

Lochia alba: Dominated by leukocytes, epithelial cells, cholesterol crystals and fat granules.

Bacteriology of Lochia

Normally non-sterile, containing saprophytic bacteria such as:

Streptococci (non-hemolytic)

Staphylococci

E. coli

Diphtheroids

These are non-pathogenic in a healthy woman with proper asepsis.

However, if pathogenic bacteria (e.g., hemolytic streptococci, anaerobes) invade → may lead to puerperal sepsis.

Abnormalities of Lochia (Lochial Disorders)

Abnormality	Definition/Description	Possible Cause	Clinical Significance
Lochiometra	Retention of lochia in uterine cavity due to obstruction of cervical canal	Cervical spasm, blood clot, or infection	Uterus enlarged, tender, no discharge; may lead to infection
Lochiorrhea	Excessive or prolonged lochial discharge beyond normal duration	Subinvolution, retained bits of placenta or membranes	May indicate delayed uterine involution
Lochiostasis	Intermittent cessation of lochial flow with distension of uterus	Obstruction by membrane, blood clot, or uterine atony	Pain, tenderness, and sudden gush when obstruction relieved
Foul-smelling Lochia	Offensive odor due to infection	Puerperal sepsis (usually anaerobic infection)	Must investigate and treat urgently

Clinical Assessment of Lochia

During postpartum rounds or examinations, the following aspects should be assessed:

1. Color and Type → Progression from rubra → serosa → alba
2. Amount → Should gradually decrease
3. Odor → Foul smell indicates infection
4. Presence of clots → Large clots may indicate atony or retained tissue
5. Associated symptoms → Fever, uterine tenderness, or abdominal pain suggest infection

Factors Affecting Lochial Discharge

Increase in Lochia	Decrease in Lochia
Breastfeeding (oxytocin release)	Obstruction of cervix
Physical activity	Uterine atony
Multiparity	Infection with endometrial edema
Retained products	Retained clots causing lochiometra

Care and Management of Lochia

Perineal hygiene: Clean vulva and perineum regularly; change pads frequently.

Observation: Note color, quantity and odor daily.

Avoid tampons:

Risk of ascending infection.

Promote uterine involution:

Encourage breastfeeding (stimulates oxytocin).

Early ambulation.

Investigate abnormalities:

If foul-smelling or excessive lochia → culture, ultrasound (for retained products).

Pathological Conditions Related to Lochia

1. Subinvolution of Uterus

Definition: Failure of uterus to return to normal size.

Lochial feature: Prolonged lochia rubra or serosa, excessive discharge.

Causes: Retained tissue, infection, anemia.

2. Puerperal Sepsis

Definition: Infection of genital tract within 6 weeks postpartum.

Lochial feature: Foul-smelling, purulent discharge, fever, uterine tenderness.

3. Retained Placental Tissue

Lochial feature: Persistent red lochia, sometimes with clots, subinvolution.

Duration Summary

Day	Type of Lochia	Color	Main Components
1–4	Rubra	Red	Blood, decidua, tissue debris
5–10	Serosa	Brownish-pink	Serum, leukocytes, mucus
11–21 (up to 6 weeks)	Alba	Whitish	Mucus, leukocytes, epithelial cells

Clinical Significance

Indicator of uterine involution: Normal progression indicates healthy recovery.

Diagnostic clue: Abnormal color, odor, or duration may signal infection or subinvolution.

Monitoring tool: Essential component of postpartum care.

Summary

Lochia represents uterine cleansing and endometrial regeneration.

Progresses from bloody (rubra) → serous (serosa) → mucoid (alba).

Normally lasts up to 4–6 weeks.

Offensive odor, prolonged bleeding, or absence of discharge = abnormal.

Proper asepsis, observation and breastfeeding help ensure normal lochial pattern.

11.3 Lactation

(*Rada'at*)

Definition

Lactation is the physiological process of secretion and ejection of milk from the mammary glands after childbirth.

It involves development of the breast, initiation of milk secretion and maintenance of milk production and ejection, under the influence of complex hormonal and neural mechanisms.

Phases (Stages) of Lactation

Lactation occurs in four physiological stages:

1. Mammogenesis – Development of mammary glands during pregnancy
2. Lactogenesis – Initiation of milk secretion after delivery
3. Galactokinesis – Ejection of milk from the alveoli to the nipple
4. Galactopoiesis – Maintenance of milk secretion during lactation

1. Mammogenesis (Development of the Breast)

Definition: Structural and functional preparation of the breast for milk secretion.

Timing: Occurs mainly during puberty and pregnancy.

Hormonal Regulation:

Hormone	Function
Estrogen	Growth and proliferation of ductal system and fat deposition.
Progesterone	Development of lobules and alveoli (secretory units).
Prolactin	Differentiation of alveolar epithelial cells into secretory cells.
Human Placental Lactogen (hPL)	Contributes to lobulo-alveolar growth.
Cortisol, Insulin, Thyroid Hormones	Support metabolic and enzymatic activity of mammary cells.

Structural Changes in Pregnancy

Breasts enlarge and become tender.

Nipple and areola become more pigmented.

Montgomery's tubercles (sebaceous glands) become prominent.

Colostrum may be secreted during late pregnancy.

2. Lactogenesis (Initiation of Milk Secretion)

Definition: Process of starting milk secretion from the mammary alveolar cells.

Timing: Begins after the expulsion of placenta.

Mechanism:

During pregnancy: High estrogen and progesterone inhibit milk secretion despite high prolactin levels.

After delivery: Sudden fall in estrogen and progesterone (due to placental expulsion) removes inhibition. Prolactin (from anterior pituitary) becomes dominant and initiates milk secretion.

Phases of Lactogenesis

Phase	Time	Description
Lactogenesis I (Secretory Differentiation)	Mid-pregnancy	Breast develops ability to secrete colostrum (inhibited by high E & P)
Lactogenesis II (Secretory Activation)	2–4 days postpartum	Rapid increase in milk volume after hormonal shift (↓E, ↓P, ↑Prolactin)

3. Galactokinesis (Milk Ejection or Let-Down Reflex)

Definition: Expulsion of milk from alveoli and ducts into the nipple, allowing the infant to suckle.

Mechanism: Mediated by neuroendocrine reflex involving oxytocin.

Steps:

1. Suckling → sensory impulses from nipple to hypothalamus.
2. Posterior pituitary releases oxytocin.
3. Oxytocin causes contraction of myoepithelial cells around alveoli and ducts.
4. Milk is ejected through the nipple.

Factors Stimulating Reflex:

Suckling

Infant's cry or sight/sound of baby (psychic stimuli)

Breast massage

Inhibition Factors:

Anxiety, fear, pain or fatigue → inhibit oxytocin release → milk ejection failure.

4. Galactopoiesis (Maintenance of Milk Secretion)

Definition: Continued secretion of milk to meet the nutritional demand of the infant.

Mechanism: Maintained by regular suckling and sustained prolactin secretion.

Hormone	Role in Galactopoiesis
Prolactin (Anterior Pituitary)	Maintains milk synthesis; secretion increases after each suckling.
Oxytocin (Posterior Pituitary)	Enables milk ejection; indirectly supports continued suckling.
Cortisol, Insulin, Thyroid Hormones	Maintain metabolic functions and nutrient supply for milk synthesis.

Suckling Reflex:

→ Stimulates hypothalamus → inhibits dopamine (prolactin-inhibiting factor) → ↑ prolactin → sustained milk production.

Feedback Mechanism:

The frequency and completeness of milk removal regulate production.

If milk accumulates → inhibitory peptides suppress further secretion.

Composition of human milk

Constituent	Human Milk	Cow's Milk (Comparison)	Remarks
Water	87–88%	87%	Keeps baby hydrated
Energy	~70 kcal/100 mL	~66 kcal/100 mL	Easily digestible
Protein	1.0–1.2 g/100 mL	3.3 g/100 mL	Mainly lactalbumin (easily digestible)
Fat	3.5–4.0 g/100 mL	3.5–4.0 g/100 mL	High in polyunsaturated fatty acids
Carbohydrate (Lactose)	6.8–7.0 g/100 mL	4.5 g/100 mL	Promotes growth of Lactobacillus bifidus
Calcium/Phosphate Ratio	2:1	1:1	Better absorption and bone mineralization
Vitamins	Rich in A, E, C; low in D and K	Variable	Vitamin D supplementation may be needed
Immunoglobulins	High (especially IgA)	Absent	Provides passive immunity
Enzymes	Amylase, lipase, lysozyme	Absent	Aid digestion and antibacterial defense

Types of milk

1. Colostrum

Duration: Secreted during first 3–5 days postpartum.

Characteristics: Thick, yellowish fluid. High in proteins (10%), immunoglobulins, and vitamin A. Low in fat and lactose. Rich in antibodies (IgA, IgG, IgM) — provides passive immunity to newborn.

Functions:

Laxative effect (helps meconium expulsion).

Protects against infections (gastrointestinal and respiratory).

Builds immunity and gut flora.

2. Transitional Milk

Duration: 6th to 10th day postpartum.

Composition: Intermediate between colostrum and mature milk.

3. Mature Milk

From 2 weeks onwards.

Composition: Stable; adapted to infant's nutritional needs.

Hormonal control of lactation

Hormone	Source	Function
Estrogen	Placenta → Ovaries	Ductal growth (inhibits secretion during pregnancy)
Progesterone	Placenta → Ovaries	Lobulo-alveolar development (inhibits secretion during pregnancy)
Oxytocin	Posterior Pituitary	Milk ejection reflex
Prolactin	Anterior Pituitary	Milk synthesis (main lactogenic hormone)
Human Placental Lactogen (hPL)	Placenta	Mammary growth during pregnancy
Cortisol, Insulin, Thyroid Hormones	Adrenal, Pancreas, Thyroid	Provide metabolic support for milk production

Advantages of breastfeeding

Baby

Ideal nutrition — balanced, easily digestible.

Provides immunological protection (IgA, lysozyme, lactoferrin).

Reduces risk of diarrhea, respiratory infections, otitis media, necrotizing enterocolitis.

Promotes bonding and emotional security.

Decreases risk of allergies, obesity, and diabetes later in life.

Mother

Promotes uterine involution (oxytocin release).

Reduces postpartum hemorrhage.

Acts as natural contraception (lactational amenorrhea).

Lowers risk of breast and ovarian cancer.

Economical and convenient.

Lactational amenorrhea

Definition: Temporary suppression of ovulation and menstruation during breastfeeding.

Mechanism:

Suckling → ↑ prolactin → inhibits hypothalamic GnRH → ↓ FSH & LH → no ovulation.

Duration: Up to 6 months (variable).

Effectiveness: 98% effective as contraception if:

1. Exclusive breastfeeding,
2. Amenorrheic,
3. Baby < 6 months.

Disorders of lactation

Condition	Description	Management
Agalactia	Complete absence of milk secretion	Reassurance, promote suckling, evaluate endocrine causes
Hypogalactia	Insufficient milk secretion	Frequent suckling, adequate nutrition, fluids, rest, domperidone/metoclopramide if needed
Engorgement	Painful overfilling of breasts due to poor drainage	Express milk, hot fomentation before feeding, cold after feeding
Cracked Nipples	Fissures due to improper latching	Proper positioning, nipple care, avoid soap, use lanolin
Mastitis	Inflammation (often Staph. aureus)	Antibiotics, continue feeding, warm compress
Breast Abscess	Collection of pus	Surgical drainage, continue feeding from opposite breast

Suppression of lactation

Indicated when breastfeeding is contraindicated (e.g., maternal HIV infection, neonatal galactosemia, maternal death, or certain drugs).

Methods:

Non-pharmacological: Firm breast binding, ice packs, analgesics.

Pharmacological: Dopamine agonists (e.g., Cabergoline 0.25 mg BD × 2 days, or Bromocriptine 2.5 mg BD × 14 days).

(Hormonal suppression is used cautiously due to side effects.)

Contraindications to breastfeeding

Maternal

HIV infection (in high-resource settings)

Active pulmonary tuberculosis (until treated)

Breast carcinoma, abscess (temporary)

Use of cytotoxic drugs, radioactive isotopes, lithium

Severe maternal illness (sepsis, psychosis)

Neonatal

Galactosemia

Phenylketonuria (partial contraindication)

Maple syrup urine disease

Summary table

Stage	Time	Main Hormones	Effect
Mammogenesis	Pregnancy	Estrogen, Progesterone, hPL	Duct and alveoli development
Lactogenesis	After delivery	↓E, ↓P, ↑Prolactin	Initiation of milk secretion
Galactokinesis	During feeding	Oxytocin	Milk ejection reflex
Galactopoiesis	Ongoing	Prolactin, Oxytocin	Maintenance of secretion

Key points

Prolactin → Production, Oxytocin → Ejection.

Milk secretion starts when estrogen and progesterone fall after delivery.

Suckling is the most potent stimulus for both prolactin and oxytocin release.

Colostrum is the ideal first food — rich in antibodies and vitamin A.

Breastfeeding benefits both mother and baby — physiologically, immunologically and psychologically.

11.4 Management of normal puerperium

(*Taba'I Zamana-i-Nifas ka Mu'alajah*)

Definition

Puerperium (postpartum period) is the period following childbirth during which the maternal body — particularly the genital organs — returns to its pre-pregnant state, both anatomically and physiologically.

Duration: ~6 weeks (42 days).

Objectives of management

1. Ensure smooth physiological recovery.
2. Detect and prevent complications.
3. Promote physical, emotional, and social well-being.
4. Support successful breastfeeding and neonatal care.

Aims of puerperal management

1. Facilitate normal involution of uterus and other organs.
2. Promote lactation and breastfeeding.
3. Maintain maternal nutrition and hygiene.
4. Prevent infection, thrombosis, and hemorrhage.
5. Provide psychological reassurance and health education.

1. Immediate puerperium (first 24 hours)

Observations Immediately After Delivery

After delivery of placenta, the mother must be observed carefully for the first 2–4 hours — the most critical period for postpartum complications.

(a) General Observations

Pulse, blood pressure and temperature every 15–30 minutes for first 2 hours.

Watch for postpartum hemorrhage (PPH) — most common immediate danger.

Observe for uterine tone and contraction — uterus should be firm, central, and below umbilicus.

Examine perineum and repair any lacerations or episiotomy under aseptic precautions.

Ensure bladder is empty — encourage micturition or use catheter if necessary.

(b) Position and Rest

Keep mother in semi-recumbent position after first few hours.

Avoid pillow initially if spinal anesthesia was used.

(c) Emotional Support

Reassure and comfort the mother; explain physiological changes to reduce anxiety.

2. General management during hospital stay

Usually 3–5 days after normal vaginal delivery.

A. General Condition and Vital Signs

Parameter	**Normal Findings / Action**
Temperature	Slight rise (<38°C) in first 24 h due to dehydration or breast engorgement. Persistent fever → infection.
Pulse	60–70 bpm; bradycardia common due to increased vagal tone. Tachycardia may indicate hemorrhage or infection.
Blood Pressure	Usually stable. Hypotension → blood loss; Hypertension → postpartum preeclampsia.
Respiration	Normal; monitor for pulmonary embolism if dyspnea develops.

B. Uterine Involution

Palpate fundal height daily:

After delivery: midway between symphysis and umbilicus.

Day 1: at umbilicus → decreases by 1 cm/day.

Day 10: no longer palpable.

Uterus should remain firm and midline.

Massage uterus gently if soft (boggy) to prevent atony and hemorrhage.

C. Lochia Observation

Note color, amount and odor daily.

Lochia rubra (1–4 days) → serosa (5–10 days) → alba (11–21 days).

Foul smell or excessive discharge indicates infection or subinvolution.

D. Perineal Care

Keep perineum clean and dry; change pads frequently.

Wash with warm antiseptic solution after each voiding or defecation.

If episiotomy/laceration present: inspect for healing, redness, or discharge.

Sitz baths after 24 hours help comfort and healing.

Advise pelvic floor (Kegel) exercises from 2nd week to restore tone.

E. Bladder Care

Encourage voiding within 6 hours after delivery.

Catheterize if retention persists.

Observe for dysuria or frequency → possible infection.

Adequate hydration (2–3 L/day) helps prevent UTI.

F. Bowel Care

Bowel movement usually delayed for 2–3 days due to atony, dehydration, or pain.

Encourage:

Adequate fluid and fiber intake.

Mild laxatives (lactulose or bisacodyl suppository) if needed.

Check for hemorrhoids and provide stool softeners if necessary.

G. Breast Care and Lactation Support

Initiate breastfeeding within ½–1 hour after birth.

Promotes uterine contraction (oxytocin release) and bonding.

Ensure proper latch and position to prevent nipple cracks.

Breast examination:

Soft and non-tender initially.

Engorgement on 3rd–4th day → feed frequently, express milk, apply warm compresses.

Cracked nipples: avoid soap; apply lanolin or expressed milk.

Mastitis: continue breastfeeding, apply warm compress, start antibiotics if needed.

H. Diet and Nutrition

Diet should be high in calories, protein, calcium, and iron.

Encourage liberal fluids (2–3 L/day), milk, fruits, and vegetables.

Lactating mothers require additional:

500 kcal/day energy

25 g/day protein

Iron, folic acid, and calcium supplements.

I. Rest and Ambulation

First day: Bed rest with gentle leg movements to prevent thrombosis.

After 24 hours: Encourage sitting up and walking.

Early ambulation prevents DVT, constipation, and promotes uterine drainage.

Adequate sleep and rest periods are essential.

J. Hygiene

Daily bath permitted after 24 hours.

Clean breasts before feeds with plain water.

Maintain hand hygiene before touching perineal or breast area.

Avoid vaginal douching or tampons.

K. Psychological Care

Emotional reassurance and family support are vital.

Explain normal physiological changes and importance of rest and breastfeeding.

Watch for postpartum blues (transient emotional lability), which usually resolves within 1–2 weeks.

If persistent sadness, insomnia or disinterest → suspect postpartum depression and refer for evaluation.

L. Uterotonic Support (if required)

Routine uterotonics (e.g., oxytocin 10 units IM after delivery) are given immediately after placenta expulsion to prevent PPH.

No routine continuation beyond first day unless uterus subinvoluted or bleeding excessive.

M. Hematological and Laboratory Follow-up

Hemoglobin estimation before discharge to assess anemia.

Urine examination for infection if symptoms appear.

Continue iron and calcium supplements for 3 months.

3. Postnatal check-up and counselling

A. Discharge Criteria

Mother can be discharged (after normal vaginal delivery) when:

Afebrile for 24 hours.

Normal pulse, BP and uterine tone.

No excessive or foul-smelling lochia.

Episiotomy/lacerations healed.

Breastfeeding well established.

Passing urine and stool normally.

B. Postnatal Visit Schedule

First visit: At 2 weeks postpartum.

Second visit: At 6 weeks postpartum.

Assess:

Uterine involution and lochia.

Breast and nipple condition.

Episiotomy/perineal healing.

Blood pressure and signs of anemia.

Emotional and psychological adjustment.

Infant health and feeding adequacy.

4. Contraceptive advice

Discuss postpartum family planning before discharge.

Timing	Method	Comments
Immediate postpartum (within 48 h)	Postpartum IUCD (CuT 380A)	Safe and effective
After 6 weeks	Barrier methods (condoms)	No hormonal interference
After 6 months (if non-lactating)	Combined oral contraceptives	Contraindicated in early lactation
During lactation	Lactational Amenorrhea Method (LAM)	Effective if exclusive breastfeeding
Permanent	Tubal ligation (interval sterilization)	If family complete

5. Immunization

Tetanus toxoid: If not completed antenatally, give second dose postpartum.

Rubella vaccine: If mother non-immune and not pregnant again, vaccinate before discharge (advise contraception for 3 months).

6. Warning signs during puerperium

Mother must be instructed to report immediately if any of the following occur:

Warning Sign	Possible Indication
Excessive vaginal bleeding	Secondary PPH or retained products
Foul-smelling discharge	Puerperal sepsis
Fever, chills, abdominal pain	Infection
Painful swollen leg	Deep vein thrombosis

Warning Sign	Possible Indication
Difficulty in breathing or chest pain	Pulmonary embolism
Breast redness, pain, abscess	Mastitis
Depression, suicidal thoughts	Postpartum depression

7. Education and counselling

Importance of exclusive breastfeeding for 6 months.

Nutrition and hygiene practices.

Rest and gradual resumption of household activities.

Sexual intercourse to be avoided until lochia ceases and perineum healed (~4–6 weeks).

Family planning and child spacing importance.

Routine postnatal check-up adherence.

Summary table

Aspect	Observation / Advice	Purpose
Vital signs	Monitor daily	Detect infection or hemorrhage
Uterus	Palpate for firmness and descent	Ensure proper involution
Lochia	Observe color, amount, odor	Detect sepsis or subinvolution
Perineum	Inspect daily	Detect infection, promote healing
Breast	Examine for engorgement/mastitis	Promote lactation
Bladder/Bowel	Encourage regular voiding	Prevent retention/constipation
Nutrition	Balanced diet with supplements	Promote recovery and lactation
Rest/Ambulation	Early ambulation, adequate rest	Prevent thrombosis, restore strength
Psychological care	Reassurance, support	Prevent postpartum depression
Contraception	Discuss before discharge	Family planning
Follow-up	2 and 6 weeks	Assess recovery

Key points

First 24 hours postpartum are most critical for hemorrhage and shock.

Uterine involution, lochia and breast condition must be checked daily.

Encourage early breastfeeding to promote oxytocin-mediated uterine contraction.

Maintain strict hygiene to prevent puerperal sepsis.

Educate about contraception, nutrition and postnatal follow-up.

11.5 Post Natal Care

(*Nighdast bad Wilada*)

Definition

Postnatal care (PNC) refers to the comprehensive care given to the mother and her newborn baby immediately after childbirth and during the first 6 weeks (42 days) following delivery, which constitutes the puerperium.

It encompasses supervision, support, prevention, detection and management of complications, ensuring physical and psychological recovery of the mother and the healthy adaptation of the newborn.

Postnatal care aims to:

Ensure safe recovery of the mother,

Establish successful lactation and

Ensure the health, nutrition and safety of the newborn.

Postnatal care of the mother

1. Objectives

   1. To facilitate normal involution of uterus and other organs.
   2. To detect and manage complications early.
   3. To support breastfeeding and nutrition.
   4. To promote psychological well-being.
   5. To provide health education and family planning advice.

2. Duration of Care

Immediate postnatal period: 0–24 hours after delivery

Early postnatal period: 1–7 days

Late postnatal period: 8–42 days

3. Immediate Postnatal Care (First 24 Hours)

A. Observations

Parameter	Findings / Management
Pulse & BP	Every 15–30 min for first 2 h; monitor for hemorrhage or shock
Temperature	Slight rise may occur due to dehydration; persistent fever → infection
Uterus	Firm, central, below umbilicus; massage if boggy
Bleeding	Observe amount and color; heavy bleeding → postpartum hemorrhage
Bladder	Encourage micturition; catheterize if retention
Perineum	Inspect for lacerations or hematoma; ensure proper suturing
General condition	Watch for pallor, restlessness, pain, or distress

B. Comfort and Position

Semi-recumbent position after first few hours.

Avoid pillows if spinal anesthesia used.

Reassure and provide emotional support.

C. Early Breastfeeding

Initiate within 30–60 minutes after birth.

Stimulates oxytocin → uterine contraction → reduces bleeding.

Promotes bonding and early lactation.

4. Early and Late Postnatal Care

A. Uterine Involution

Fundal height decreases by 1 cm/day.

By 10th day, uterus not palpable abdominally.

Monitor daily; soft uterus → massage and give uterotonics.

B. Lochia

Observe daily:

Lochia rubra: Day 1–4 (red)

Lochia serosa: Day 5–10 (pinkish/brown)

Lochia alba: Day 11–21 (whitish)

Foul smell or prolonged discharge → infection or subinvolution.

C. Bladder and Bowel

Encourage voiding within 6 hours.

Prevent constipation by high-fiber diet, fluids, and mild laxatives if needed.

D. Perineal Care

Wash perineum with antiseptic solution after each voiding.

Change sanitary pads frequently.

Sitz baths after 24 hours relieve pain and promote healing.

Inspect for infection or gaping sutures.

E. Breast Care

Examine for engorgement, nipple cracks, or mastitis.

Feed frequently and correctly.

Apply warm compresses before feeding; cold compresses after feeding to relieve engorgement.

Maintain hygiene — no soap on nipples.

F. Nutrition

Diet should include:

High protein (80–100 g/day)

High calories (+500 kcal/day)

Iron, calcium, folate supplements

Plenty of fluids (2–3 L/day)

G. Rest and Ambulation

Bed rest for first day; early ambulation thereafter.

Promotes uterine drainage, prevents thrombosis, and aids recovery.

Encourage mild pelvic floor exercises (Kegel's) after 2 weeks.

H. Psychological Care

Provide reassurance, family support, and counseling.

Watch for:

Postpartum blues (transient sadness, tearfulness – resolves in 1 week)

Postpartum depression (persistent low mood – requires referral)

I. Immunization and Medications

Complete TT vaccination if pending.

Rubella vaccine if non-immune (avoid pregnancy for 3 months).

Continue iron and calcium supplements for 3 months.

J. Contraceptive Advice

Method	Time to Start	Remarks
LAM (Lactational Amenorrhea)	Immediate	Effective if exclusive breastfeeding
Condoms	Anytime	Safe during lactation
IUCD (PPIUCD or Interval)	Within 48 h / After 6 weeks	Long-term
Progestin-only pills/injections	After 6 weeks	Safe during lactation
Combined OCPs	After 6 months	May reduce milk
Tubal ligation	At cesarean / After 6 weeks	Permanent

K. Follow-up Visits

First visit: 48–72 hours

Second visit: 1–2 weeks

Third visit: 6 weeks

Assess:

Uterine involution

Lochia

Breast/nipple condition

Episiotomy healing

Blood pressure and anemia

Contraceptive counselling

Postnatal care of the newborn

1. Objectives

Ensure smooth physiological adaptation to extrauterine life.

Prevent infection, hypothermia and hypoglycemia.

Support breastfeeding and growth.

Monitor for neonatal jaundice or sepsis.

Educate mother about hygiene and danger signs.

2. Immediate care at birth

Airway, Breathing and Circulation (ABC)

Clear airway: Suction mouth → nose (if needed).

Dry and stimulate baby to cry.

Assess Apgar score at 1 and 5 minutes.

If baby doesn't cry, follow neonatal resuscitation steps.

Thermal Care

Prevent heat loss (hypothermia):

Dry the baby immediately.

Keep under radiant warmer or on mother's chest (skin-to-skin).

Cover with warm clothes and cap.

Room temperature: ~26–28°C.

Cord Care

Clamp and cut umbilical cord under aseptic precautions.

Keep stump clean and dry — no ointments or coverings.

Watch for redness, discharge or bleeding.

Eye Care

Clean eyelids with sterile cotton swabs.

Apply antibiotic eye drops (e.g., erythromycin 0.5%) to prevent ophthalmia neonatorum.

Vitamin K Administration

1 mg Vitamin K1 (IM) immediately after birth — prevents hemorrhagic disease of newborn.

3. Early neonatal care (first week)

Feeding

Initiate exclusive breastfeeding within 30 minutes of birth.

Feed on demand (8–12 times/day).

No pre-lacteal feeds (honey, sugar water, etc.).

Colostrum should never be discarded — it's rich in antibodies and nutrients.

Monitoring

Parameter	Normal Range / Observation
Temperature	36.5–37.5°C
Respiration	30–60/min
Heart rate	120–160/min
Urine	Within 24 hours
Meconium	Within 24–48 hours

C. Hygiene

Keep cord clean and dry.

Bathe only after 24 hours if room warm.

Keep baby wrapped and warm.

Use clean clothes and bedding.

D. Sleep

Baby sleeps 16–20 hours/day.

Always place baby on back (supine position) to prevent SIDS.

E. Immunization

At birth, administer:

1. BCG vaccine – for tuberculosis
2. Oral Polio Vaccine (OPV-0) – birth dose
3. Hepatitis B vaccine – within 24 hours

F. Growth Monitoring

Birth weight recorded; average 2.5–3.5 kg.

5–10% weight loss normal in first week; regained by 10–14 days.

Record length and head circumference.

G. Detection of Danger Signs

Mother should be educated to report immediately if:

Baby not feeding or weak suckling

Fever or hypothermia

Fast breathing, chest in-drawing, or grunting

Convulsions or lethargy

Yellow discoloration of skin before 24 h or after 7 days (pathological jaundice)

Pus from umbilical stump or eyes

Persistent vomiting or abdominal distension

4. Late neonatal care (day 8–28)

Continue exclusive breastfeeding.

Observe for adequate weight gain (~25–30 g/day).

Continue keeping baby warm and clean.

Attend immunization as per schedule.

Follow-up visits at 2 weeks and 6 weeks for both mother and baby.

Postnatal care must extend beyond hospital stay into the community.

Role of Health Workers (ANM / ASHA):

Conduct home visits:

1st day, 3rd day, 7th day, 14th day, and 42nd day.

Monitor for maternal or neonatal danger signs.

Ensure immunizations and breastfeeding.

Promote hygiene and family planning.

Refer to higher center if complications detected.

Postnatal care of mother and baby

Aspect	**Mother**	**Newborn**
Duration	6 weeks (puerperium)	28 days (neonatal period)
Observation	Vitals, uterus, lochia, perineum	Temp, respiration, feeding, weight
Nutrition	High-calorie, high-protein diet	Exclusive breastfeeding
Hygiene	Perineal care, handwashing	Cord care, clean clothes
Immunization	TT, Rubella (if needed)	BCG, OPV, Hepatitis B
Rest	Adequate rest, early ambulation	Sleep 16–20 hours/day
Psychological care	Prevent depression	Bonding and attachment
Contraception	Postpartum family planning	—

Follow-up	48 h, 2 wks, 6 wks	2 wks, 6 wks
Danger signs	Fever, bleeding, foul lochia	Poor feeding, fever, jaundice, difficulty breathing

Key points

Postnatal period = 6 weeks after delivery.

Uterus descends 1 cm/day → not palpable after 10 days.

Lochia changes color from red → brown → white.

Breastfeeding should start within 30–60 min.

Exclusive breastfeeding for 6 months.

Postnatal check-ups: 48 h, 2 weeks, 6 weeks.

Newborn vaccines: BCG, OPV-0, Hepatitis B.

Danger signs (mother): Excessive bleeding, fever, foul lochia.

Danger signs (baby): Not feeding, fever, jaundice, respiratory distress.

11.6 Puerperal Pyrexia

(*Humma Nefasiyah*)

Definition

According to the World Health Organization (WHO) and DC Dutta,

> Puerperal pyrexia is defined as a rise in temperature to 38°C (100.4°F) or more, maintained for 24 hours or recurring during any two of the first ten days following childbirth or abortion (excluding the first 24 hours).

Incidence

Occurs in about 5–10% of deliveries in developing countries.

Incidence is higher after cesarean section, prolonged labor, premature rupture of membranes, and instrumental deliveries.

Significance

Puerperal pyrexia is an important cause of maternal morbidity and mortality.

It is usually due to infection introduced during or after labor, and hence, it reflects quality of obstetric care and asepsis.

Etiology (Causes)

Puerperal pyrexia can be caused by infective or non-infective factors.

A. Infective Causes (Most Common)

Infection may occur at various anatomical sites:

Site of Infection	Condition	Common Causative Organisms
Genital tract	Puerperal sepsis (endometritis, parametritis, pelvic cellulitis, pelvic abscess, septic thrombophlebitis)	Streptococcus pyogenes (Group A), Staphylococcus aureus, E. coli, Clostridium welchii, anaerobes
Urinary tract	Cystitis, pyelitis	E. coli, Proteus, Klebsiella
Breast	Mastitis, breast abscess	Staphylococcus aureus
Respiratory tract	Atelectasis, pneumonia (esp. after cesarean or anesthesia)	Pneumococci, Staphylococci
Wound site	Episiotomy wound infection, cesarean wound infection	Staphylococcus aureus, Streptococci
Systemic infection	Malaria, typhoid, urinary sepsis	Depending on endemic area

B. Non-infective Causes

Condition	Mechanism
Breast engorgement	Milk stasis causing mild temperature rise
Dehydration or exhaustion	Especially after prolonged labor
Drug reactions or blood transfusion reaction	Pyrogenic or immunologic
Thrombophlebitis (non-septic)	Pelvic or leg vein thrombosis
Aseptic pelvic hematoma	Resorptive fever

Pathophysiology

1. Source of Infection

Infection is commonly introduced during labor or delivery via:

Contaminated hands or instruments,

Prolonged rupture of membranes,

Retained products of conception, or

Unhygienic environment.

2. Spread of Infection

Ascending infection from lower genital tract → uterus → parametrium → pelvic peritoneum → general peritonitis → septicemia.

Venous spread via pelvic veins → thrombophlebitis → emboli → secondary infections (lungs, kidneys).

Lymphatic spread → pelvic cellulitis and abscess.

Risk Factors

1. Prolonged labor (>18 hours)
2. Premature rupture of membranes (PROM)
3. Multiple vaginal examinations

4. Operative delivery (forceps, vacuum, cesarean)
5. Retained products of conception
6. Poor perineal hygiene
7. Anemia, malnutrition, diabetes
8. Unsterile instruments or delivery conditions
9. History of genital tract infection before labor

Clinical Features

The presentation depends on the underlying cause and site of infection.

General Symptoms

Fever ≥ 38°C (100.4°F)

Malaise, chills, rigors

Headache, myalgia, anorexia

Tachycardia, sweating

Occasionally, delirium in severe infection

Local Symptoms and Signs

Site	**Findings**
Uterus (Endometritis)	Tender, subinvoluted uterus; foul-smelling lochia (offensive, scanty, or absent); suprapubic pain
Parametritis / Pelvic cellulitis	Pelvic pain, tenderness in lateral fornices; fever; may lead to abscess
Pelvic thrombophlebitis	Spiking fever with chills despite antibiotics; tender cord-like veins on lateral pelvic wall
Peritonitis	Severe abdominal pain, rigidity, distension, absent bowel sounds
Wound infection (episiotomy/ cesarean)	Local redness, discharge, gaping wound, tenderness
Breast (mastitis)	Painful, swollen, red, indurated area; may progress to abscess
Urinary tract infection	Dysuria, frequency, suprapubic discomfort
Respiratory tract infection	Cough, crepitations, chest pain, tachypnea

Investigations

A. General Investigations

Complete Blood Count (CBC): Leukocytosis with neutrophilia (↑WBC, ↑Neutrophils)

Urine analysis: For pus cells, bacteria, culture and sensitivity

Blood culture: To identify septicemia

Culture of lochia, wound discharge, or breast milk

Ultrasound pelvis: To detect retained products or abscess

Chest X-ray: If pneumonia or embolism suspected

CT / MRI pelvis: For deep pelvic abscess or thrombophlebitis

Diagnosis

1. Clinical Diagnosis

Fever ≥ 38°C on 2 occasions within 10 days postpartum (excluding first 24 h).

Foul-smelling lochia, uterine tenderness, and subinvolution → suggest genital tract infection.

2. Confirmatory Diagnosis

Based on laboratory evidence of infection and exclusion of non-infective causes.

Differential Diagnosis

Condition	**Distinguishing Features**
Breast engorgement	Mild fever (<38.4°C), no chills, subsides after feeding
Mastitis	Localized breast pain, redness, fever
Urinary tract infection	Dysuria, frequency, positive urine culture
Malaria / Viral infection	Specific systemic symptoms
Drug or transfusion reaction	Related to timing after medication/transfusion

Management

Management involves general, specific and supportive measures.

1. General Measures

1. Isolation: Prevent cross infection.
2. Strict asepsis: Perineal hygiene, handwashing, sterile dressing.
3. Monitoring: Temperature, pulse, BP, lochia, uterine involution.
4. Hydration: Oral or IV fluids to prevent dehydration.
5. Nutrition: High-protein, high-calorie diet with vitamins and iron.
6. Rest: Absolute bed rest in acute phase.
7. Analgesics/Antipyretics: Paracetamol for fever and pain relief.

2. Specific Measures

A. Antibiotic Therapy

Start broad-spectrum antibiotics empirically, then modify based on culture report.

Example regimen:

Ampicillin (2 g IV 6-hourly)

Gentamicin (80 mg IV 8-hourly)

Metronidazole (500 mg IV 8-hourly)

→ Continue for 7–10 days or until afebrile for 48 hours.

→ In severe cases: use third-generation cephalosporins (Ceftriaxone, Cefotaxime).

B. Evacuation of Retained Products

If ultrasound shows retained placental tissue → Evacuation and curettage under antibiotic cover.

C. Drainage of Abscess

For pelvic, perineal, or breast abscess → surgical drainage required.

D. Management of Specific Sites

Condition	**Treatment**
Endometritis	Triple antibiotic therapy; uterotonics if subinvolution
Parametritis	Broad-spectrum antibiotics; analgesics; hot fomentations
Pelvic abscess	Surgical drainage (posterior colpotomy or laparotomy)
Pelvic thrombophlebitis	IV heparin + antibiotics
Mastitis	Continue breastfeeding; antibiotics (Cloxacillin); abscess drainage if needed
UTI	Antibiotics based on urine culture
Wound infection	Daily dressing, debridement, secondary suturing if required

3. Supportive Therapy

IV fluids for dehydration or toxemia

Blood transfusion if anemia or septicemia

Oxygen therapy if hypoxia

Psychological support to anxious mothers

Prevention

A. Antenatal Period

Treat anemia, malnutrition, and infections.

Educate on perineal hygiene.

B. Intrapartum Period

Strict asepsis in labor ward.

Avoid unnecessary vaginal examinations.

Use sterile instruments.

Prevent prolonged labor and PROM.

C. Postnatal Period

Maintain perineal hygiene and proper care of wounds.

Encourage early ambulation.

Avoid retained products (ensure complete delivery of placenta).

Early recognition of fever and prompt treatment.

Complications

1. Pelvic abscess
2. Septic pelvic thrombophlebitis

3. General peritonitis
4. Septicemia and septic shock
5. Disseminated intravascular coagulation (DIC)
6. Death (if untreated)

Prognosis

With early diagnosis and adequate antibiotic therapy, prognosis is excellent.

Delay in treatment → risk of sepsis, septic shock, and death.

Summary

Feature	Description
Definition	Temperature ≥38°C on 2 occasions within 10 days postpartum (excluding first 24 h)
Common cause	Genital tract infection (endometritis)
Main organisms	Streptococci, Staphylococci, E. coli, anaerobes
Symptoms	Fever, malaise, pelvic pain, foul lochia
Signs	Tender uterus, subinvolution, tachycardia
Investigations	CBC, urine culture, lochia/wound culture, USG pelvis
Treatment	Broad-spectrum antibiotics, uterotonics, drainage if abscess
Prevention	Aseptic delivery, perineal hygiene, early detection
Complications	Pelvic abscess, thrombophlebitis, septicemia

Key Points

Definition: ≥38°C on ≥2 occasions within 10 days postpartum (excluding first 24 h).

Most common cause → Genital tract infection.

Most common organism → Streptococcus pyogenes (Group A).

Characteristic feature → Foul-smelling lochia and tender subinvoluted uterus.

Triple antibiotic regimen: Ampicillin + Gentamicin + Metronidazole.

Prevention = Aseptic technique during delivery and proper postnatal hygiene.

11.7 Puerperal Sepsis

(Enten-e-nafasi)

Definition

Puerperal sepsis is a life-threatening infection of the genital tract or related structures occurring within the first 6 weeks postpartum (puerperium), typically presenting with fever (≥38°C) and other systemic or localized symptoms. It is a subset of puerperal pyrexia and is defined by the WHO as a genital tract infection occurring from the time of rupture of membranes or labor to 42 days postpartum, often involving endometritis (infection of the endometrium/myometrium). Puerperal sepsis is a leading cause of maternal morbidity and mortality, particularly in low-resource settings like India.

Epidemiology

Global Incidence: 4–10% of postpartum women, with higher rates (10–20%) in low-resource settings.

India: Incidence ranges from 10–15%, contributing to 20–30% of maternal deaths (National Family Health Survey-5, 2020). Higher prevalence in rural areas due to unhygienic delivery practices and limited postnatal care.

Mortality: Globally, puerperal sepsis accounts for 10–15% of maternal deaths; in India, it is a leading cause, with mortality rates of 2–10% in severe cases.

Timing: Most cases occur within the first 7–10 days postpartum, peaking at days 3–5.

Etiology

Puerperal sepsis is primarily caused by bacterial infections, often polymicrobial, involving the genital tract or related structures. Common pathogens and sources include:

1. Pathogens:

Gram-Positive: Group B Streptococcus(GBS), Staphylococcus aureus (including MRSA), Streptococcus pyogenes.

Gram-Negative: Escherichia coli, Klebsiella pneumoniae, Enterobacter spp.

Anaerobes: Bacteroides fragilis, Peptostreptococcus, Clostridium spp.

Others: Chlamydia trachomatis, Mycoplasma, or rarely Neisseria gonorrhoeae.

Polymicrobial: Common in endometritis, involving a mix of aerobic and anaerobic bacteria from vaginal flora.

2. Sources of Infection:

Endometritis (60–70% of cases): Infection of the endometrium/myometrium, often following vaginal or cesarean delivery.

Wound Infection (15–20%): Cesarean section incision or episiotomy/perineal lacerations.

Retained Placental Tissue: Provides a nidus for infection.

Ascending Infection: From vaginal flora, exacerbated by prolonged rupture of membranes (PROM) or multiple vaginal examinations.

Hematogenous Spread: Rare, from systemic infections (e.g., urinary tract, respiratory).

Iatrogenic: Contamination from unsterile instruments or poor hygiene during delivery.

Pathophysiology

Mechanism:

Invasion: Bacteria ascend from the vagina or are introduced during delivery (e.g., via instruments, manual placental removal), colonizing the endometrium or surgical wounds.

Inflammatory Response: Pathogens trigger a local inflammatory response, releasing cytokines (e.g., IL-6, TNF-α), leading to fever, tissue damage, and systemic symptoms.

Tissue Necrosis: Polymicrobial infections cause endometrial necrosis or abscess formation, particularly in severe endometritis.

Systemic Spread: Bacteremia or endotoxins lead to sepsis, characterized by systemic inflammatory response syndrome (SIRS), organ dysfunction, or septic shock.

Coagulopathy: Severe cases may trigger disseminated intravascular coagulation (DIC) due to endotoxin-mediated endothelial damage.

Predisposing Factors:

Disruption of the endometrial barrier during delivery.

Retained placental tissue or blood clots provide a culture medium.

Immunosuppression from anemia, malnutrition, or labor stress (common in India).

Risk Factors

Maternal:

Anemia (50–60% prevalence in India), malnutrition, or immunosuppression (e.g., HIV).

Pre-existing infections (e.g., bacterial vaginosis, UTI, chorioamnionitis).

Chronic diseases (e.g., diabetes, obesity, tuberculosis).

Obstetric:

Cesarean delivery (10–20% infection risk vs. 1–2% for vaginal delivery).

Prolonged labor (>24 hours) or PROM (>18 hours).

Multiple vaginal examinations (>5), manual placental removal, or retained products of conception.

Episiotomy, perineal lacerations, or operative delivery.

Socioeconomic:

Unhygienic delivery practices (common in rural India).

Limited access to sterile equipment, antibiotics, or postnatal care.

Low socioeconomic status, increasing malnutrition and infection risk.

Environmental:

Poor sanitation in delivery settings.

Endemic infections (e.g., malaria, typhoid) increasing systemic sepsis risk.

Clinical Presentation

General Symptoms

Fever (≥38°C, often >38.5°C), chills, or rigors.

Tachycardia (>100 bpm), hypotension (sepsis), or tachypnea.

Malaise, fatigue, or myalgia.

Specific Symptoms

Endometritis (most common):

Foul-smelling lochia (purulent or bloody).

Heavy vaginal bleeding or large clots.

Lower abdominal pain or uterine tenderness on palpation.

Subinvoluted uterus (enlarged, boggy, above expected level).

Wound Infection

Erythema, warmth, discharge, or dehiscence at cesarean or episiotomy site.

Localized pain or swelling.

Systemic Sepsis

High fever, hypotension (systolic BP <90 mmHg), or altered mental status.

Organ dysfunction: Oliguria, respiratory distress, or jaundice.

Other

Mastitis: Unilateral breast pain, redness, or fever (if secondary infection).

UTI: Dysuria, frequency, or suprapubic pain (if concurrent).

Neonatal Signs:

Poor feeding, lethargy, or neonatal sepsis (e.g., GBS transmission) in 5–10% of cases.

Diagnosis

Diagnosis requires a high index of suspicion, combining clinical assessment, laboratory tests, and imaging to identify the infection source and severity.

1. Clinical Assessment:

History

Onset and pattern of fever (e.g., persistent vs. intermittent).

Associated symptoms: Foul lochia, abdominal pain, wound issues, or systemic complaints.

Risk factors: Cesarean delivery, PROM, unhygienic delivery, or anemia.

Physical Examination

Vital signs: Fever (≥38°C), tachycardia, hypotension (sepsis), or tachypnea.

Abdomen: Uterine tenderness, subinvolution (fundus above expected level).

Perineum/Wound: Erythema, discharge, or dehiscence.

Pelvic exam (sterile speculum): Foul lochia, cervical motion tenderness, or adnexal masses.

Breasts/Lungs: Rule out mastitis or pneumonia.

2. Laboratory Tests:

Complete Blood Count (CBC)

Leukocytosis (>15,000/µL) with left shift or leukopenia (sepsis).

Anemia (hemoglobin <11 g/dL, common in India) worsens outcomes.

Blood Cultures: Positive in 10–20% of cases; identify bacteremia or specific pathogens.

Endometrial Swab: Culture for pathogens, though vaginal flora contamination limits specificity.

Urine Analysis/Culture: Rule out UTI (pyuria, bacteriuria).

Coagulation Profile: PT, aPTT, fibrinogen, D-dimer for DIC (if sepsis or retained tissue).

Infection Screen

C-Reactive Protein (CRP) or procalcitonin: Elevated in sepsis.

Malaria smear/rapid test or tuberculosis testing (India-specific).

HIV or TORCH serology if systemic infection suspected.

3. Imaging

Ultrasound

Pelvic: Detect retained placental tissue, hematoma, or abscess.

Transvaginal: Assess endometrial cavity or adnexal masses.

CT/MRI: For suspected septic pelvic thrombophlebitis or deep pelvic abscess (rare).

Chest X-Ray: Rule out pneumonia or pulmonary edema in severe sepsis.

4. Sepsis Criteria (SIRS or qSOFA for severe cases)

SIRS: ≥2 of: Temperature >38°C or <36°C, heart rate >90 bpm, respiratory rate >20/min, WBC >12,000 or <4,000/μL.

qSOFA: ≥2 of: Respiratory rate ≥22/min, altered mentation, systolic BP <100 mmHg.

Positive criteria indicate need for urgent management.

5. Differential Diagnosis

Other causes of puerperal pyrexia: Mastitis, UTI, wound infection, thromboembolism, or non-puerperal infections (e.g., appendicitis, malaria).

Non-infectious: Physiological fever (first 24 hours, <38°C), drug reaction, or hematoma.

Management

Management of puerperal sepsis focuses on rapid antibiotic therapy, source control, supportive care, and prevention of complications. Severe cases require hospitalization and multidisciplinary care.

1. General Principles:

Stabilization

IV fluids (1–2 L crystalloids) to correct hypovolemia; monitor urine output (>0.5 mL/kg/hour).

Oxygen if SpO2 <94% or respiratory distress.

Paracetamol (1 g IV/oral every 6–8 hours) for fever and pain.

Hospitalization

Admit all women with suspected puerperal sepsis (fever >38.5°C, systemic symptoms, or organ dysfunction).

ICU for septic shock, DIC, or multi-organ failure.

Supportive Care

Nutrition: High-protein diet (2,500–3,000 kcal/day), iron (60–120 mg/day) for anemia (critical in India).

Continue breastfeeding unless contraindicated (e.g., severe sepsis requiring maternal separation).

Monitor vital signs, urine output, and response to treatment every 4–6 hours.

2. Antibiotic Therapy

Empiric Treatment (initiate within 1 hour of suspicion):

Broad-spectrum to cover polymicrobial infection:

Preferred: Clindamycin (900 mg IV every 8 hours) + gentamicin (5 mg/kg IV daily).

Alternative: Ampicillin (2 g IV every 6 hours) + metronidazole (500 mg IV every 8 hours) or piperacillin-tazobactam (4.5 g IV every 8 hours).

Adjust based on culture results (if available) and local resistance patterns.

Duration: IV antibiotics until afebrile for 24–48 hours (typically 3–5 days), followed by oral antibiotics (e.g., amoxicillin-clavulanate 625 mg thrice daily) for a total of 7–14 days.

Cesarean Wound Infection: Add vancomycin (15–20 mg/kg IV every 12 hours) if MRSA suspected.

3. Source Control

Retained Placental Tissue:

Ultrasound to confirm retained products.

Dilation and curettage (D&C) under antibiotic cover; risks include Asherman syndrome.

Abscess:

Ultrasound-guided drainage for pelvic or wound abscess.

Surgical exploration for deep abscess or wound dehiscence.

Necrotic Tissue: Debride cesarean or perineal wounds if infected.

4. Management of Severe Sepsis/Septic Shock

Sepsis Bundle (per WHO/Surviving Sepsis Campaign):

Blood cultures before antibiotics.

Broad-spectrum antibiotics within 1 hour.

IV fluids (30 mL/kg crystalloids within 3 hours).

Vasopressors (e.g., norepinephrine) if hypotension persists (mean arterial pressure <65 mmHg).

Monitor: Lactate levels, urine output, and organ function (renal, hepatic, respiratory).

Supportive: Mechanical ventilation for respiratory failure, dialysis for renal failure, or blood transfusion for severe anemia (<7 g/dL).

DIC: Fresh frozen plasma (15–20 mL/kg), cryoprecipitate (if fibrinogen <1 g/L), or platelets (if <50,000/µL).

5. Neonatal Care

Evaluate infant for sepsis (e.g., GBS, *E. coli*) if maternal infection confirmed.

Pediatric consultation for antibiotics (e.g., ampicillin + gentamicin) and monitoring.

Complications

1. Maternal

Sepsis/Septic Shock: 1–2% mortality; multi-organ failure (renal, hepatic, respiratory).

Pelvic Abscess: Requires drainage; may lead to chronic pain or infertility.

Septic Pelvic Thrombophlebitis: Persistent fever despite antibiotics; treat with heparin and prolonged antibiotics.

DIC: Hemorrhage or thromboembolism; 10–20% risk in severe sepsis.

Infertility: Endometrial scarring (Asherman syndrome) or tubal damage post-endometritis.

Chronic Pelvic Pain: From unresolved infection or adhesions.

2. Neonatal

Vertical transmission of infection (5–10% risk of neonatal sepsis, e.g., GBS).

Poor feeding, growth failure, or neonatal death.

3. Psychosocial

Maternal anxiety or PPD (10–20% risk) from prolonged illness or hospitalization.

Stigma in India may delay recovery or care-seeking.

Prevention

1. Antenatal

Screen and treat infections (e.g., GBS, UTI, bacterial vaginosis).

Correct anemia (iron 60–120 mg/day, folate) to improve immunity, critical in India (50–60% prevalence).

Educate on hygiene, nutrition, and warning signs (fever, foul lochia).

2. Intrapartum

Use sterile techniques: Sterile gloves, instruments, and delivery kits.

Minimize vaginal examinations (<5) and avoid manual placental removal unless necessary.

Prophylactic antibiotics for cesarean delivery (cefazolin 1 g IV) or prolonged PROM (>18 hours).

Active management of the third stage of labor (AMTSL): Oxytocin (10 IU IM), controlled cord traction, uterine massage to prevent retained tissue.

3. Postpartum

Promote perineal hygiene: Warm water cleansing, frequent pad changes, handwashing.

Monitor for fever, foul lochia, or wound issues in the first 24 hours and at discharge.

Encourage early ambulation to reduce thromboembolism risk, countering prolonged bed rest practices in India.

Support breastfeeding to enhance uterine involution and reduce endometritis risk.

Ensure postnatal visits (within 24 hours, 3 days, 10–14 days) per WHO guidelines.

Post-Management Care

Immediate:

Monitor response to antibiotics: Afebrile within 48–72 hours, normalized vital signs, and improved symptoms.

Continue supportive care: Nutrition, hydration, pain relief, and anemia correction.

Assess neonatal health for signs of infection or poor feeding; coordinate with pediatricians.

Follow-Up:

1–2 Weeks:

Confirm resolution of infection (no fever, normal lochia, healing wounds).

Repeat CBC for anemia or leukocytosis; continue iron if hemoglobin <11 g/dL.

Screen for PPD (EPDS score >10), as sepsis increases psychological stress.

6 Weeks:

Comprehensive exam: BP, pelvic exam (confirm involution, cervical closure), cervical smear if due.

Assess for long-term complications: Infertility, chronic pelvic pain, or Asherman syndrome.

Contraception counseling: Progesterone-only methods or IUDs for breastfeeding women; combined oral contraceptives for non-breastfeeding women.

Key points

Puerperal sepsis is a life-threatening genital tract infection within 6 weeks postpartum, often presenting with fever (≥38°C), foul lochia, and uterine tenderness.

Common pathogens include GBS, E. coli and anaerobes; endometritis is the primary source (60–70%).

Risk factors include cesarean delivery, PROM, anemia (50–60% in India), and unhygienic practices.

Diagnosis involves clinical assessment, CBC, blood/endometrial cultures, and ultrasound to identify retained tissue or abscess.

Management includes broad-spectrum antibiotics (clindamycin + gentamicin), source control (D&C, abscess drainage), and supportive care; severe sepsis requires ICU management.

Prevention relies on sterile delivery, AMTSL, hygiene, and early postnatal monitoring, with focus on anemia and access barriers in India.

11.8 Subinvolution of the Uterus

(*Aubur-Rahim Juz'i*)

Subinvolution of the uterus is the delayed or incomplete return of the uterus to its pre-pregnancy size and state during the puerperium, the 6–8-week period following childbirth. Normally, the uterus reduces from approximately 1,000 g post-delivery to 50–100 g by 6 weeks through myometrial contraction and autolysis. Subinvolution is characterized by a persistently enlarged, boggy uterus beyond the expected timeline (typically >2–3 weeks postpartum), often associated with prolonged or heavy lochia and an increased risk of complications such as secondary postpartum hemorrhage (PPH) or infection.

Epidemiology

Incidence: Occurs in 1–5% of postpartum women globally; higher in low-resource settings like India (5–10%) due to risk factors such as anemia, infection, and limited postnatal care.

India: Contributes to 10–20% of secondary PPH cases, a significant cause of maternal morbidity, particularly in rural areas with poor access to care.

Timing: Typically diagnosed between 2–6 weeks postpartum, with symptoms peaking at 10–14 days.

Etiology

Subinvolution results from factors that impair uterine contraction, endometrial regeneration, or tissue clearance. Common causes include:

1. Retained Placental Tissue or Products of Conception (30–40%):

Incomplete expulsion of placental fragments, blood clots, or decidual tissue.

Provides a nidus for infection or inhibits myometrial contraction.

2. Infection (Endometritis) (20–30%):

Polymicrobial infection (Escherichia coli, Group B Streptococcus, anaerobes) causes inflammation, delaying involution.

3. Uterine Fibroids (10–15%):

Submucosal or intramural fibroids interfere with myometrial contraction.

4. Uterine Atony:

Poor myometrial tone, often due to multiparity, overdistension, or inadequate oxytocin release.

5. Hormonal Factors:

Reduced oxytocin (e.g., limited breastfeeding) or persistent high progesterone levels (rare).

6. Other:

Adenomyosis, endometrial hyperplasia, or coagulation disorders (e.g., von Willebrand disease).

Chronic systemic conditions (e.g., anemia, hypothyroidism) impairing tissue repair.

Pathophysiology

Normal Involution:

Post-delivery, oxytocin-mediated myometrial contractions compress blood vessels, reducing bleeding and uterine size.

Autolysis (lysosomal degradation) reduces myometrial cell size, and endometrial regeneration replaces the decidual layer.

Lochia (blood, mucus, tissue) is expelled as the uterus shrinks, completing involution by 6–8 weeks.

Subinvolution:

Impaired myometrial contraction leads to a boggy, enlarged uterus, prolonging lochia and increasing bleeding risk.

Retained placental tissue or infection causes local inflammation, edema, and delayed endometrial healing.

Fibroids or adenomyosis mechanically hinder contraction, perpetuating subinvolution.

Systemic factors (e.g., anemia, malnutrition) reduce tissue repair capacity, common in India (50–60% anemia prevalence).

Risk Factors

Maternal:

Anemia (50–60% in India), malnutrition, or hypothyroidism.

Multiparity (weaker myometrial tone).

Obesity or diabetes, increasing infection risk.

Obstetric:

Cesarean delivery (delayed involution due to surgical trauma).

Prolonged labor (>24 hours), prolonged rupture of membranes (PROM >18 hours).

Manual placental removal, retained placenta, or multiple gestation.

Episiotomy or perineal lacerations, increasing infection risk.

Socioeconomic:

Unhygienic delivery practices (common in rural India).

Limited access to postnatal care or antibiotics.

Malnutrition, exacerbating anemia and poor healing.

Environmental:

Poor sanitation, increasing infection risk.

Lack of sterile delivery kits in low-resource settings.

Clinical Presentation

Symptoms:

Prolonged or Heavy Lochia: Persistent lochia rubra or serosa beyond 2–3 weeks, or heavy bleeding (soaking pads in <1–2 hours).

Lower Abdominal Pain: Dull, aching pain due to uterine distension or infection.

Fever: If infection (endometritis) is present; temperature ≥38°C.

General Symptoms: Fatigue, malaise, or weakness, often exacerbated by anemia.

Physical Examination:

Uterus: Enlarged, boggy, and higher than expected (e.g., palpable above pelvis after day 10–14).

Lochia: Heavy, prolonged, or foul-smelling (if infected).

Pelvic Exam: Uterine tenderness, cervical motion tenderness (endometritis), or palpable masses (fibroids).

Vital Signs: Fever, tachycardia (>100 bpm), or hypotension if secondary PPH or sepsis occurs.

Associated Signs:

Wound infection (cesarean/episiotomy): Erythema, discharge, or dehiscence.

Systemic: Pallor (anemia), chills, or rigors (infection).

Diagnosis

Diagnosis is based on clinical findings, supported by laboratory tests and imaging to identify the underlying cause.

1. Clinical Assessment

History:

Duration and nature of lochia (e.g., heavy, prolonged, foul-smelling).

Associated symptoms: Pain, fever, or bleeding.

Risk factors: Cesarean delivery, PROM, anemia, or multiparity.

Physical Examination:

Fundal height: Above expected level (e.g., >pelvis after day 10).

Uterine consistency: Boggy, tender if infected.

Lochia: Assess volume, color, and odor.

General: Check for anemia (pallor), fever, or tachycardia.

2. Laboratory Tests

Complete Blood Count (CBC):

Leukocytosis (>15,000/µL) or left shift suggests infection.

Anemia (hemoglobin <11 g/dL, common in India) contributes to poor healing.

Blood Cultures: Positive in 10–20% of endometritis cases; identify bacteremia.

Endometrial Swab: Culture for pathogens (limited by vaginal flora contamination).

Coagulation Profile: PT, aPTT, fibrinogen for DIC if secondary PPH or sepsis.

C-Reactive Protein (CRP)/Erythrocyte Sedimentation Rate (ESR): Elevated in infection.

3. Imaging

Ultrasound:

Transvaginal or abdominal: Detect retained placental tissue, blood clots, or endometrial thickening.

Assess uterine size and presence of abscess or hematoma.

CT/MRI(rare): For suspected fibroids, adenomyosis, or deep pelvic collections.

4. Differential Diagnosis

Secondary PPH (without subinvolution): Due to coagulopathy or trauma.

Endometritis (without subinvolution): Fever and foul lochia but normal uterine size.

Uterine fibroids or adenomyosis: Pre-existing conditions mimicking subinvolution.

Systemic infections: Malaria, typhoid, or tuberculosis (India-specific).

Management

Management aims to treat the underlying cause, promote uterine involution, and prevent complications such as secondary PPH or sepsis.

1. General Principles

Hospitalization:

Admit women with heavy bleeding, fever, or suspected infection/retained tissue.

Monitor vital signs, lochia, and uterine size every 4–6 hours.

Supportive Care:

IV fluids (1–2 L crystalloids) for hydration, especially if bleeding or fever.

Paracetamol (1 g IV/oral every 6–8 hours) for pain or fever.

Nutrition: High-protein diet (2,500–3,000 kcal/day), iron (60–120 mg/day), and calcium to support recovery, critical in India due to anemia.

Encourage breastfeeding to stimulate oxytocin release and promote involution.

2. Cause-Specific Management

Retained Placental Tissue:

Ultrasound: Confirm presence of tissue or clots.

Dilation and Curettage (D&C): Perform under antibiotic cover (e.g., clindamycin 900 mg IV) to remove retained products.

Risks: Uterine perforation, Asherman syndrome (endometrial scarring).

Uterotonics: Oxytocin (10–20 IU IV) or methylergometrine (0.2 mg IM every 6 hours, max 5 doses) to enhance contraction post-D&C.

Endometritis

Antibiotics: Broad-spectrum: Clindamycin (900 mg IV every 8 hours) + gentamicin (5 mg/kg IV daily) for 48–72 hours, then oral (e.g., amoxicillin-clavulanate 625 mg thrice daily) for 7–10 days.

Alternative: Ampicillin (2 g IV every 6 hours) + metronidazole (500 mg IV every 8 hours).

Continue until afebrile for 24–48 hours.

Supportive: Analgesics, hydration, and monitor for abscess formation.

Uterine Fibroids

Uterotonics: Methylergometrine or misoprostol (400–600 µg orally) to promote contraction.

Surgical: Myomectomy or uterine artery embolization for large fibroids (rare in puerperium).

Uterine Atony

Uterotonics: Oxytocin (10–40 IU IV infusion) or methylergometrine (0.2 mg IM).

Manual Massage: To stimulate contraction.

Anemia

Iron supplementation (60–120 mg/day oral; parenteral if severe, e.g., iron sucrose 200 mg IV).

Blood transfusion if hemoglobin <7 g/dL with symptoms (e.g., tachycardia, fatigue).

3. Secondary PPH

Stabilization: IV fluids, blood transfusion if hemoglobin <7 g/dL or significant bleeding.

Uterotonics: Oxytocin, misoprostol (600–1,000 µg rectally), or carboprost (250 µg IM every 15 minutes, max 8 doses).

Surgical:

D&C for retained tissue.

Uterine tamponade (Bakri balloon) for persistent bleeding.

Uterine artery ligation or hysterectomy (1–2% of severe cases) if uncontrollable.

4. Monitoring Response

Expect reduced lochia, uterine firmness, and size decrease within 48–72 hours of treatment.

Persistent symptoms require re-evaluation for abscess, resistant infection, or other causes.

Complications

1. Secondary Postpartum Hemorrhage (20–30%):

Heavy bleeding due to retained tissue or poor myometrial tone; may require transfusion or hysterectomy.

2. Puerperal Sepsis (10–20%):

Progression of endometritis to systemic infection, septic shock, or multi-organ failure (1–2% mortality).

3. Infertility:

Endometrial scarring (Asherman syndrome) post-D&C or severe endometritis.

Tubal damage from pelvic infection.

4. Chronic Pelvic Pain:

Due to adhesions or unresolved inflammation.

5. Anemia:

Worsened by prolonged bleeding; increases fatigue and infection risk.

6. Psychosocial:

Maternal anxiety or postpartum depression (10–20% risk) from prolonged recovery or hospitalization.

Prevention

1. Antenatal:

Correct anemia (iron 60–120 mg/day, folate) to improve tissue repair, critical in India.

Screen and treat infections (e.g., bacterial vaginosis, UTI).

Educate on hygiene and warning signs (heavy bleeding, foul lochia, fever).

2. Intrapartum:

Use sterile techniques: Sterile gloves, instruments, and delivery kits.

Minimize vaginal examinations (<5) and avoid manual placental removal unless necessary.

Prophylactic antibiotics for cesarean delivery (cefazolin 1 g IV) or prolonged PROM (>18 hours).

Active management of the third stage of labor (AMTSL): Oxytocin (10 IU IM), controlled cord traction, uterine massage to prevent retained tissue.

3. Postpartum:

Promote perineal hygiene: Warm water cleansing, frequent pad changes, handwashing.

Encourage breastfeeding to enhance oxytocin release and involution.

Monitor uterine size, lochia, and vital signs in the first 24 hours and at discharge.

Schedule postnatal visits (within 24 hours, 3 days, 10–14 days) per WHO guidelines to detect subinvolution early.

Post-Management Care

Immediate: Monitor response to treatment: Reduced lochia, uterine firmness, and size within 48–72 hours. Continue antibiotics until afebrile for 24–48 hours; complete oral course (7–10 days).

Supportive care: Iron supplementation, hydration, and pain relief.

Assess neonatal health for signs of infection or poor feeding.

Follow-Up

1–2 Weeks:

Confirm uterine involution (non-palpable abdominally), normal lochia (serosa/alba), and no fever.

Repeat CBC for anemia; continue iron if hemoglobin <11 g/dL.

Screen for postpartum depression (EPDS score >10), as subinvolution increases psychological stress.

6 Weeks:

Comprehensive exam: BP, pelvic exam (confirm uterine size, cervical closure), cervical smear if due.

Assess for long-term complications: Infertility, chronic pain, or Asherman syndrome.

Contraception counseling: Progesterone-only methods or IUDs for breastfeeding women; combined oral contraceptives for non-breastfeeding women.

Key points

Subinvolution is the delayed return of the uterus to pre-pregnancy size, typically >2–3 weeks postpartum, causing prolonged/heavy lochia and an enlarged, boggy uterus.

Common causes include retained placental tissue, endometritis, fibroids, or uterine atony.

Risk factors include cesarean delivery, PROM, anemia (50–60% in India), and unhygienic practices.

Diagnosis involves clinical assessment (uterine size, lochia), ultrasound, and laboratory tests (CBC, cultures).

Management includes uterotonics (oxytocin, methylergometrine), antibiotics for infection, D&C for retained tissue, and supportive care (iron, nutrition).

Prevention relies on AMTSL, sterile delivery, hygiene, and early postnatal monitoring, with focus on anemia and access barriers in India.

11.9 Urinary Tract Complications

(*Awaridat-e-Majra Bawl*)

Urinary tract complications are common in obstetrics due to the physiological and anatomical changes of pregnancy, labor, and the postpartum period, as well as the impact of obstetric interventions such as episiotomy, forceps delivery, vacuum delivery, cesarean section, and destructive operations. These complications include urinary tract infections (UTIs), urinary retention, bladder injuries, ureteral injuries, and fistulae, which can significantly affect maternal morbidity. Antenatal assessments, such as cardiotocography (CTG) and non-stress tests (NST), may indirectly identify conditions like preterm labor or sepsis associated with urinary complications, guiding timely interventions.

The goals of managing urinary tract complications in obstetrics are:

To prevent and treat infections that can lead to maternal and fetal morbidity.

To identify and repair injuries caused by obstetric procedures.

To manage voiding dysfunction and prevent chronic complications like fistulae.

To integrate findings from fetal well-being assessments (e.g., NST, ultrasonography) with maternal care to ensure comprehensive management.

Pathophysiology

Pregnancy induces significant changes in the urinary tract, predisposing women to complications:

1. Anatomical Changes

Ureteral Dilatation: Progesterone-mediated smooth muscle relaxation and uterine compression cause hydroureter and hydronephrosis, particularly on the right side, increasing the risk of urinary stasis and infection.

Bladder Displacement: The enlarging uterus elevates the bladder, reducing its capacity and altering voiding dynamics.

Urethral Compression: In late pregnancy, the fetal head may compress the urethra, contributing to urinary retention.

2. Physiological Changes

Increased Glomerular Filtration Rate (GFR): Enhanced renal blood flow increases urine output, potentially diluting urinary defenses against infection.

Glycosuria: Common in pregnancy, it promotes bacterial growth, increasing UTI risk.

Immunosuppression: Relative immunosuppression of pregnancy increases susceptibility to infections.

3. Obstetric Interventions

Episiotomy/Instrumental Delivery: Trauma to the perineum or pelvic floor during forceps or vacuum delivery can impair bladder function or cause fistulae.

Cesarean Section: Surgical manipulation near the bladder or ureters increases the risk of injury.

Destructive Operations: Invasive procedures in rare cases of fetal demise may cause direct trauma to the urinary tract.

Catheterization: Routine use during labor or cesarean section increases infection risk.

4. Labor and Postpartum

Prolonged labor or obstructed labor (detected via CTG or clinical assessment) can compress the bladder or ureters, leading to ischemia or retention.

Postpartum edema or pelvic nerve trauma may impair bladder sensation and voiding.

Types of Urinary Tract Complications

1. Urinary Tract Infections (UTIs)

UTIs are the most common urinary tract complications in pregnancy, encompassing asymptomatic bacteriuria (ASB), cystitis, and pyelonephritis.

Asymptomatic Bacteriuria (ASB)

Definition: Presence of ≥10^5 colony-forming units (CFU)/mL of a single bacterial species in urine without symptoms.

Prevalence: 2–10% of pregnant women.

Pathophysiology: Urinary stasis, glycosuria, and immunosuppression promote bacterial growth (e.g., *Escherichia coli* [80%], *Klebsiella*, *Proteus*).

Risk: Untreated ASB progresses to pyelonephritis in 20–40% of cases, increasing risks of preterm labor, low birth weight, and sepsis.

Diagnosis: Routine urine culture screening at 12–16 weeks or first prenatal visit. Midstream clean-catch urine sample showing ≥10^5 CFU/mL.

Management:

Antibiotics safe in pregnancy (e.g., nitrofurantoin 100 mg BID for 5–7 days, amoxicillin 500 mg TID, or cephalexin 500 mg QID). Repeat culture 1–2 weeks post-treatment to confirm clearance.

Prevention: Encourage hydration, frequent voiding, and perineal hygiene.

Cystitis

Definition: Symptomatic lower UTI with dysuria, urgency, frequency, or suprapubic pain.

Prevalence: 1–2% of pregnant women.

Pathophysiology: Similar to ASB, with bacterial invasion of the bladder mucosa.

Diagnosis: Clinical symptoms plus urine dipstick (positive for nitrites/leukocytes) or culture. Urinalysis showing pyuria (>10 white blood cells/high-power field).

Management:

Antibiotics as for ASB, tailored to culture sensitivities. Analgesics (e.g., phenazopyridine for symptom relief, used cautiously).

Complications: Progression to pyelonephritis if untreated.

Pyelonephritis

Definition: Upper UTI involving the kidneys, characterized by fever, flank pain, nausea, and systemic symptoms.

Prevalence: 0.5–2% of pregnant women.

Pathophysiology: Ascending infection from the bladder or hematogenous spread, often complicating untreated ASB or cystitis.

Diagnosis:

Clinical: Fever (>38°C), flank pain, costovertebral angle tenderness, nausea/vomiting.

Laboratory: Positive urine culture, pyuria, leukocytosis, elevated C-reactive protein (CRP).

Imaging: Renal ultrasound if atypical presentation or no response to treatment.

Management:

Hospitalization for IV antibiotics (e.g., ceftriaxone 1–2 g daily or ampicillin/gentamicin until afebrile for 48 hours). Transition to oral antibiotics (e.g., cephalexin) for 10–14 days.

Supportive care: IV fluids, antipyretics, antiemetics.

Fetal monitoring (e.g., NST, ultrasonography) to assess for preterm labor or fetal distress.

Complications: Sepsis, acute respiratory distress syndrome (ARDS), preterm delivery, fetal demise.

2. Urinary Retention

Definition: Inability to void completely, leading to residual urine in the bladder (>150 mL post-void).

Prevalence: Common postpartum (5–15%), rare antenatally.

Pathophysiology:

Antenatal: Uterine compression of the bladder/urethra, especially in retroverted uterus or with large fibroids.

Intrapartum: Prolonged labor, epidural anesthesia, or pelvic nerve trauma (e.g., during forceps/ vacuum delivery) impair bladder sensation.

Postpartum: Perineal edema, pain from episiotomy, or pelvic floor trauma disrupts voiding reflexes.

Risk Factors:

Instrumental delivery (forceps/vacuum), episiotomy, prolonged second stage, epidural use. Cesarean section with prolonged catheterization.

Primiparity, perineal trauma, or postpartum hemorrhage.

Diagnosis:

Clinical: Inability to void within 6 hours postpartum, lower abdominal pain, palpable bladder. Post-void residual volume >150 mL via ultrasound or catheterization.

Management:

Intermittent Catheterization: Preferred for short-term retention to reduce infection risk.

Indwelling Catheter: For persistent retention (24–48 hours), removed after trial of voiding.

Pain Management: Analgesics for perineal pain (e.g., NSAIDs) to facilitate voiding.

Pelvic Floor Exercises: Kegel exercises to restore bladder function.

Urology Referral: For persistent retention (>1 week) or suspected neurological injury.

Complications: Recurrent UTIs, bladder overdistension, chronic voiding dysfunction.

3. Bladder and Ureteral Injuries

Definition: Iatrogenic trauma to the bladder or ureters during obstetric procedures, particularly cesarean section or destructive operations.

Prevalence: Bladder injury (0.1–1% of cesareans), ureteral injury (<0.1%).

Pathophysiology:

Bladder Injury: Occurs during cesarean section (e.g., dissection of bladder flap), forceps delivery, or destructive operations due to proximity to the uterus.

Ureteral Injury: Rare, associated with cesarean hysterectomy, extensive adhesions, or destructive procedures involving pelvic manipulation.

Risk Factors:

Repeat cesarean sections (adhesions increase risk).

Emergency cesarean or destructive operations with poor visualization.

Prolonged labor or abnormal fetal presentations requiring complex interventions.

Diagnosis:

Intraoperative: Visible bladder laceration, urine leakage, or hematuria during cesarean.

Postoperative: Abdominal pain, hematuria, oliguria, or urinary leakage (suspect fistula).

Imaging: Cystoscopy, CT urography, or retrograde pyelography to confirm injury.

Management:

Bladder Injury:

Intraoperative repair with two-layer closure using absorbable sutures (e.g., polyglactin 3-0). Indwelling catheter for 7–14 days to allow healing.

Ureteral Injury:

Ureteral reimplantation or stenting by a urologist.

Prolonged catheterization and monitoring for obstruction or leakage.

Follow-Up: Imaging (e.g., ultrasound, cystogram) to confirm healing.

Complications: Fistulae (vesicovaginal, ureterovaginal), chronic urinary incontinence, renal dysfunction.

4. Vesicovaginal and Ureterovaginal Fistulae

Definition: Abnormal communications between the bladder/ureter and vagina, leading to continuous urinary leakage.

Prevalence: Rare in high-resource settings (<0.1%), more common in low-resource settings due to prolonged obstructed labor.

Pathophysiology:

Obstructed Labor: Prolonged compression of the bladder or ureters against the pelvic bones causes ischemic necrosis, leading to fistula formation.

Iatrogenic: Trauma during cesarean section, destructive operations, or instrumental delivery (forceps/vacuum).

Risk Factors:

Prolonged labor (detected via CTG Category II/III tracings), neglected shoulder dystocia, or failed instrumental delivery.

Emergency cesarean or destructive operations in low-resource settings.

Lack of skilled obstetric care or delayed access to cesarean section.

Diagnosis:

Clinical: Continuous urinary leakage postpartum, vaginal pooling of urine.

Methylene Blue Test: Instill dye into the bladder; vaginal leakage confirms vesicovaginal fistula.

Imaging: Cystoscopy, CT urography, or MRI to identify fistula tract.

Management:

Conservative: Small fistulae (<1 cm) may heal with prolonged catheterization (4–6 weeks).

Surgical: Fistula repair via transvaginal or transabdominal approach by a urologist or gynecologist.

Supportive Care: Skin protection, psychological support, and infection prevention.

Complications: Chronic incontinence, social stigma, recurrent infections, infertility.

Diagnosis of Urinary Tract Complications

History:

Antenatal: Dysuria, frequency, flank pain, or decreased voiding.

Intrapartum/Postpartum: Inability to void, perineal pain, or continuous leakage.

Risk factors: Prolonged labor, instrumental delivery, cesarean, or maternal comorbidities.

Physical Examination:

Abdominal: Palpable bladder, suprapubic tenderness.

Pelvic: Perineal edema, episiotomy site infection, or vaginal leakage.

Costovertebral angle tenderness for pyelonephritis.

Laboratory Tests:

Urinalysis: Pyuria, hematuria, nitrites, or bacteriuria.

Urine culture: Identifies causative organisms and antibiotic sensitivities.

Blood tests: Leukocytosis, elevated CRP, or renal function tests for pyelonephritis or ureteral injury.

Imaging:

Ultrasound: Assesses bladder volume, hydronephrosis, or post-void residual.

CT urography or cystoscopy: For suspected bladder/ureteral injuries or fistulae.

Fetal Monitoring:

NST/CTG or ultrasonography to assess fetal well-being in cases of pyelonephritis or suspected preterm labor.

Management and Prevention

Management

UTIs: Prompt antibiotic treatment based on culture sensitivities. Hospitalization for pyelonephritis with IV antibiotics and fetal monitoring.

Urinary Retention: Intermittent or indwelling catheterization, pain management, and pelvic floor rehabilitation.

Bladder/Ureteral Injuries: Intraoperative repair by skilled surgeons, with urology consultation for complex cases. Postoperative catheterization and imaging follow-up.

Fistulae: Conservative management for small fistulae; surgical repair for persistent cases. Multidisciplinary care involving urologists, gynecologists, and psychologists.

Prevention

Antenatal: Routine screening for ASB at 12–16 weeks to prevent pyelonephritis. Encourage hydration, frequent voiding, and perineal hygiene. Monitor high-risk pregnancies (e.g., diabetes, preeclampsia) with NST/CTG and ultrasound to detect complications early.

Intrapartum: Avoid prolonged labor through timely CTG monitoring and intervention (e.g., cesarean for Category III tracings). Use episiotomy judiciously to minimize perineal trauma during instrumental delivery. Ensure proper surgical technique during cesarean to avoid bladder/ureteral injury. Limit catheterization duration to reduce infection risk.

Postpartum: Monitor voiding within 6 hours post-delivery; catheterize if necessary. Provide pain relief for perineal trauma to facilitate voiding. Educate patients on signs of UTI or retention.

Guidelines ACOG (2020):

Recommends routine screening for ASB at 12–16 weeks with urine culture.

Advises prompt treatment of UTIs to prevent pyelonephritis and preterm labor.

Supports bladder catheterization during cesarean but recommends removal within 24 hours to reduce infection risk.

Conclusion

Urinary tract complications in obstetrics, including UTIs, urinary retention, bladder/ureteral injuries, and fistulae, are significant contributors to maternal morbidity, particularly when associated with obstetric interventions like episiotomy, forceps, vacuum, cesarean section, or destructive operations. Pregnancy-related anatomical and physiological changes, combined with the trauma of labor and delivery, predispose women to these complications. Antenatal fetal assessments (e.g., NST, CTG, ultrasonography) play a critical role in detecting maternal conditions like pyelonephritis that affect fetal well-being, guiding timely interventions.

11.10 Breast Complications

(*Aridat-e-Thad I*)

Introduction

The breast undergoes marked physiological and structural changes during pregnancy, lactation, and the puerperium under the influence of estrogen, progesterone, prolactin, and oxytocin. These changes, though essential for lactation, predispose the breast to a variety of complications. Breast complications are common in the early postpartum period and may adversely affect maternal comfort, continuation of breastfeeding, and neonatal nutrition. Prompt recognition and appropriate management are therefore of considerable clinical importance in obstetric practice.

Physiological basis of breast complications

During pregnancy and lactation, the breast shows:

Proliferation of ducts and lobules

Increased vascularity and lymphatic drainage

Milk secretion and accumulation within alveoli

Failure of effective milk removal or breach in nipple integrity may lead to milk stasis, inflammation, and infection, forming the basis of most breast complications.

Classification of breast complications

Breast complications in obstetrics may be classified as:

Non-infective breast conditions

Infective breast conditions

Nipple abnormalities and disorders

Miscellaneous conditions

1. Non-infective breast complications

Breast Engorgement

Definition

Breast engorgement is a condition characterized by painful distension of the breasts due to accumulation of milk, interstitial edema, and increased vascularity, commonly occurring between the 2nd and 5th day postpartum.

Etiology

Delay in initiation of breastfeeding

Infrequent or ineffective suckling

Improper attachment of the baby

Sudden cessation of breastfeeding

Clinical Features

Bilateral breast enlargement

Firm, tense, and tender breasts

Shiny skin with flattened nipples

Difficulty in milk expression

Management

Early initiation and frequent breastfeeding

Correction of positioning and latch

Manual expression or breast pump usage

Warm fomentation before feeding

Cold compresses after feeding

Analgesics for pain relief

Blocked Milk Duct

Definition

A blocked duct results from obstruction of milk flow in a segment of the breast, leading to localized milk stasis.

Etiology

Incomplete emptying of the breast

Pressure from tight clothing or brassiere

Skipped feeds

Clinical Features

Localized tender lump

Mild erythema

Absence of fever or systemic symptoms

Management

Frequent feeding from the affected breast

Gentle breast massage towards the nipple

Warm compresses

Ensuring effective emptying of the breast

2. Infective breast complications

Mastitis

Definition

Mastitis is an acute inflammation of breast tissue, usually associated with infection, occurring most commonly during the first six weeks of lactation.

Etiology

Milk stasis

Cracked or fissured nipples

Ascending bacterial infection

Causative Organisms

Staphylococcus aureus (most common)

Streptococcus species

Clinical Features

Unilateral breast pain and swelling

Localized redness and warmth

Fever, chills, and malaise

Flu-like symptoms

Diagnosis

Diagnosis is primarily clinical. Breast milk culture may be considered in recurrent or non-responding cases.

Management

Continuation of breastfeeding or milk expression

Effective drainage of the breast

Antibiotic therapy (e.g., dicloxacillin, cephalexin)

Analgesics and antipyretics

Adequate rest and hydration

Breast Abscess

Definition

A breast abscess is a localized collection of pus within the breast tissue, usually resulting from inadequately treated mastitis.

Risk Factors

Delayed treatment of mastitis

Diabetes mellitus

Poor personal hygiene

Clinical Features

Localized, fluctuant, tender swelling

Severe pain

Fever and systemic toxicity

Overlying skin erythema

Diagnosis

Clinical examination

Ultrasonography of the breast

Management

Incision and drainage or ultrasound-guided aspiration

Broad-spectrum antibiotics

Breastfeeding may be continued from the unaffected breast; milk expression from the affected side is encouraged

3. Nipple abnormalities and disorders

Cracked (Fissured) Nipples

Definition

Cracked nipples are linear breaks in the epithelium of the nipple, commonly seen during early lactation.

Etiology

Improper attachment of the baby

Prolonged suckling

Dryness and lack of nipple care

Clinical Features

Severe pain during feeding

Bleeding or oozing from the nipple

Increased risk of mastitis

Management

Correction of breastfeeding technique

Application of expressed breast milk or lanolin

Short, frequent feeds

Temporary use of nipple shields if required

Inverted and Flat Nipples

These conditions may interfere with effective breastfeeding.

Management

Antenatal counseling and nipple exercises

Use of breast pump prior to feeding

Nipple shields when necessary

Sore Nipples

May result from improper latch, excessive moisture, or candidal infection.

Management

Improvement of positioning

Keeping nipples clean and dry

Topical antifungal therapy if indicated

4. Miscellaneous breast conditions

Galactocele

Definition

A galactocele is a retention cyst filled with milk, caused by obstruction of a lactiferous duct.

Clinical Features

Painless, soft, cystic breast lump

Absence of inflammation

Management

Usually conservative

Aspiration if symptomatic

Candidal Infection of the Breast

Clinical Features

Burning nipple pain

Shiny, erythematous nipples

Pain persisting after feeds

Management

Topical antifungal therapy to the mother

Simultaneous treatment of the infant

Prevention of breast complications

Early initiation of breastfeeding

Proper positioning and attachment

Regular and complete emptying of breasts

Maintenance of nipple hygiene

Early treatment of nipple trauma

Conclusion

Breast complications constitute an important group of disorders encountered during the puerperium. Most complications arise from milk stasis or nipple trauma and can be prevented by appropriate breastfeeding practices. Early diagnosis, continuation of breastfeeding and timely medical or surgical intervention ensure favorable maternal and neonatal outcomes.

11.11 Puerperal venous Thrombosis & Pulmonary embolism

(*Khusar-e-Waridi Nefasi aur insed-e-Ri'wi*)

Puerperal venous thrombosis and pulmonary embolism represent the most serious manifestations of venous thromboembolism (VTE) in obstetrics. These conditions occur predominantly during the postpartum period, particularly within the first six weeks following delivery, and constitute a major cause of maternal morbidity and mortality worldwide. Despite advances in obstetric care, pulmonary embolism remains one of the leading causes of sudden maternal death.

Pregnancy and the puerperium are physiologically hypercoagulable states. When combined with additional risk factors such as operative delivery, infection, prolonged immobilization, or inherited thrombophilia, the risk of venous thrombosis increases substantially. Early recognition, appropriate investigation, and prompt anticoagulant therapy are crucial for preventing fatal outcomes.

Epidemiology

Incidence of VTE in pregnancy and puerperium: approximately 1–2 per 1000 pregnancies

Risk is 5–10 times higher in pregnancy and 20–80 times higher in the puerperium compared to non-pregnant women

Majority of fatal pulmonary emboli occur postpartum, especially after cesarean section

Etiopathogenesis

The pathogenesis of puerperal venous thrombosis is best explained by Virchow's triad, all three components of which are exaggerated during pregnancy and puerperium.

1. Hypercoagulability

Pregnancy induces a physiological hypercoagulable state to prevent excessive bleeding during childbirth.

Increased fibrinogen levels

Increased clotting factors: VII, VIII, IX, X, XII

Reduced anticoagulant activity:

Decreased protein S

Resistance to activated protein C

Suppressed fibrinolysis due to increased plasminogen activator inhibitors (PAI-1, PAI-2)

This hypercoagulable state persists for several weeks postpartum.

2. Venous Stasis

Compression of pelvic veins and inferior vena cava by the gravid uterus

Reduced venous tone due to progesterone

Prolonged recumbency during labor and postpartum period

Decreased mobility after cesarean section

Venous stasis is more pronounced in the left lower limb due to compression of the left iliac vein by the right iliac artery (May–Thurner phenomenon).

3. Endothelial Injury

Trauma to pelvic veins during labor and vaginal delivery

Surgical trauma during cesarean section

Endometritis and puerperal sepsis

Instrumental deliveries

Risk factors for puerperal venous thromboembolism

Obstetric Risk Factors

Cesarean section (highest risk)

Prolonged labor

Instrumental delivery

Postpartum hemorrhage

Puerperal sepsis

Multiple pregnancy

Pre-eclampsia

Maternal Risk Factors

Obesity

Advanced maternal age (>35 years)

Multiparity

Prolonged immobilization

Dehydration

Medical and Genetic Risk Factors

Previous history of VTE

Inherited thrombophilias:

Factor V Leiden mutation

Prothrombin gene mutation

Antithrombin III deficiency

Protein C and S deficiency

Acquired thrombophilia (antiphospholipid syndrome)

Classification of puerperal venous thrombosis

1. Superficial venous thrombosis
2. Deep vein thrombosis (DVT)
   Lower limb DVT
   Pelvic vein thrombosis
   Ovarian vein thrombosis
3. Septic pelvic thrombophlebitis
4. Pulmonary embolism

Deep vein thrombosis (DVT)

Definition

Deep vein thrombosis is the formation of a thrombus within the deep venous system, most commonly involving the iliofemoral veins during the puerperium.

Sites of Thrombosis

Femoral vein

Popliteal vein

Iliac veins

Ovarian veins (especially right ovarian vein)

Clinical Features

Unilateral swelling of the leg

Pain and tenderness along the course of veins

Increased local temperature

Pitting edema

Cyanosis of limb in severe cases (phlegmasia cerulea dolens)

Dilated superficial veins

Low-grade fever

Homan's sign is neither sensitive nor specific and is of limited clinical value.

Complications

Pulmonary embolism

Post-thrombotic syndrome

Chronic venous insufficiency

Recurrence in future pregnancies

Diagnosis

Clinical suspicion remains paramount

Compression Doppler ultrasonography – investigation of choice

MRI venography for pelvic vein thrombosis

D-dimer levels are physiologically elevated and unreliable in puerperium

Venography is rarely performed due to invasiveness

Management of DVT

Anticoagulant Therapy:

Low molecular weight heparin (LMWH) is the drug of choice

Unfractionated heparin in renal impairment or high bleeding risk

Transition to oral anticoagulants (warfarin) postpartum with overlap

Duration of therapy: minimum 6 months, including at least 6 weeks postpartum

Supportive Measures:

Initial bed rest with limb elevation

Graduated compression stockings

Adequate hydration

Analgesics

Septic pelvic thrombophlebitis

Definition

Septic pelvic thrombophlebitis is characterized by infected thrombus formation in pelvic veins, usually following puerperal infection, especially after cesarean section.

Clinical Features

Persistent high spiking fever

Failure to respond to antibiotics

Minimal abdominal or pelvic signs

Tachycardia

Diagnosis

Diagnosis of exclusion

CT or MRI may show thrombosed pelvic veins

Management

Broad-spectrum intravenous antibiotics

Anticoagulation therapy

Surgical intervention rarely indicated

Pulmonary embolism (PE)

Definition

Pulmonary embolism occurs when a thrombus, most commonly originating from the deep veins of the legs or pelvis, dislodges and embolizes to the pulmonary arterial circulation.

Pathophysiology

Obstruction of pulmonary arteries

Ventilation-perfusion mismatch

Hypoxemia

Increased pulmonary vascular resistance

Right ventricular strain and failure in massive PE

Clinical Features

Mild to Moderate PE

Sudden onset dyspnea

Pleuritic chest pain

Tachypnea

Tachycardia

Anxiety

Massive PE

Severe hypoxia

Hypotension

Syncope

Cyanosis

Sudden collapse and death

Diagnosis

High index of suspicion is critical

Arterial blood gases: hypoxemia, respiratory alkalosis

ECG: sinus tachycardia, right heart strain

Chest X-ray: often normal

CT pulmonary angiography – investigation of choice

V/Q scan in selected cases

Echocardiography for massive PE

Management of Pulmonary Embolism

Emergency Management

Oxygen therapy

Hemodynamic support

Immediate anticoagulation

Anticoagulation

LMWH or unfractionated heparin

Oral anticoagulants after stabilization

Thrombolytic Therapy

Indicated in life-threatening massive PE

Agents: alteplase

Inferior Vena Cava (IVC) Filter

Considered when anticoagulation is contraindicated

Prevention of puerperal venous thromboembolism

Risk assessment in antenatal and postpartum period

Early mobilization after delivery

Adequate hydration

Graduated compression stockings

Prophylactic LMWH in high-risk women

Prognosis

Early diagnosis significantly improves outcome

Mortality is high in untreated massive PE

Recurrence risk exists in subsequent pregnancies

Long-term anticoagulation may be required in thrombophilia

Conclusion

Puerperal venous thrombosis and pulmonary embolism remain life-threatening obstetric emergencies. The hypercoagulable state of pregnancy, combined with venous stasis and endothelial injury, predisposes postpartum women to thromboembolic events. A high index of suspicion, prompt diagnostic evaluation, and early initiation of anticoagulation are essential to reduce maternal mortality. Preventive strategies and thromboprophylaxis play a pivotal role in high-risk patients.

11.12 Psychiatric Disorders

(*Nafsiyati khlal*)

Psychiatric disorders during pregnancy and the puerperium constitute an important cause of maternal morbidity and, in severe cases, mortality. The puerperium is a period of profound biological, psychological, and social transition. Sudden hormonal withdrawal, sleep deprivation, emotional stress, and altered social roles predispose women to a wide spectrum of mental disorders. These disorders adversely affect maternal health, mother–infant bonding, breastfeeding, and child development. Severe conditions such as puerperal psychosis are medical emergencies and may result in suicide or infanticide if not treated promptly.

Etiopathogenesis

The etiology of psychiatric disorders in pregnancy and puerperium is multifactorial.

1. Biological Factors

Sudden fall in estrogen and progesterone after delivery

Dysregulation of hypothalamic–pituitary–adrenal axis

Neurotransmitter imbalance (serotonin, dopamine, norepinephrine)

Sleep deprivation

Anemia, nutritional deficiencies

2. Psychological Factors

Anxiety related to childbirth

Fear of maternal inadequacy

Body image disturbance

Previous psychiatric illness

3. Social Factors

Poor family and social support

Marital conflict

Domestic violence

Low socioeconomic status

Unwanted pregnancy

Classification

Psychiatric disorders associated with pregnancy and puerperium include:

Postpartum blues

Postpartum depression

Puerperal (postpartum) psychosis

Anxiety disorders

Psychiatric disorders complicating pregnancy

Substance use disorders

1. Postpartum blues

Definition

A transient emotional disturbance occurring within the first week postpartum, characterized by mild depressive symptoms without functional impairment.

Incidence

Occurs in 50–80% of postpartum women.

Clinical Features

Tearfulness

Emotional lability

Irritability

Anxiety

Insomnia

Management

Reassurance regarding self-limiting nature

Emotional support

Adequate rest

No pharmacological treatment

2. Postpartum depression

Definition

A non-psychotic depressive disorder occurring within 4 weeks to 12 months postpartum, associated with significant impairment of functioning.

Incidence

10–15% of postpartum women.

Clinical Features

Persistent low mood

Anhedonia

Fatigue

Sleep and appetite disturbance

Guilt and worthlessness

Poor bonding with infant

Suicidal ideation

Management of postpartum depression

A. General Principles

Early diagnosis through screening

Individualized treatment

Protection of mother and infant

Preservation of breastfeeding

B. Non-Pharmacological Management

Cognitive behavioral therapy

Interpersonal therapy

Supportive psychotherapy

Family counseling

Used alone in mild cases or combined with drugs in moderate to severe cases.

C. Pharmacological Management

Indicated in moderate to severe depression.

Antidepressants

SSRIs are first-line (sertraline, fluoxetine)

Drugs compatible with breastfeeding preferred

Lowest effective dose used

Monitoring

Suicide risk assessment

Regular follow-up

3. Puerperal (postpartum) psychosis

Definition

A severe psychiatric emergency characterized by acute onset of psychotic symptoms, usually within 2 weeks of delivery.

Incidence

1–2 per 1000 deliveries.

Risk Factors

Bipolar disorder

Previous psychosis

Family history

Primiparity

Clinical Features

Delusions and hallucinations

Severe mood swings

Disorganized behavior

Insomnia

Suicidal or infanticidal thoughts

Management of puerperal psychosis

A. Emergency Measures

Immediate hospitalization

Constant supervision

Separation of mother from infant if risk exists

B. Pharmacological Management

Antipsychotics (haloperidol, atypical antipsychotics)

Mood stabilizers (lithium with caution)

Benzodiazepines for agitation

C. Electroconvulsive Therapy (ECT)

Safe and effective

Indicated in severe depression, catatonia, or suicidal risk

D. Long-Term Management

Psychiatric follow-up

Prophylaxis in future pregnancies

Counseling regarding recurrence risk

4. Anxiety disorders

Types

Generalized anxiety disorder

Panic disorder

Obsessive–compulsive disorder

Post-traumatic stress disorder

Management

Psychological therapy (first-line)

SSRIs if severe

Avoid benzodiazepines unless necessary

5. Psychiatric disorders complicating pregnancy

Women with pre-existing psychiatric illness may relapse due to drug discontinuation.

Avoid abrupt cessation of medication

Risk–benefit analysis

Close obstetric–psychiatric collaboration

6. Substance use disorders

Substances

Alcohol

Tobacco

Opioids

Management

Counseling and behavioral therapy

Gradual withdrawal

Neonatal monitoring

Special management issues

Breastfeeding Considerations

Prefer drugs compatible with lactation

Monitor infant for sedation

Medico-Legal Aspects

Consent issues in psychotic patients

Mandatory psychiatric referral

Safeguarding infant welfare

Prevention

Antenatal mental health screening

Identification of high-risk women

Adequate social support

Postpartum follow-up

Prognosis

Postpartum blues resolves spontaneously

Depression responds well to treatment

Psychosis has high recurrence risk

Conclusion

Psychiatric disorders in pregnancy and puerperium represent a significant challenge in obstetric care. Early identification, appropriate management, and multidisciplinary collaboration are essential to reduce maternal morbidity and mortality. Integration of mental health services into routine obstetric care is crucial for optimal maternal and neonatal outcomes.

Long Answer Questions (LAQs)

Describe normal puerperium and the physiological changes occurring during this period.

Discuss postnatal care and management of a normal puerperium.

Explain puerperal sepsis with causes, clinical features, and management.

Describe breast complications during puerperium and their management.

Discuss psychiatric disorders in puerperium with classification and management.

Short Answer Questions (SAQs)

Define puerperium.

What is lochia?

Define subinvolution of uterus.

What is puerperal pyrexia?

List causes of puerperal venous thrombosis.

Multiple Choice Questions (MCQs)

1. Duration of puerperium is approximately:

A. 2 weeks B. 4 weeks

C. 6 weeks D. 8 weeks

Answer: C

2. Normal lochia rubra lasts for about:

A. 24 hours B. 3–4 days

C. 7–10 days D. 2 weeks

Answer: B

3. Normal involution of uterus is complete by:

A. 2 weeks   B. 4 weeks

C. 6 weeks   D. 8 weeks

Answer: C

4. Puerperal pyrexia is defined as temperature ≥38°C after:

A. First 12 hours   B. First 24 hours

C. First 24 hours on two occasions   D. First 48 hours

Answer: C

5. Most common cause of puerperal sepsis is:

A. Staphylococcus   B. Polymicrobial infection

C. Clostridium   D. Gonococcus

Answer: B

6. Subinvolution of uterus commonly occurs due to:

A. Early ambulation   B. Breastfeeding

C. Retained products of conception   D. Oxytocin use

Answer: C

7. Most common breast complication in puerperium is:

A. Breast abscess   B. Breast engorgement

C. Mastitis   D. Galactocele

Answer: B

8. Puerperal venous thrombosis most commonly involves:

A. Femoral vein   B. Ovarian vein

C. Popliteal vein   D. Inferior vena cava

Answer: B

9. Most common urinary complication in puerperium is:

A. Hematuria   B. Urinary retention

C. Renal failure   D. Incontinence

Answer: B

10. Most common psychiatric disorder in puerperium is:

A. Puerperal psychosis   B. Postpartum blues

C. Severe depression   D. Schizophrenia

Answer:

12

Obstetrical Procedures & Operations

(Taulidi Amaliyat wa Jaraheyat)

12.1 *Qata-ul-Ejaan* (Episiotomy)
12.2 *Gardish/Tahweel* (Version)
12.3 *Milqt aur mehjm ke zriyah wiladat* (Forceps and vacuum Delivery)
12.4 *Shigaaf-e-Qaisree* (Caesarean Section)
12.5 *Takhreebi dastkariyan* (Destructive Operations)

Learning Objective (At the end of the session, the students should be able to)

Explain Episiotomy & Discuss the Indications, advantages, types, procedure & complications of *Qata-Ul- Ejaan* (Episiotomy)
Describe the process of the *Gardish* (Version)
Elaborate the Forceps & Ventouse Delivery
Summarise the *Takhreesi Dastkariya* (Destructive Operations)
Identify the types of perineal tears and Explain post-repair care & techniques for suturing & repairing.
Identify the *Shigaaf-e-Qaisree* (Caesarean Section) & Enlist risk factors.
Explain pre-operative care & Identify surgical instruments used in C-sections.
Summarise the *Takhreesi Dastkariya* (Destructive Operations).
Demonstrate the steps of stitch removal.

Obstetrical Procedures and Operations

(*Taulidi Amaliyat wa Jaraheyat*)

Obstetrical procedures and operations encompass a range of medical interventions performed during pregnancy, labor and delivery to ensure the safety and well-being of both the mother and the fetus. These procedures are needed for managing complications, facilitating safe delivery, and addressing emergencies that may arise during childbirth. They range from non-invasive techniques, such as external cephalic version, to invasive surgical interventions, like cesarean sections. The choice of procedure depends on clinical indications, maternal and fetal conditions, and evidence-based guidelines. Key obstetrical procedures include episiotomy, forceps delivery, vacuum extraction, cesarean section and cervical cerclage, among others. Each procedure requires precise indications, skilled execution and careful consideration of risks and benefits.

12.1 Episiotomy

(*Qata-ul-Ejaan*)

Definition

Episiotomy is a deliberate surgical incision made in the perineum—the fibromuscular tissue between the vaginal introitus and the anus—during the second stage of labor to enlarge the vaginal opening and facilitate delivery. Historically, episiotomy was performed routinely to prevent severe perineal lacerations, expedite delivery, and reduce pelvic floor trauma. However, contemporary evidence has shifted toward restrictive use, limiting episiotomy to specific clinical scenarios where benefits outweigh risks.

Historical Context

Episiotomy gained widespread use in the early 20th century, driven by the belief that it prevented severe perineal tears, protected the pelvic floor, and reduced neonatal trauma. Routine episiotomy rates in some regions exceeded 80% of vaginal deliveries by the mid-20th century. However, landmark studies in the 1990s and 2000s, including randomized controlled trials and meta-analyses, challenged these assumptions, demonstrating that routine episiotomy offered no significant benefits over spontaneous tearing and was associated with increased morbidity. This led to a paradigm shift toward selective, or restrictive, episiotomy practices.

Indications

Episiotomy is now reserved for specific clinical situations where it is likely to improve maternal or fetal outcomes. Indications include:

1. Fetal Distress

Non-reassuring fetal heart rate patterns (e.g., bradycardia, late decelerations) necessitating expedited delivery.

Episiotomy may reduce delivery time by a few minutes, critical in preventing fetal hypoxia.

2. Shoulder Dystocia

To provide additional space for maneuvers (e.g., McRoberts maneuver, suprapubic pressure) to deliver the fetal shoulders.

3. Instrumental Delivery

During forceps or vacuum-assisted deliveries, episiotomy may reduce perineal resistance and the risk of uncontrolled tears.

4. Prolonged Second Stage of Labor

When maternal exhaustion, ineffective pushing, or failure to progress prolongs the second stage, episiotomy may facilitate delivery.

5. Prevention of Severe Perineal Tears

In cases of suspected macrosomia, a large fetal head, or rigid perineal tissues (e.g., in primigravidas), episiotomy may reduce the risk of third- or fourth-degree tears.

6. Breech Delivery

To allow adequate space for delivery of the aftercoming head in vaginal breech births.

7. Maternal Medical Conditions

In rare cases, to minimize maternal effort during pushing in patients with cardiovascular or respiratory compromise (e.g., severe hypertension, heart failure).

8. Other Rare Indications

Abnormal perineal anatomy (e.g., scarring from previous trauma) or cultural preferences in specific settings.

Types of Episiotomy

Two primary types of episiotomy are performed, distinguished by the direction of the incision:

1. Midline (Median) Episiotomy

Description: A vertical incision from the posterior vaginal fourchette toward the anus, typically 2–4 cm in length.

- Advantages

Easier and faster to repair due to linear alignment.

Less postoperative pain compared to mediolateral episiotomy.

Reduced blood loss due to fewer vessels in the midline.

Better cosmetic outcomes with minimal scarring.

- Disadvantages

Higher risk of extension into the anal sphincter (third-degree tear) or rectum (fourth-degree tear), particularly in uncontrolled deliveries.

Less suitable for instrumental deliveries or cases with high risk of perineal trauma.

Indications: Preferred in settings with low risk of severe tearing, such as multiparous women with elastic perineal tissues.

2. Mediolateral Episiotomy

Description: An incision made at a 45–60-degree angle from the posterior vaginal fourchette, directed laterally to avoid the anal sphincter.

- Advantages

Lower risk of extension into the anal sphincter or rectum, making it safer in high-risk deliveries (e.g., macrosomia, instrumental delivery).

Preferred in settings where severe perineal trauma is a concern.

- Disadvantages

More challenging to repair due to the angled incision.

Increased postoperative pain and blood loss due to transection of more muscle fibers and blood vessels.

Potential for poorer cosmetic outcomes due to irregular scarring.

Indications: Preferred in primigravidas, instrumental deliveries, or cases with anticipated perineal resistance.

Technique

Performing an episiotomy requires precision, adherence to aseptic technique, and careful consideration of maternal and fetal status. The procedure is typically performed during the second stage of labor, when the perineum is stretched by the presenting part.

1. Preparation

Informed Consent: Obtain verbal or written consent when possible, explaining the procedure, indications, risks, and alternatives. In emergencies, implied consent may apply.

Analgesia: Ensure adequate pain control, typically through:

Local anesthesia (e.g., 5–10 mL of 1% lidocaine infiltrated into the perineum).

Regional anesthesia (e.g., epidural or spinal, if already in place).

In some cases, pudendal nerve block may be used.

Positioning: The patient is typically in the lithotomy position, with the perineum accessible and well-visualized.

Asepsis: Use sterile gloves, drapes, and instruments to minimize infection risk.

2. Procedure

Timing: Perform the incision during a contraction, when the perineum is maximally stretched by the fetal head, to minimize tissue trauma.

Incision

Use sharp, straight surgical scissors or a scalpel.

For midline episiotomy, make a 2–4 cm incision directly posterior from the vaginal fourchette, stopping short of the anal sphincter.

For mediolateral episiotomy, make a 2–4 cm incision at a 45–60-degree angle from the midline, directed toward the ischial tuberosity, avoiding the anal sphincter.

The incision should extend through the vaginal mucosa, subcutaneous tissue, and superficial perineal muscles (e.g., bulbospongiosus, transverse perineal).

Depth Control: Avoid deep incisions that risk the anal sphincter or rectum.

Hemostasis: Ensure bleeding is controlled, as the perineum is vascularized by branches of the pudendal artery.

3. Repair

Repair is performed post-delivery, after the placenta is expelled, to ensure maternal stability.

Materials: Use absorbable sutures, such as polyglactin 910 (Vicryl) or chromic catgut (2-0 or 3-0 gauge), to minimize the need for suture removal.

Technique

1. Vaginal Mucosa: Close with a continuous running suture, starting above the apex of the incision to ensure hemostasis and prevent hematoma formation.

2. Perineal Muscles: Reapproximate the bulbospongiosus and transverse perineal muscles with interrupted sutures to restore anatomical integrity.

3. Skin: Close with a subcuticular suture for cosmetic results or interrupted sutures for added strength.

Anatomical Alignment: Ensure proper alignment to prevent tension, asymmetry, or long-term complications like dyspareunia.

Post-Repair Check: Inspect for hemostasis, symmetry, and patency of the vaginal introitus.

Complications

Episiotomy, while generally safe, is associated with potential complications, particularly when performed unnecessarily or improperly. These include:

1. Infection

The perineum is prone to contamination by vaginal and fecal flora, increasing the risk of wound infection.

Signs include erythema, swelling, discharge, or fever.

Prevention involves aseptic technique and postoperative perineal hygiene.

2. Hematoma

Bleeding into the perineal tissues can form a hematoma, causing pain and swelling.

Large hematomas may require surgical drainage.

3. Perineal Pain

Common in the immediate postpartum period, particularly with mediolateral episiotomy due to greater tissue disruption.

May persist in cases of poor repair or infection.

4. Extension of the Incision

Midline episiotomies are at higher risk of extending into the anal sphincter (third-degree tear) or rectum (fourth-degree tear).

These tears are associated with anal incontinence, with reported rates of 0.5–5% for third-degree tears and 0.1–0.8% for fourth-degree tears.

5. Wound Dehiscence

Breakdown of the suture line, often due to infection, hematoma, or excessive tension.

May require secondary repair or conservative management with wound care.

6. Dyspareunia

Painful intercourse due to scar tissue, poor healing, or altered perineal anatomy.

Reported in 10–20% of women post-episiotomy, particularly with mediolateral incisions.

7. Pelvic Floor Dysfunction

Long-term complications include urinary incontinence, fecal incontinence, or pelvic organ prolapse, particularly with anal sphincter involvement.

Risk is higher with midline episiotomy or severe tears.

8. Psychological Impact

Women may experience dissatisfaction or trauma if episiotomy is performed without consent or results in prolonged recovery.

Guidelines

The shift from routine to restrictive episiotomy is supported by robust evidence:

- Cochrane Reviews (2017, updated 2020):

A meta-analysis of randomized controlled trials found that restrictive episiotomy policies (performing episiotomy only when clinically indicated) result in

Fewer severe perineal tears (third- or fourth-degree).

Less posterior perineal trauma.

Reduced need for suturing.No significant difference in neonatal outcomes compared to routine episiotomy.

- American College of Obstetricians and Gynecologists (ACOG, 2018)

Recommends restrictive use of episiotomy, emphasizing clinical judgment over routine practice. Notes that midline episiotomy is associated with a higher risk of anal sphincter injury and should be avoided in high-risk cases.

- World Health Organization (WHO, 2018)

Advises against routine episiotomy, recommending its use only for specific indications like fetal distress or instrumental delivery.

Emphasizes hands-on perineal support and controlled delivery to minimize trauma.

- Royal College of Obstetricians and Gynaecologists (RCOG, 2020)

Supports mediolateral episiotomy over midline in settings with high risk of severe tearing. Recommends training in perineal repair techniques to reduce complications.

Postoperative Care

Effective postpartum care is essential to minimize complications and promote recovery

1. Pain Management

Administer nonsteroidal anti-inflammatory drugs (NSAIDs) or acetaminophen for pain relief. Recommend warm sitz baths (2–3 times daily) to reduce discomfort and promote healing. In severe cases, short-term opioid analgesics may be considered.

2. Wound Care

Advise perineal hygiene, including gentle cleansing with water after urination or defecation and patting dry to prevent infection. Avoid harsh soaps or douches that may irritate the wound.

3. Monitoring

Assess for signs of infection (e.g., redness, swelling, discharge), hematoma, or dehiscence during postpartum visits (typically at 1–2 weeks and 6 weeks).

Evaluate for anal sphincter function in cases of suspected severe tears.

4. Pelvic Floor Rehabilitation

Encourage Kegel exercises starting 2–4 weeks postpartum to strengthen pelvic floor muscles and reduce the risk of incontinence.

5. Patient Education

Counsel on expected recovery timelines (typically 2–6 weeks for complete healing).

Address concerns about sexual activity, recommending a delay of 4–6 weeks or until pain-free.

Conclusion

Episiotomy remains a valuable tool in obstetrics when used judiciously, but its routine application is no longer supported by evidence. A thorough understanding of its indications, anatomical considerations, techniques and potential complications is essential for obstetricians to optimize maternal and fetal outcomes.

12.2 Version

(*Gardish/Tahweel*)

Introduction

Malpresentations such as breech, transverse lie, and oblique lie are associated with increased maternal and perinatal morbidity and mortality. Version is an obstetric maneuver aimed at correcting these abnormal presentations to facilitate safer vaginal delivery or reduce the need for cesarean section. Though its role has diminished with the increased safety of cesarean delivery, version still holds important clinical relevance, especially external cephalic version (ecv).

Definition

Version is defined as an obstetric procedure in which the fetus is deliberately turned from one presentation to another by manual manipulation, either through the maternal abdominal wall or by introducing the hand into the uterus.

Historical aspect

Version is one of the oldest obstetric procedures, described by Hippocrates.

Internal podalic version was widely practiced before the advent of safe cesarean section.

With modern imaging, anesthesia, and surgical safety, **external cephalic version** remains the only commonly practiced form today.

Classification of version

1. Based on method

External version

Internal version

Combined version

2. Based on timing

Antepartum version

Intrapartum version

3. Based on resulting presentation

Cephalic version

Podalic version

EXTERNAL CEPHALIC VERSION (ECV)

Definition

External cephalic version is a procedure in which the fetus is turned from breech or transverse lie into cephalic presentation by gentle manipulation through the maternal abdomen, with the uterus intact.

Objectives of ECV

To convert breech or transverse lie into vertex

To reduce cesarean section rate

To allow vaginal delivery when conditions are favorable

Indications of ECV

Singleton pregnancy

Breech presentation

Transverse or oblique lie

Live fetus

Gestational age ≥ 36–37 weeks

Adequate amniotic fluid

No contraindication to vaginal delivery

Contraindications

Absolute contraindications

Placenta previa

Previous classical cesarean section

Uterine rupture or scar dehiscence

Multiple pregnancy (except after delivery of first twin)

Major uterine anomaly

Fetal compromise

Relative contraindications

Oligohydramnios

Pre-eclampsia

Iugr

Anterior placenta

Rh-negative pregnancy (requires anti-d)

Optimal timing of ECV

Nulliparous women: 36–37 weeks

Multiparous women: 37–38 weeks

Rationale:

Earlier attempts → high reversion rate

Later attempts → reduced success due to engagement

Prerequisites for ecv

Informed consent

Ultrasound confirmation of:

Presentation

Placental location

Amniotic fluid index

Reactive NST

Empty bladder

Availability of emergency cesarean section

Tocolysis (e.g., beta-agonists)

Continuous fetal monitoring

Mechanism (principle) of ECV

The fetus behaves like a mobile object floating in fluid.

Rotation is achieved using:

Pressure on fetal breech

Pressure on fetal head

Counter-resistance of uterine wall

This creates a controlled rotational movement.

Technique of External Cephalic Version

1. Mother placed in supine position with left lateral tilt
2. Uterine relaxation achieved using tocolytics
3. One hand dislodges breech from pelvis
4. Other hand guides fetal head toward pelvis
5. Fetus rotated by forward roll or backward flip
6. Continuous ultrasound and fetal heart monitoring
7. Confirmation of cephalic presentation after procedure

Success rate

Overall success: 40–60%

Higher success in:

Multiparity

Adequate liquor

Non-engaged breech

Posterior placenta

Causes of failure

Oligohydramnios

Frank breech

Anterior placenta

Obesity

Uterine tone increased

Engaged breech

Complications of ECV

(usually rare)

Fetal

Transient fetal bradycardia

Cord entanglement

Placental abruption

Emergency cesarean

Maternal

Abdominal discomfort

Anxiety

Rare uterine rupture

Post-procedure care

Fetal heart rate monitoring for at least 30 minutes

Anti-d immunoglobulin for rh-negative women

Advice regarding labor signs

Repeat attempt may be considered if safe

INTERNAL VERSION

Definition

Internal version is a procedure where the obstetrician introduces a hand into the uterus to grasp and turn the fetus to achieve a desired presentation.

Types

Internal podalic version

Cephalic internal version (rare)

Indications

Second twin with transverse or breech lie

Fully dilated cervix

Ruptured membranes

Fetus alive or dead

Contraindications

Incompletely dilated cervix

Uterine scar

Contracted pelvis

Live singleton pregnancy

Technique of internal podalic version

1. General or regional anesthesia
2. Hand introduced into uterus
3. Identify fetal feet
4. Grasp and bring feet down
5. Convert into breech extraction

Complications

Uterine rupture

Cord prolapse

Fetal trauma

Infection

Combined version

One hand inside uterus, one on abdomen, rarely used, mainly historical importance.

Comparison: External vs Internal version

Feature	External version	Internal version
Route	Abdominal	Intrauterine
Timing	Antepartum	Intrapartum
Risk	Low	High
Use	Common	Rare
Indication	Breech	Second twin

Current status in modern obstetrics

External cephalic version is recommended by WHO, RCOG, ACOG

Internal version is limited to special situations

Cesarean section has replaced most dangerous versions

Conclusion

Version is a valuable obstetric maneuver when performed with proper case selection, adequate facilities, and skilled hands. External cephalic version remains a safe and effective method to reduce cesarean delivery in breech presentation, while internal version has limited but specific indications.

12.3 Forceps and vacuum Delivery

(*Milqt aur mehjm ke zriyah wiladat*)

Forceps Delivery

Forceps delivery is an operative vaginal delivery technique in which specialized metal instruments (obstetric forceps) are used to grasp the fetal head and assist its passage through the birth canal during the second stage of labor. Forceps are designed to mimic the natural curve of the maternal pelvis and facilitate traction or rotation of the fetal head to achieve vaginal delivery.

Historical Context

Forceps were first introduced in the 16th century by the Chamberlen family and have since evolved into various designs tailored for specific clinical scenarios. While once a common intervention, the use of forceps has declined in favor of vacuum extraction and cesarean section due to the technical skill required and the potential for maternal and fetal trauma. However, forceps remain a critical tool in skilled hands for specific indications.

Types of Forceps

Forceps are classified based on their design and intended use:

1. Low (Outlet) Forceps

Used when the fetal head is at or below the +2 station (relative to the ischial spines) and the scalp is visible at the introitus without separating the labia. Requires minimal rotation (≤45 degrees).

2. Mid-Forceps

Used when the fetal head is engaged but above the +2 station, often requiring rotation to correct malposition (e.g., occiput posterior to occiput anterior). Associated with higher risks and requires greater expertise.

3. High Forceps

Applied when the fetal head is not engaged, above the 0 station. Rarely performed in modern obstetrics due to high risks of maternal and fetal injury; cesarean section is preferred.

4. Rotational Forceps

Specialized forceps (e.g., Kielland forceps) designed to rotate the fetal head from occiput posterior or transverse to occiput anterior positions. Used in mid-cavity deliveries by experienced operators.

Common forceps designs include:

Simpson Forceps: For molded fetal heads (common in primigravidas).

Tucker-McLane Forceps: For less molded heads (common in multiparas).

Kielland Forceps: For rotational deliveries.

Piper Forceps: For breech deliveries, to deliver the aftercoming head.

Indications

Forceps delivery is indicated when expedited vaginal delivery is necessary due to maternal or fetal conditions, provided vaginal delivery is feasible. Indications include:

1. Fetal Distress

Non-reassuring fetal heart rate patterns (e.g., prolonged bradycardia, late decelerations) requiring urgent delivery.

2. Prolonged Second Stage of Labor

In primigravidas: >3 hours with epidural or >2 hours without epidural.

In multiparas: >2 hours with epidural or >1 hour without epidural.

Caused by maternal exhaustion, inadequate pushing, or failure to progress.

3. Maternal Conditions

Medical conditions necessitating reduced maternal pushing effort (e.g., cardiac disease, severe hypertension, respiratory compromise).

4. Fetal Malposition

Persistent occiput posterior or transverse positions requiring rotation for delivery.

5. Breech Delivery (Piper forceps)

To assist delivery of the aftercoming head in vaginal breech births.

Prerequisites

Before performing forceps delivery, the following conditions must be met:

Cervix fully dilated (10 cm).

Membranes ruptured

Fetal head engaged (at least 0 station for mid-forceps, +2 for low forceps).

Fetal position known (e.g., occiput anterior, posterior, or transverse).

Adequate maternal pelvis (no cephalopelvic disproportion).

Adequate analgesia (epidural, spinal, or local anesthesia).

Bladder emptied to prevent injury.

Informed consent obtained, except in emergencies.

Experienced operator available, particularly for mid or rotational forceps.

Backup plan for cesarean section in case of failure.

Technique

1. Preparation

Confirm indication and prerequisites.

Obtain informed consent, explaining risks, benefits, and alternatives.

Ensure adequate analgesia (epidural, spinal, or pudendal block).

Position the patient in the lithotomy position with legs supported.

Empty the bladder via catheterization if necessary.

Use aseptic technique with sterile gloves, drapes, and instruments.

2. Application

Select appropriate forceps based on fetal position and pelvic anatomy.

Check forceps for proper alignment and function (blades lock securely).

Identify the fetal head's position using landmarks (e.g., fontanelles, sutures).

Apply the left blade first (maternal right side), guiding it along the pelvic curve, then the right blade, ensuring the blades grasp the fetal head symmetrically over the parietal bones.

Lock the forceps to ensure a secure grip without excessive pressure.

3. Traction and Delivery

Apply gentle, intermittent traction during maternal contractions, mimicking the natural curve of the pelvis (J-shaped trajectory).

For rotational forceps, rotate the fetal head (e.g., occiput posterior to anterior) before traction.

Deliver the head slowly to minimize perineal trauma.

Remove forceps once the head is delivered, and complete delivery per standard vaginal delivery protocol.

4. Post-Delivery

Inspect the vagina and perineum for lacerations or extensions.

Repair any tears or perform episiotomy repair if performed concurrently.

Monitor the mother and neonate for complications.

Complications

Forceps delivery carries risks for both mother and fetus, particularly with mid or rotational forceps

Maternal Complications

Perineal trauma: Lacerations, third- or fourth-degree tears (2–10% risk).

Vaginal or cervical lacerations.

Postpartum hemorrhage due to trauma or uterine atony.

Infection or hematoma at the repair site.

Urinary or fecal incontinence, particularly with anal sphincter injury.

Chronic perineal pain or dyspareunia.

Fetal Complications

Facial bruising, lacerations, or nerve injury (e.g., facial palsy, 0.1–0.5% risk).

Skull fracture or cephalhematoma (0.5–1% risk).

Intracranial hemorrhage (rare, <0.1%).

Neonatal jaundice due to bruising.

Procedure Failure

Inability to deliver vaginally, necessitating cesarean section.

Guidelines

ACOG (2020): Recommends forceps delivery only by trained operators, with low forceps preferred over mid-forceps due to lower complication rates. Cesarean section is favored over high forceps.

RCOG (2020): Emphasizes restrictive use of instrumental delivery, with clear documentation of indications and informed consent.

Cochrane Review (2017): Found forceps delivery effective for expediting delivery but associated with higher maternal perineal trauma compared to vacuum extraction.

Vacuum Delivery

Vacuum extraction, or ventouse delivery, is an operative vaginal delivery technique using a suction cup applied to the fetal head to assist delivery through traction during maternal contractions. It is less invasive than forceps in terms of maternal trauma but requires careful technique to avoid fetal complications.

Historical Context

Vacuum extraction was introduced in the 1950s as an alternative to forceps, with modern soft silicone or plastic cups replacing earlier metal cups to reduce fetal trauma. Vacuum delivery has become more common than forceps in many settings due to its ease of use and lower maternal morbidity.

Types of Vacuum Devices

Soft Cups

Made of silicone or plastic, flexible, and less traumatic to the fetal scalp.

Used for low or outlet deliveries.

Rigid Cups

Made of metal or hard plastic, providing stronger suction.

Used for mid-cavity or rotational deliveries.

Handheld vs. Pump Systems

Handheld devices allow manual suction control.

Pump systems provide consistent suction pressure.

Indications

Vacuum delivery shares similar indications with forceps:

1. Fetal Distress: Non-reassuring fetal heart rate patterns requiring urgent delivery.
2. Prolonged Second Stage of Labor: Due to maternal exhaustion or failure to progress.
3. Maternal Conditions: To reduce pushing effort in medical conditions.
4. Fetal Malposition: To assist rotation (e.g., occiput posterior to anterior) with appropriate vacuum devices.

Prerequisites

Identical to forceps delivery, with additional considerations:

Gestational age ≥34 weeks: To minimize risk of fetal scalp injury or hemorrhage.

No contraindications: Avoid in suspected cephalopelvic disproportion, face presentation, or fetal intracranial hemorrhage.

Technique

1. Preparation

Confirm prerequisites (full cervical dilation, ruptured membranes, engaged head, known position).

Obtain informed consent and ensure adequate analgesia.

Position the patient in lithotomy and empty the bladder.

Use aseptic technique.

2. Application

Select an appropriate vacuum cup (soft for outlet, rigid for mid-cavity).

Apply the cup to the fetal head, ideally over the posterior fontanelle, avoiding the face or anterior fontanelle.

Create suction (typically 0.8 bar or 600 mmHg) using a hand pump or vacuum system.

Check for secure placement to prevent cup detachment ("pop-off").

3. Traction and Delivery

Apply gentle traction during contractions, following the pelvic curve.

Limit traction to 3–5 pulls over 15–20 minutes to avoid prolonged suction.

Deliver the head slowly and remove the cup once the head is delivered.

4. Post-Delivery

Inspect for maternal trauma and repair lacerations or episiotomy if performed.

Examine the neonate for scalp injuries or bruising.

Complications

Maternal Complications

Lower risk of perineal trauma compared to forceps (1–5% risk of third-degree tears).

Vaginal or cervical lacerations.

Postpartum hemorrhage or infection.

Fetal Complications

Scalp bruising, lacerations, or cephalhematoma (5–15% risk).

Subgaleal hemorrhage (0.1–1%, potentially life-threatening).

Intracranial hemorrhage (rare, <0.1%).

Neonatal jaundice due to scalp trauma.

Procedure Failure

Cup detachment ("pop-off") requiring repeat application or alternative delivery method.

Guidelines

ACOG (2020): Recommends vacuum extraction as a first-line instrumental delivery for low or outlet procedures due to ease of use and lower maternal morbidity.

RCOG (2020): Advises limiting vacuum attempts to prevent fetal scalp injury and monitoring neonates post-delivery for complications.

Comparative Analysis: Forceps vs. Vacuum vs. Episiotomy

Maternal Trauma: Forceps > Vacuum > Episiotomy (in terms of perineal trauma risk).

Fetal Trauma: Vacuum (higher cephalhematoma risk) > Forceps (higher facial injury risk) > Episiotomy (minimal fetal impact).

Ease of Use: Vacuum is simpler to apply; forceps require greater skill.

Indications Overlap: All three are used for fetal distress or prolonged second stage, but episiotomy is often an adjunct to instrumental delivery.

Training: Forceps require extensive training; vacuum is more accessible to less experienced operators.

Conclusion

Forceps delivery, vacuum extraction, and episiotomy are critical obstetrical procedures for managing complicated vaginal deliveries. Forceps offer precise control for complex cases but carry higher maternal trauma risks. Vacuum extraction is less invasive but requires careful monitoring for fetal scalp injuries. Episiotomy, when used restrictively, facilitates instrumental deliveries and reduces severe perineal tears.

12.4 Caesarean Section

(*Shigaaf-e-Qaisree*)

A cesarean section (C-section) is a surgical procedure in which the fetus is delivered through incisions in the maternal abdominal wall and uterus. It is one of the most common major surgical procedures worldwide, performed when vaginal delivery poses risks to the mother or fetus or is not feasible. Cesarean sections can be planned (elective) or performed emergently based on clinical circumstances.

Historical Context

The term "cesarean" is derived from the Latin caedere (to cut), with historical references to deliveries through abdominal incisions, though often posthumously in ancient times. Modern cesarean section techniques emerged in the 19th century with advancements in anesthesia, antisepsis and surgical methods. Today, cesarean section rates vary globally, ranging from 10–20% in some regions to over 50% in others, influenced by medical, cultural and socioeconomic factors. The World Health Organization (WHO) suggests an optimal cesarean rate of 10–15% for populations, though higher rates may be justified in high-risk settings.

Indications

Cesarean section is indicated when vaginal delivery is contraindicated or unsafe. Indications are categorized as maternal, fetal or labor-related, and may be elective (planned) or emergent:

1. Maternal Indications

Cephalopelvic Disproportion (CPD): Inadequate pelvic dimensions relative to the fetal head, confirmed by clinical or imaging assessment.

Previous Cesarean Section: Particularly with a classical (vertical) uterine incision or multiple prior cesareans, increasing the risk of uterine rupture.

Maternal Medical Conditions: Severe preeclampsia, eclampsia, cardiac disease, or other conditions where vaginal delivery poses significant risk.

Obstructive Lesions: Fibroids, ovarian masses, or cervical abnormalities blocking the birth canal.

Maternal Request: In some cases, after counseling, for non-medical reasons (controversial and varies by region).

Pelvic Abnormalities: Deformities or trauma affecting pelvic capacity.

2. Fetal Indications

Fetal Distress: Non-reassuring fetal heart rate patterns (e.g., prolonged bradycardia, late decelerations) requiring urgent delivery.

Malpresentation: Breech, transverse lie, or face presentation unsuitable for vaginal delivery.

Fetal Macrosomia: Estimated fetal weight >4,500 g in non-diabetic mothers or >4,000 g in diabetic mothers, increasing the risk of shoulder dystocia.

Multiple Gestations: Non-vertex presentation of the first twin or complications in twin pregnancies.

Congenital Anomalies: Conditions like hydrocephalus requiring alternative delivery methods.

Cord Prolapse: Umbilical cord prolapse with risk of compression and fetal hypoxia.

3. Labor-Related Indications

Failure to Progress: Arrest of dilation (no cervical change despite adequate contractions) or arrest of descent (no progress in the second stage).

Failed Instrumental Delivery: Inability to achieve vaginal delivery with forceps or vacuum extraction.

Placental Abnormalities: Placenta previa (covering the cervical os) or placental abruption with maternal or fetal compromise.

Uterine Rupture: A life-threatening emergency requiring immediate cesarean delivery.

Infection: Active genital herpes or HIV with high viral load, to reduce vertical transmission risk.

4. Elective Indications

Scheduled repeat cesareans, often at 39 weeks to avoid labor onset.

Planned delivery for maternal or fetal conditions (e.g., placenta previa, severe preeclampsia).

Classification

Cesarean sections are classified based on urgency and incision type:

Urgency (Lucas Classification):

Category 1 (Emergent): Immediate threat to maternal or fetal life (e.g., cord prolapse, uterine rupture). Target delivery within 30 minutes.

Category 2: Urgent but no immediate threat (e.g., fetal distress, failure to progress). Target delivery within 60–75 minutes.

Category 3: Early delivery needed but no immediate risk (e.g., scheduled repeat cesarean).

Category 4 (Elective): Planned at a time convenient for the patient and team.

Uterine Incision Type

Low Transverse (Kerr): Most common, made horizontally in the lower uterine segment. Associated with lower blood loss and reduced risk of rupture in future pregnancies.

Classical (Vertical): Vertical incision through the uterine fundus, used in preterm deliveries, anterior placenta previa, or abnormal fetal presentations. Higher risk of rupture in subsequent pregnancies.

Low Vertical: Less common, used when transverse incision is inadequate.

T or J-Shaped: Extensions of a transverse incision, used in complex cases but increase rupture risk.

Prerequisites

Before performing a cesarean section, the following must be ensured:

Informed Consent: Obtained for elective procedures, explaining risks, benefits and alternatives. In emergencies, implied consent may apply.

Anesthesia: Regional (spinal or epidural) preferred for most cases; general anesthesia used for emergencies or contraindications to regional.

Fetal Viability: Confirmed unless the procedure is for maternal indications (e.g., severe preeclampsia).

Surgical Team: Includes obstetrician, anesthesiologist, neonatologist (if fetal distress) and operating room staff.

Blood Availability: Cross-matched blood for high-risk cases (e.g., placenta previa, abruption).

Bladder Catheterization: To prevent bladder injury and improve visualization.

Antibiotics: Prophylactic antibiotics (e.g., cefazolin 2 g IV) administered 30–60 minutes before incision to reduce infection risk.

Technique

Cesarean section requires meticulous surgical technique to ensure maternal and fetal safety. The procedure is performed in an operating room under sterile conditions.

1. Preparation

Position the patient supine with a left lateral tilt (15–30 degrees) to prevent aortocaval compression.

Administer anesthesia (spinal, epidural, or general).

Catheterize the bladder and prep the abdomen with antiseptic solution.

Ensure fetal heart rate monitoring until the start of surgery.

2. Abdominal Incision

Pfannenstiel Incision: Most common, a curved transverse incision 2–3 cm above the pubic symphysis. Provides good cosmetic results and less postoperative pain.

Midline Vertical Incision: Used in emergencies, obese patients, or when extensive access is needed. Associated with more pain and poorer cosmesis.

Incise through skin, subcutaneous tissue, fascia, and rectus muscles, then enter the peritoneal cavity.

3. Uterine Incision

Identify the lower uterine segment (thinner, less vascular).

Make a low transverse incision (preferred) or classical incision based on clinical needs.

Extend the incision manually or with scissors, avoiding the bladder and uterine arteries.

Rupture the amniotic membranes and deliver the fetus.

4. Fetal Delivery

Deliver the fetal head through the uterine incision, applying gentle fundal pressure if needed.

Suction the neonate's mouth and nose to clear airways.

Clamp and cut the umbilical cord, then hand the neonate to the pediatric team.

Deliver the placenta manually or spontaneously, ensuring complete removal to prevent postpartum hemorrhage.

5. Closure

Close the uterine incision in two layers with absorbable sutures (e.g., polyglactin 910) to ensure hemostasis and strength.

Inspect for bleeding and repair any extensions (e.g., to the cervix or broad ligament).

Close the peritoneum (optional), rectus fascia (with non-absorbable or long-lasting absorbable sutures), and skin (subcuticular sutures or staples).

Remove the bladder catheter post-procedure unless prolonged monitoring is needed.

6. Postoperative Care

Monitor vital signs, uterine tone, and vaginal bleeding in the recovery room.

Administer oxytocin (10–40 IU IV) to promote uterine contraction and prevent hemorrhage.

Provide pain management (e.g., NSAIDs, opioids, patient-controlled analgesia).

Encourage early ambulation (within 6–12 hours) to reduce thromboembolism risk.

Monitor for signs of infection, hemorrhage, or thromboembolism.

Counsel on wound care, activity restrictions, and breastfeeding.

Complications

Cesarean section is a major surgical procedure with potential maternal and fetal complications:

Maternal Complications

Infection: Endometritis, wound infection (5–10% risk). Prophylactic antibiotics reduce this risk.

Hemorrhage: From uterine atony, lacerations, or placenta accreta (2–5% risk). May require blood transfusion or hysterectomy.

Thromboembolism: Deep vein thrombosis or pulmonary embolism (0.1–0.5% risk). Early ambulation and prophylactic anticoagulants (e.g., heparin) mitigate this.

Bladder or Bowel Injury: Rare (<1%), but higher in repeat cesareans or emergencies.

Adhesions: Intra-abdominal adhesions increasing the risk of complications in future surgeries.

Uterine Rupture in Future Pregnancies: Higher with classical incisions (4–9% risk) vs. low transverse (0.5–1%).

Anesthesia Complications: Hypotension, headache (post-spinal), or rare anaphylaxis.

Long-Term Risks: Placenta previa or accreta in subsequent pregnancies, chronic pain.

Fetal Complications

Respiratory Distress: Transient tachypnea of the newborn or respiratory distress syndrome, particularly in elective cesareans before 39 weeks (1–5% risk).

Fetal Injury: Lacerations from scalpel (0.1–0.5%).

Delayed Bonding: Due to separation from the mother post-delivery.

Other

Longer recovery time (4–6 weeks) compared to vaginal delivery.

Increased healthcare costs and hospital stay (typically 2–4 days).

Guidelines

WHO (2018)

Recommends cesarean sections only when medically necessary, as rates above 10–15% do not improve maternal or neonatal outcomes.

ACOG (2020)

Supports vaginal birth after cesarean (VBAC) for women with one prior low transverse cesarean, with success rates of 60–80%. Advises against elective cesareans before 39 weeks unless medically indicated, to reduce neonatal respiratory complications. Recommends prophylactic antibiotics and thromboembolism prophylaxis.

RCOG (2015, updated 2020)

Emphasizes informed consent and counseling on risks of repeat cesareans.

Supports enhanced recovery protocols to reduce hospital stay and complications.

Cochrane Review (2018): Found that low transverse incisions have lower complication rates than classical incisions. Skin closure with subcuticular sutures improves cosmetic outcomes compared to staples.

Conclusion

Cesarean section is a cornerstone of operative obstetrics, providing a safe alternative to vaginal delivery when indicated. It requires meticulous surgical technique, comprehensive preoperative preparation, and vigilant postoperative care to minimize complications. When integrated with forceps delivery, vacuum extraction and episiotomy, these procedures form a spectrum of interventions to address the complexities of childbirth.

12.5 Destructive Operations

(*Takhreebi dastkariya*)

Destructive Operations

Definition

Destructive operations are obstetric procedures performed to reduce the size of a non-viable fetus to facilitate its delivery through the vaginal route, thereby preserving maternal life or health in situations where other delivery methods (e.g., cesarean section, instrumental delivery) are not feasible or pose significant risks. These procedures are exceedingly rare in modern obstetrics due to advancements in cesarean section techniques and perinatal care but remain relevant in resource-limited settings, extreme emergencies, or cases of confirmed fetal demise.

Historical Context

Destructive operations were historically common in obstetrics before the advent of safe cesarean sections and modern anesthesia in the 19th and 20th centuries. Procedures such as craniotomy, embryotomy, and cleidotomy were used to manage obstructed labor in cases of fetal demise or severe maternal compromise. With improvements in surgical techniques, anesthesia, and infection control, the need for destructive operations has significantly declined in high-resource settings. However, they are still occasionally performed in low-resource settings where access to cesarean section is limited or in emergencies where maternal survival is prioritized.

Indications

Destructive operations are performed only in exceptional circumstances where the fetus is confirmed to be non-viable (e.g., intrauterine fetal demise, IUFD) and vaginal delivery is obstructed, posing a significant risk to maternal life or health. Specific indications include:

1. Obstructed Labor with Fetal Demise

Cephalopelvic disproportion (CPD) or abnormal fetal presentation (e.g., transverse lie, neglected shoulder presentation) preventing vaginal delivery.

Prolonged labor with a non-viable fetus, where cesarean section is not feasible due to maternal instability, lack of surgical facilities, or cultural barriers.

2. Fetal Anomalies Incompatible with Life

Severe congenital anomalies (e.g., anencephaly, hydrocephalus) causing obstruction, with confirmed fetal demise.

3. Maternal Life-Threatening Conditions

Severe maternal compromise (e.g., hemorrhagic shock, sepsis) where immediate delivery is required, and cesarean section carries excessive risk or is unavailable.

4. Failed Alternative Methods

Inability to deliver the fetus via forceps, vacuum, or cesarean section due to anatomical constraints, maternal instability, or resource limitations.

5. Resource-Limited Settings

Lack of access to surgical facilities, anesthesia, or blood transfusion services, necessitating vaginal delivery despite obstruction.

Destructive operations are contraindicated when:

The fetus is viable and has a reasonable chance of survival.

Cesarean section or instrumental delivery is feasible and safer for the mother.

Maternal condition allows for alternative interventions.

Types of Destructive Operations

Destructive operations are classified based on the anatomical structure targeted to reduce fetal size and facilitate delivery. The main types include:

1. Craniotomy

Definition: Perforation and decompression of the fetal skull to reduce its diameter and allow vaginal delivery.

Indications: Obstructed labor due to a large fetal head (e.g., hydrocephalus, CPD) with confirmed fetal demise.

Technique

Confirm fetal demise via ultrasound or absent fetal heart tones.

Ensure adequate anesthesia (regional or general) and maternal stabilization.

Use a perforator (e.g., Simpson's perforator) to puncture the fetal skull through the fontanelles or sutures.

Collapse the skull by removing cerebral contents and applying traction with forceps or manual pressure.

Deliver the fetus vaginally, ensuring careful extraction to avoid maternal trauma.

Complications: Risk of uterine or cervical lacerations, infection, or maternal psychological trauma.

2. Embryotomy (Decapitation, Evisceration)

Definition: Dismemberment of the fetal body (e.g., removal of the head, limbs, or thoracic contents) to relieve obstruction.

Indications: Neglected transverse lie, locked twins, or severe obstruction with fetal demise.

Technique

Use specialized instruments (e.g., decapitation hook, embryotomy scissors) under direct visualization or ultrasound guidance.

For decapitation, sever the fetal neck to release a trapped head or shoulder.

For evisceration, open the fetal thorax or abdomen to reduce bulk, followed by vaginal delivery.

Ensure meticulous removal of all fetal parts to prevent retained products of conception.

Complications: High risk of maternal soft tissue injury, hemorrhage, or infection.

3. Cleidotomy

Definition: Division of the fetal clavicles to reduce shoulder width and facilitate delivery.

Indications: Shoulder dystocia or transverse lie with fetal demise, where other maneuvers fail.

Technique

Use heavy scissors or a scalpel to cut one or both clavicles under anesthesia. Apply traction to deliver the fetus vaginally.

Complications: Risk of maternal perineal or vaginal trauma and infection.

4. Spondylotomy

Definition: Division of the fetal spine to collapse the torso and relieve obstruction.

Indications: Rare, used in extreme cases of transverse lie or locked twins with fetal demise.

Technique: Similar to embryotomy, using scissors or a saw-like instrument to section the spine.

Complications: Similar to embryotomy, with high maternal trauma risk.

Prerequisites

Destructive operations are high-risk procedures requiring strict adherence to clinical and ethical standards:

Confirmed Fetal Demise: Verified by ultrasound or absent fetal heart tones to avoid harm to a viable fetus.

Informed Consent: Obtained whenever possible, explaining the procedure, indications, risks, and alternatives. In emergencies, implied consent may apply.

Adequate Anesthesia: Regional (epidural/spinal) or general anesthesia to ensure maternal comfort and safety.

Skilled Operator: Performed by an experienced obstetrician familiar with destructive techniques.

Sterile Conditions: To minimize infection risk, using aseptic technique and sterile instruments.

Maternal Stabilization: Address maternal shock, sepsis, or hemorrhage before proceeding.

Backup Plan: Availability of cesarean section or surgical facilities in case of complications or failure.

Psychological Support: Counseling for the mother and family due to the traumatic nature of the procedure.

Technique (General Approach)

The specific technique varies by procedure (e.g., craniotomy, embryotomy), but general steps include:

1. Preparation

Confirm fetal demise and maternal indications via clinical assessment and imaging.

Obtain informed consent and provide psychological support.

Administer prophylactic antibiotics (e.g., cefazolin 2 g IV) to reduce infection risk.

Position the patient in the lithotomy position and ensure adequate anesthesia.

Empty the bladder to prevent injury and improve access.

2. Procedure

Use specialized instruments (e.g., perforator, decapitation hook, embryotomy scissors) under direct visualization or ultrasound guidance.

Perform the destructive procedure (e.g., skull perforation, dismemberment) to reduce fetal size.

Apply gentle traction with forceps or manual pressure to deliver the fetus, avoiding excessive force to minimize maternal trauma.

Ensure complete removal of fetal parts and placenta to prevent retained products.

3. Post-Procedure

Inspect the vagina, cervix, and uterus for lacerations or extensions.

Repair any maternal trauma using absorbable sutures (e.g., polyglactin 910).

Administer oxytocin (10–40 IU IV) to promote uterine contraction and prevent hemorrhage.

Monitor for signs of infection, hemorrhage, or psychological distress.

Provide postpartum care, including antibiotics, pain management, and counseling.

Complications

Destructive operations carry significant risks due to their invasive nature and the underlying maternal or fetal conditions:

Maternal Complications

Soft Tissue Injury: Lacerations to the vagina, cervix, or uterus (5–15% risk), potentially leading to fistula formation.

Hemorrhage: From uterine or cervical trauma, retained products, or atony (10–20% risk).

Infection: Endometritis, sepsis, or wound infection, exacerbated by prolonged labor or non-sterile conditions (10–25% risk).

Uterine Rupture: Rare but catastrophic, particularly in prolonged obstructed labor.

Psychological Trauma: Grief, guilt, or post-traumatic stress disorder due to fetal loss and the nature of the procedure.

Procedure-Related Complications

Incomplete removal of fetal parts, leading to infection or hemorrhage.

Failure to relieve obstruction, necessitating cesarean section or further intervention.

Long-Term Risks

Asherman's syndrome (intrauterine adhesions) from aggressive curettage.

Infertility or obstetric complications in future pregnancies due to uterine or cervical scarring.

Guidelines

WHO (2018): Emphasizes that destructive operations should be a last resort, performed only when fetal demise is confirmed and cesarean section is not feasible. Training in these techniques is recommended for providers in resource-limited settings.

RCOG (2020): Notes that destructive operations are rarely indicated in high-resource settings due to the availability of cesarean section but may be necessary in emergencies or low-resource contexts.

FIGO (International Federation of Gynecology and Obstetrics, 2019): Advocates for improved access to cesarean section and skilled obstetric care to reduce the need for destructive operations.

Limited Evidence: Due to their rarity in modern practice, there are few contemporary studies on destructive operations. Historical data and case reports highlight their risks and the need for skilled operators.

Conclusion

Destructive operations are rare and extreme interventions in obstetrics, reserved for cases of confirmed fetal demise and obstructed labor where maternal survival is at risk, and other methods (e.g., cesarean section, instrumental delivery) are not feasible. These procedures require exceptional technical skill, strict adherence to ethical principles, and comprehensive maternal support. In contrast, cesarean section, forceps delivery, vacuum extraction, and episiotomy are more commonly used to manage obstetric complications while preserving fetal viability when possible. Evidence-based guidelines emphasize minimizing invasive interventions, improving access to cesarean section, and ensuring skilled obstetric care to reduce the need for destructive operations. Obstetricians must balance clinical judgment, technical expertise, and compassion to optimize maternal outcomes in these challenging scenarios.

Long Answer Questions (LAQs)

Define version in obstetrics. Describe its types, indications, contraindications, technique, complications and present status in modern obstetrics.

Describe episiotomy with reference to its definition, indications, types, technique, complications and repair.

Define caesarean section. Discuss its indications, types, steps of lower segment caesarean section (LSCS), complications and postoperative care.

Describe forceps delivery. Discuss indications, prerequisites, types of forceps, technique and complications.

What are destructive obstetric operations? Describe types, indications, contraindications and ethical considerations.

Short Answer Questions (SAQs)

Indications of external cephalic version.

Types of episiotomy.

Indications of vacuum extraction.

Complications of caesarean section.

Indications for destructive operations.

Multiple Choice Questions (MCQs)

1. Best time to perform external cephalic version is:

A. 28 weeks B. 32 weeks

C. 37 weeks D. During second stage

Answer: C

2. Most common complication of episiotomy is:

A. Uterine rupture B. Perineal pain

C. PPH D. Fistula

Answer: B

3. Which is an absolute contraindication to ECV?
A. Multiparity B. Breech presentation
C. Placenta previa D. Adequate liquor
Answer: C
4. Forceps delivery requires all EXCEPT:
A. Fully dilated cervix B. Engaged head
C. Ruptured membranes D. Undilated cervix
Answer: D
5. Vacuum extraction works by:
A. Traction on limbs B. Compression of skull
C. Negative pressure on fetal scalp D. Uterine contraction
Answer: C
6. Most common indication for caesarean section is:
A. Breech presentation B. Fetal distress
C. Previous caesarean section D. Twin pregnancy
Answer: C
7. Lower segment caesarean section is preferred because:
A. More bleeding B. Poor healing
C. Less blood loss and better healing D. More adhesions
Answer: C
8. Internal podalic version is mainly done for:
A. Singleton breech B. Placenta previa
C. Second twin D. Preterm labor
Answer: C
9. Destructive operations are indicated when:
A. Fetus is alive and viable B. Fetus is dead and vaginal delivery is obstructed
C. Pelvis is adequate D. Cervix is closed
Answer: B
10. Most serious complication of forceps delivery is:
A. Perineal pain B. Vaginal tear
C. Intracranial hemorrhage D. Cephalhematoma
Answer: C

13

Fetal Surveillance / Antenatal Assessment of Fetal Wellbeing

(Janeen ki nighdasht Qbl az weladaat./ Janeeen ki sehtmndi ka jayeza)

13.1 *Saririyyati jayeza* (Clinical Assessment)
13.2 *Kemyawi jayeza* (Biochemical Assessment)
13.3 *Bayu phizikal jayeza* (Biophysical Assessment)
13.4 *Ehsay-e-hrkt-e-jneen* (Fetal movement Count)
13.5 *Altrasonography* (Ultrasonography)
13.6 *Murakabatu qlbel jneen* (CardioTocography)
13.7 *Ikhtebare adm-e-jihad* (Non-stress test)
13.8 *Janeeni bayaphysikal profayil* (Fetal Biophysical Profile)
13.9 Doppler altrasound (Doppler Ultrasound)
13.10Ikhtebar-e-ehterzi sautu (Vibroacoustic Stimulation Test)
13.11Ikhteabr-e- tqllus-e-jiahd (Contraction stress test)
13.12Hijam-e-Rutubat-i-Aminusiyya (Amniotic Fluid Volume)

Learning Objective (At the end of the session, the students should be able to)

Evaluate the Clinical Assessment of fetal growth
Discuss the Biochemical tests for pulmonary maturity
Evaluate the Biophysical Tests (Fetal Movement Count, Ultrasonography, Cardiotocography, Non-stress test (NST), Fetal Biophysical Profile (BPP), Doppler Ultrasound, Vibroacoustic Stimulation Test Contraction Stress Test, Amniotic Fluid Volume) for fetal well-being.

Antenatal Assessment of Fetal Well-Being

Introduction

Antenatal assessment of fetal well-being is a cornerstone of modern obstetric care, aimed at monitoring fetal health throughout pregnancy to optimize maternal and neonatal outcomes. These assessments identify fetuses at risk of hypoxia, growth restriction, or other complications, enabling timely interventions such as induction of labor, cesarean section or instrumental delivery. Fetal well-being is evaluated through a combination of clinical, biochemical, biophysical, and imaging modalities, each providing complementary insights into fetal status. These assessments are critical in high-risk pregnancies (e.g., maternal hypertension, diabetes, or fetal growth restriction) but are also used in low-risk pregnancies to ensure optimal outcomes.

The primary goals of antenatal fetal assessment are:

To detect fetal distress or hypoxia early, preventing adverse outcomes such as stillbirth or neonatal morbidity.

To guide clinical management, including timing and mode of delivery (e.g., vaginal delivery with episiotomy, forceps, vacuum, or cesarean section).

To avoid unnecessary interventions in healthy fetuses, minimizing maternal and fetal risks.

13.1 Clinical Assessment

(*Saririyyati jayeza*)

Clinical assessment involves non-invasive evaluations performed during antenatal visits to monitor fetal well-being through maternal history, physical examination, and simple measurements. It is the first step in identifying potential risks and guiding further testing.

Components

1. Maternal History:

Symptoms of Concern: Decreased fetal movements, vaginal bleeding, abdominal pain, or symptoms of preeclampsia (e.g., headache, visual changes).

Risk Factors: Maternal conditions (e.g., hypertension, diabetes, thyroid disorders), smoking, substance use, or previous adverse pregnancy outcomes (e.g., stillbirth, preterm birth).

Obstetric History: Parity, previous cesarean sections, or instrumental deliveries (e.g., forceps, vacuum) that may influence current pregnancy management.

2. Physical Examination:

Symphysio-Fundal Height (SFH):

Measured from the pubic symphysis to the uterine fundus using a tape measure.

Normal SFH approximates gestational age in centimeters (e.g., 28 cm at 28 weeks).

Discrepancies (SFH $<10^{th}$ or $>90^{th}$ percentile) suggest intrauterine growth restriction (IUGR), macrosomia, or polyhydramnios, prompting further evaluation (e.g., ultrasonography).

Abdominal Palpation (Leopold Maneuvers):

Assesses fetal lie (longitudinal, transverse, oblique), presentation (cephalic, breech), and position (e.g., occiput anterior).

Identifies malpresentations that may necessitate cesarean section or instrumental delivery.

Fetal Heart Rate (FHR) Auscultation:

Performed using a Pinard stethoscope or handheld Doppler device.

Normal FHR: 110–160 beats per minute (bpm).

Abnormalities (e.g., tachycardia >160 bpm, bradycardia <110 bpm) indicate potential fetal distress, requiring biophysical or ultrasonographic assessment.

3. Maternal Vital Signs:

Blood pressure monitoring to detect hypertensive disorders (e.g., preeclampsia), which can compromise fetal well-being.

Weight gain assessment to identify excessive or inadequate gain, associated with macrosomia or IUGR, respectively.

Indications for Further Testing

Discrepant SFH or abnormal FHR.

Maternal symptoms (e.g., reduced fetal movements).

High-risk conditions (e.g., gestational diabetes, post-term pregnancy).

13.2 Biochemical Assessment

(*Kemyawi jayeza*)

Biochemical assessment involves analyzing maternal or fetal biomarkers to evaluate placental function and fetal well-being, particularly in high-risk pregnancies. These tests are used in conjunction with clinical and biophysical assessments to identify fetuses at risk of hypoxia or growth restriction.

Key Biochemical Tests

1. Maternal Serum Markers:

Alpha-Fetoprotein (AFP):

Measured in the second trimester (15–20 weeks) as part of maternal serum screening.

Elevated AFP may indicate neural tube defects, placental dysfunction, or fetal demise.

Low AFP is associated with Down syndrome or IUGR.

Human Chorionic Gonadotropin (hCG) and Estriol:

Part of the quadruple screen (AFP, hCG, estriol, inhibin-A).

Abnormal levels may suggest placental insufficiency or fetal anomalies, prompting further investigation.

Pregnancy-Associated Plasma Protein-A (PAPP-A):

Measured in the first trimester.

Low levels are associated with IUGR, preeclampsia, or preterm birth.

2. Amniotic Fluid Analysis:

Amniocentesis: Performed in cases of suspected fetal anomalies or genetic conditions.

Amniotic fluid bilirubin levels (in rhesus isoimmunization) or lecithin/sphingomyelin (L/S) ratio (to assess lung maturity) may be analyzed.

Rarely used for routine fetal well-being but indicated in specific high-risk cases.

3. Placental Growth Factor (PlGF) and Soluble fms-like Tyrosine Kinase-1 (sFlt-1):

Emerging biomarkers for preeclampsia and placental insufficiency.

Low PlGF or high sFlt-1/PlGF ratio indicates placental dysfunction, increasing the risk of IUGR or stillbirth.

Indications

High-risk pregnancies (e.g., preeclampsia, diabetes, previous stillbirth).

Abnormal clinical findings (e.g., reduced SFH, decreased fetal movements).

Suspected fetal anomalies or genetic conditions.

13.3 Biophysical Assessment

(*Bayu phizikal jayeza*)

Overview

Biophysical assessment uses non-invasive tests to evaluate fetal behavior, movement, and physiological responses to assess well-being. These tests focus on fetal responses to hypoxia, which manifest as changes in heart rate, breathing, or movement patterns.

Key Biophysical Tests

1. Non-Stress Test (NST):

Definition: Continuous electronic fetal monitoring to assess FHR in response to fetal movements.

Technique: Performed using a cardiotocograph (CTG) with an external FHR monitor and tocodynamometer. Conducted for 20–40 minutes, typically after 28 weeks.

A reactive NST shows ≥2 accelerations (≥15 bpm increase for ≥15 seconds) within 20 minutes, indicating fetal well-being.

A non-reactive NST (no accelerations) prompts further testing (e.g., biophysical profile).

Indications: High-risk pregnancies, decreased fetal movements, or post-term pregnancy.

Interpretation:

Reactive: Normal, reassuring.

Non-reactive: May indicate fetal hypoxia, requiring further evaluation.

Limitations: High false-positive rate for non-reactive results (up to 50%).

2. Biophysical Profile (BPP):

Definition: A composite score combining NST and ultrasound parameters to assess fetal well-being.

Components (scored 0 or 2 points each, total 10 points):

Reactive NST (2 points if reactive, 0 if non-reactive).

Fetal breathing movements (≥1 episode of rhythmic breathing for ≥30 seconds).

Fetal body movements (≥3 discrete movements in 30 minutes).

Fetal tone (≥1 episode of extension and flexion, e.g., hand opening/closing).

Amniotic fluid volume (single pocket >2 cm in two perpendicular planes).

Technique:

Performed using real-time ultrasonography and CTG. Typically takes 30–60 minutes.

Scoring:

8–10: Normal, low risk of fetal hypoxia.

6: Equivocal, repeat in 24 hours or consider delivery if near term.

4 or less: High risk of fetal hypoxia, often indicating urgent delivery (e.g., cesarean section).

Indications: Non-reactive NST, high-risk pregnancies, or suspected IUGR.

Limitations: Time-consuming, operator-dependent, and requires ultrasound expertise.

3. Contraction Stress Test (CST):

Definition: Assesses FHR response to uterine contractions, simulating labor stress.

Technique:

Administer oxytocin or nipple stimulation to induce contractions.

Monitor FHR for late decelerations (indicative of uteroplacental insufficiency).

Positive CST: Late decelerations with ≥50% of contractions, suggesting fetal compromise.

Negative CST: No late decelerations, reassuring.

Indications: Rarely used due to risks of inducing preterm labor; reserved for specific cases with equivocal NST/BPP results.

Limitations: Contraindicated in preterm labor, placenta previa, or previous cesarean section.

Guidelines

ACOG (2020):

Recommends NST and BPP as primary tools for fetal surveillance in high-risk pregnancies (e.g., IUGR, diabetes, post-term).

Suggests weekly or twice-weekly testing after 32–34 weeks in high-risk cases.

CST is rarely recommended due to risks and availability of safer alternatives.

13.4 Fetal movement Count

(*Ehsay-e-hrkt-e-jneen*)

Fetal movement counting (FMC), also known as kick counting, is a simple, non-invasive method for mothers to monitor fetal well-being by tracking fetal movements. It empowers patients to detect potential fetal distress early, prompting timely medical evaluation.

Technique

Method: The mother counts distinct fetal movements (kicks, rolls, or flutters) over a specified period.

Common protocols include:

Cardiff "Count to Ten" Method: Count 10 movements within 12 hours. Fewer than 10 movements prompts medical evaluation.

Daily Monitoring: Record the time taken to feel 10 movements, typically within 2 hours in the evening when fetal activity peaks.

Performed after 28 weeks, when fetal movements are consistent.

Instructions

Lie on the left side or sit quietly in a comfortable position.

Focus on counting distinct movements, avoiding distractions.

Report decreased movements (<10 in 12 hours or significant reduction from baseline) to a healthcare provider.

Indications

Routine monitoring in low- and high-risk pregnancies after 28 weeks.

Maternal perception of decreased fetal movements.

High-risk conditions (e.g., IUGR, maternal diabetes, hypertension).

Guidelines

ACOG (2020):

Recommends FMC as a screening tool for all pregnant women after 28 weeks.

Advises immediate evaluation (e.g., NST, ultrasound) for decreased fetal movements.

13.5 Ultrasonography

(*Altrasonography*)

Ultrasonography is the gold standard for antenatal assessment of fetal well-being, providing real-time visualization of fetal anatomy, growth and physiological parameters. It is non-invasive, widely available in high-resource settings, and integral to modern obstetric care.

Ultrasound Parameters

1. Fetal Biometry

Measures head circumference (HC), biparietal diameter (BPD), abdominal circumference (AC), and femur length (FL).

Used to assess fetal growth and detect IUGR (<10th percentile) or macrosomia (>90th percentile).

Serial measurements (every 2–4 weeks) in high-risk pregnancies to monitor growth trends.

2. Amniotic Fluid Volume

Assessed using the Amniotic Fluid Index (AFI) (sum of deepest vertical pockets in four uterine quadrants) or Single Deepest Pocket (SDP).

Normal AFI: 5–25 cm; SDP: 2–8 cm.

Oligohydramnios (AFI <5 cm or SDP <2 cm): Associated with IUGR, placental insufficiency, or post-term pregnancy.

Polyhydramnios (AFI >25 cm or SDP >8 cm): Associated with diabetes, fetal anomalies, or twin pregnancies.

Abnormalities may prompt delivery (e.g., cesarean section) or further monitoring.

3. Doppler Velocimetry

Measures blood flow in fetal and placental vessels to assess placental function and fetal adaptation to hypoxia.

Umbilical Artery Doppler:

Evaluates resistance in the umbilical artery.

Normal: Forward flow throughout the cardiac cycle.

Abnormal: Absent or reversed end-diastolic flow (AEDF/REDF), indicating severe placental insufficiency and high risk of fetal demise.

Middle Cerebral Artery (MCA) Doppler:

Assesses fetal cerebral blood flow.

Increased flow (low pulsatility index) suggests brain-sparing in response to hypoxia.

Ductus Venosus Doppler:

Assesses fetal venous return.

Absent or reversed a-wave indicates cardiac compromise, often necessitating urgent delivery.

Indications: IUGR, preeclampsia, post-term pregnancy, or suspected fetal hypoxia.

4. Fetal Anatomy Survey

Performed in the second trimester (18–22 weeks) to detect congenital anomalies (e.g., neural tube defects, cardiac anomalies).

May identify conditions affecting fetal well-being (e.g., hydrocephalus requiring cesarean or destructive operation in non-viable cases).

5. Fetal Behavior and Tone

Assessed as part of the BPP (breathing, movements, tone).

Reduced activity or tone suggests hypoxia or neurological compromise.

Indications

Routine screening (e.g., first-trimester dating, second-trimester anomaly scan).

High-risk pregnancies (e.g., IUGR, diabetes, hypertension, multiple gestations).

Suspected fetal distress (e.g., decreased movements, non-reactive NST).

Guiding delivery decisions (e.g., cesarean for placenta previa or malpresentation).

Guidelines

ACOG (2020):

Recommends routine ultrasound at 11–14 weeks (dating, nuchal translucency) and 18–22 weeks (anatomy scan).

Supports Doppler velocimetry in IUGR or high-risk pregnancies, with delivery recommended for AEDF/REDF near term.

Conclusion

Antenatal assessment of fetal well-being is a multifaceted approach combining clinical, biochemical, biophysical, and ultrasonographic methods to monitor fetal health and guide obstetric management. Clinical assessments provide initial screening, while biochemical markers offer insights into placental function. Biophysical tests (NST, BPP) and fetal movement counts detect acute fetal distress, and ultrasonography provides detailed anatomical and physiological data. These assessments inform critical decisions, such as the need for episiotomy, forceps, vacuum, cesarean section, or in rare cases, destructive operations.

13.6 CardioTocography

(*Murakabatu qlbel jneen*)

Cardiotocography (CTG) is a non-invasive method for continuously monitoring the fetal heart rate (FHR) and uterine contractions to assess fetal well-being and detect signs of hypoxia or distress. It is used antenatally (e.g., as part of the NST) and intrapartum to guide clinical management. CTG records FHR via an external Doppler ultrasound transducer and uterine activity via a tocodynamometer, producing a graphical output (tocogram) for analysis.

Principles

CTG is based on the premise that a healthy fetus responds to its environment (e.g., movements, uterine contractions) with characteristic FHR patterns. Hypoxia or placental insufficiency alters these patterns, manifesting as reduced variability, decelerations, or abnormal baseline rates. Key FHR parameters include:

Baseline FHR: The mean FHR, normally 110–160 beats per minute (bpm), sustained for ≥10 minutes.

Variability: Fluctuations in FHR (5–25 bpm), reflecting autonomic nervous system function. Reduced variability (<5 bpm) suggests fetal compromise.

Accelerations: Transient increases in FHR (≥15 bpm for ≥15 seconds), typically associated with fetal movements, indicating well-being.

Decelerations: Transient decreases in FHR, classified as early, late, or variable, which may indicate umbilical cord compression, uteroplacental insufficiency, or head compression.

Technique

1. Equipment:

External Doppler Ultrasound Transducer: Detects FHR by sensing fetal cardiac motion.

Tocodynamometer: Measures uterine contractions by detecting changes in abdominal pressure.

CTG Monitor: Displays FHR and uterine activity traces on paper or digital output.

2. Procedure:

Position the patient semi-recumbent or in a left lateral position to avoid aortocaval compression.

Apply the Doppler transducer to the maternal abdomen over the fetal heart (located via Leopold maneuvers or ultrasound).

Place the tocodynamometer over the uterine fundus to detect contractions.

Record for 20–40 minutes (antenatal) or continuously (intrapartum).

Ensure maternal comfort and explain the procedure to reduce anxiety.

3. Setting:

Antenatal: Performed in outpatient clinics, labor wards, or fetal assessment units, typically after 28 weeks.

Intrapartum: Used during labor to monitor fetal response to contractions.

Interpretation

CTG interpretation involves analyzing four key FHR features:

1. Baseline FHR:

Normal: 110–160 bpm.

Tachycardia (>160 bpm): May indicate fever, infection, or early hypoxia.

Bradycardia (<110 bpm): Suggests severe hypoxia or congenital heart block.

2. Variability:

Normal: 5–25 bpm, reflecting healthy autonomic function.

Reduced (<5 bpm for >40 minutes): Indicates hypoxia, acidosis, or fetal sleep (requires further evaluation).

Absent: High risk of fetal compromise.

3. Accelerations:

Presence of ≥2 accelerations (≥15 bpm for ≥15 seconds) in 20 minutes is reassuring.

Absence may indicate fetal hypoxia or reduced activity, prompting further tests (e.g., BPP, ultrasound).

4. Decelerations:

Early Decelerations: Synchronous with contractions, due to head compression; usually benign.

Late Decelerations: Occur after the peak of contractions, indicating uteroplacental insufficiency; concerning for hypoxia.

Variable Decelerations: Abrupt, variable in timing, due to cord compression; severe or prolonged decelerations suggest distress.

Prolonged Decelerations: FHR <110 bpm for >2 minutes, indicating urgent evaluation.

Classification Systems

ACOG (2009, updated 2020): Uses a three-tier system for intrapartum CTG:

Category I (Normal): Baseline 110–160 bpm, moderate variability, no late or variable decelerations, ±accelerations. Reassuring, no immediate intervention needed.

Category II (Indeterminate): Any tracing not clearly Category I or III (e.g., tachycardia, reduced variability, variable decelerations). Requires close monitoring and further evaluation (e.g., BPP, scalp stimulation).

Category III (Abnormal): Absent variability with recurrent late decelerations, variable decelerations, or prolonged bradycardia. Indicates high risk of fetal acidosis; urgent delivery (e.g., cesarean section, forceps, or vacuum) is often required.

FIGO (2015): Similar to ACOG, classifies tracings as normal, suspicious, or pathological, guiding intrapartum management.

Indications

Antenatal:

High-risk pregnancies (e.g., IUGR, preeclampsia, diabetes, post-term pregnancy).

Decreased fetal movements reported by the mother.

Suspected fetal distress based on clinical or ultrasound findings.

Intrapartum:

Routine monitoring in high-risk labors (e.g., induced labor, epidural use).

Suspected fetal distress or abnormal labor progression.

Clinical Applications

Antenatal: Used as part of the NST to assess fetal well-being and guide timing of delivery.

Intrapartum: Monitors fetal response to labor, informing decisions for interventions like episiotomy, forceps, vacuum, or cesarean section.

High-Risk Scenarios: Detects hypoxia in conditions like placental insufficiency or cord compression, prompting urgent delivery.

Complications

False-Positive Rates: Up to 50–60% of non-reassuring tracings (Category II) do not indicate true fetal distress, leading to unnecessary interventions.

Maternal Discomfort: Prolonged monitoring may cause discomfort or anxiety.

Technical Issues: Signal loss or artifacts (e.g., maternal heart rate mistaken for FHR) can lead to misinterpretation.

Guidelines

ACOG (2020)

Recommends CTG (via NST) for high-risk pregnancies after 32–34 weeks, typically weekly or twice-weekly. Supports intrapartum CTG in high-risk labors but cautions against overuse in low-risk labors due to increased cesarean rates without improved neonatal outcomes.

13.7 Non-stress test

(*Ikhtebare adm-e-jihad*)

Definition

The non-stress test (NST) is a specific application of cardiotocography used antenatally to assess fetal well-being by evaluating FHR accelerations in response to fetal movements. It is called "non-stress" because it does not involve inducing uterine contractions, unlike the contraction stress test (CST). The NST is a simple, non-invasive, and widely used screening tool to detect fetal hypoxia or distress.

Principles

The NST relies on the observation that a healthy fetus responds to spontaneous movements with FHR accelerations, reflecting intact autonomic and cardiovascular function. The absence of accelerations or reduced variability may indicate fetal hypoxia, acidosis, or neurological compromise, prompting further evaluation or intervention.

Technique

1. Equipment: Same as CTG (Doppler ultrasound transducer, tocodynamometer, CTG monitor).

2. Procedure:

Position the patient semi-recumbent or left lateral to optimize fetal perfusion.

Apply the Doppler transducer to monitor FHR and the tocodynamometer to detect uterine activity (though contractions are not induced).

Monitor for 20–40 minutes, noting FHR accelerations and maternal perception of fetal movements.

If no accelerations occur, extend monitoring or use vibroacoustic stimulation (VAS) to stimulate fetal movement (e.g., a sound stimulus applied to the abdomen).

In some cases, maternal glucose intake (e.g., juice) may enhance fetal activity.

3. Performed in outpatient clinics, antenatal wards, or fetal assessment units, typically after 28 weeks when FHR accelerations are reliable.

Interpretation

Reactive NST (Reassuring):

≥2 accelerations (≥15 bpm increase for ≥15 seconds) within 20 minutes, associated with fetal movements.

Normal baseline FHR (110–160 bpm) and moderate variability (5–25 bpm).

Indicates low risk of fetal hypoxia within the next 7 days.

Non-Reactive NST (Non-Reassuring):

<2 accelerations in 40 minutes, or absent/reduced variability.

May indicate fetal hypoxia, sleep cycle, or maternal factors (e.g., sedation, smoking).

Requires further evaluation with BPP, ultrasound, or extended monitoring.

Abnormal NST:

Persistent bradycardia, absent variability, or recurrent decelerations.

Indicates high risk of fetal compromise, often necessitating urgent delivery (e.g., cesarean section).

Indications

High-Risk Pregnancies:

Maternal conditions: Hypertension, diabetes, preeclampsia, renal disease.

Fetal conditions: IUGR, oligohydramnios, post-term pregnancy, multiple gesttaxations.

Maternal Complaints: Decreased fetal movements or other concerning symptoms.

Follow-Up: After abnormal clinical findings (e.g., discrepant symphysio-fundal height) or ultrasound results (e.g., reduced amniotic fluid).

Clinical Applications

Screening: Routine monitoring in high-risk pregnancies after 32–34 weeks (weekly or twice-weekly).

Triage: Evaluates maternal reports of decreased fetal movements, guiding further testing.

Delivery Planning: Non-reactive or abnormal NSTs may prompt induction, instrumental delivery (forceps/vacuum with episiotomy), or cesarean section.

Complications

False-Positives: Up to 50% of non-reactive NSTs are due to fetal sleep or maternal factors, not true distress.

Maternal Anxiety: Prolonged monitoring or non-reassuring results may cause stress.

Over-Intervention: Non-reactive NSTs may lead to unnecessary cesareans without additional testing (e.g., BPP).

Guidelines

ACOG (2020):

Recommends NST as a primary surveillance tool in high-risk pregnancies, starting at 32–34 weeks.

Suggests combining NST with BPP or ultrasound for non-reactive results to reduce false-positives.

Advises delivery for abnormal NSTs (e.g., absent variability with decelerations) in term or near-term pregnancies.

Conclusion

Cardiotocography, particularly the non-stress test, is a cornerstone of antenatal fetal surveillance, providing real-time insights into fetal well-being through FHR patterns. The NST is a simple, non-invasive screening tool to detect fetal hypoxia, guiding further evaluation with BPP, ultrasound, or delivery decisions.

13.8 Fetal Biophysical Profile

(*Janeeni bayaphysikal profayil*)

The Fetal Biophysical Profile (BPP) is a diagnostic tool used in obstetrics to assess fetal well-being, particularly in high-risk pregnancies, by evaluating multiple fetal parameters through ultrasound and cardiotocography. It provides a comprehensive evaluation of fetal health, aiding clinicians in determining the risk of fetal hypoxia or compromise and guiding decisions about delivery or continued monitoring.

The BPP, developed by Manning et al. in the 1980s, is a non-invasive prenatal test that combines ultrasound-based observations of fetal behavior and amniotic fluid volume with non-stress test (NST) results to assess fetal well-being. It is primarily used in the third trimester to identify fetuses at risk of adverse outcomes, such as intrauterine growth restriction (IUGR), stillbirth, or perinatal morbidity, particularly in high-risk pregnancies.

The BPP evaluates five parameters, each scored as 0 or 2 based on specific criteria, with a maximum score of 10. These parameters reflect acute fetal status (fetal heart rate reactivity, breathing, movement, and tone) and chronic fetal condition (amniotic fluid volume). The test helps differentiate between a healthy fetus, a fetus experiencing hypoxia, and a fetus at risk of impending compromise.

Components of the Fetal Biophysical Profile

The BPP consists of five components, each assessed over a 30-minute observation period via ultrasound, except for the NST, which may require additional time. Each parameter is scored as follows:

1. Non-Stress Test (NST) – Fetal Heart Rate (FHR) Reactivity

Definition: Measures fetal heart rate accelerations in response to fetal movement, indicating an intact autonomic nervous system and adequate oxygenation.

Criteria for Normal (Score = 2): At least two FHR accelerations, each ≥15 beats per minute (bpm) above baseline and lasting ≥15 seconds, within a 20-minute period.

Abnormal (Score = 0): Fewer than two accelerations or accelerations not meeting the criteria.

Significance: FHR reactivity is a sensitive indicator of fetal oxygenation and neurologic integrity. Absence of reactivity may suggest hypoxia or acidosis.

2. Fetal Breathing Movements

Definition: Rhythmic movements of the fetal diaphragm and chest wall observed on ultrasound, reflecting medullary function.

Criteria for Normal (Score = 2): At least one episode of fetal breathing lasting ≥30 seconds within 30 minutes.

Abnormal (Score = 0): No breathing movements or episodes lasting <30 seconds.

Significance: Fetal breathing is regulated by the central nervous system and is sensitive to hypoxia. Reduced or absent breathing may indicate fetal distress.

3. Fetal Gross Body Movements

Definition: Discrete movements of the fetal trunk or limbs, such as rolling or stretching, observed via ultrasound.

Criteria for Normal (Score = 2): At least three distinct body or limb movements within 30 minutes.

Abnormal (Score = 0): Fewer than three movements.

Significance: Fetal movements reflect neuromuscular function and oxygenation. Decreased movements may indicate hypoxia or neurologic compromise.

4. Fetal Tone

Definition: Assesses fetal muscle tone through active flexion and extension of limbs or trunk.

Criteria for Normal (Score = 2): At least one episode of active extension with return to flexion of a limb or trunk (e.g., opening and closing of the hand or flexion/extension of a limb).

Abnormal (Score = 0): No episodes of active extension/flexion or slow, incomplete movements.

Significance: Tone is a basic neuromuscular function and one of the last parameters to be affected by hypoxia. Absence of tone is a late sign of fetal compromise.

5. Amniotic Fluid Volume (AFV)

Definition: Measures the volume of amniotic fluid, which reflects placental function and fetal renal perfusion over time.

Criteria for Normal (Score = 2): At least one vertical pocket of amniotic fluid measuring ≥2 cm in two perpendicular planes (single deepest pocket method) or an Amniotic Fluid Index (AFI) ≥5 cm.

Abnormal (Score = 0): No pocket ≥2 cm or AFI <5 cm (oligohydramnios).

Significance: Amniotic fluid volume is a marker of chronic fetal status. Oligohydramnios may indicate placental insufficiency, fetal renal abnormalities, or chronic hypoxia.

Scoring and Interpretation

The BPP score ranges from 0 to 10, with each parameter contributing 0 or 2 points. The total score guides clinical management:

- 8–10 (Normal): Indicates a low risk of fetal hypoxia. Typically, no immediate intervention is required, and monitoring continues based on the clinical scenario.
- 6 (Equivocal): Suggests possible fetal compromise. If amniotic fluid volume is normal, repeat testing within 24 hours is often recommended. In cases of oligohydramnios, further evaluation or delivery may be considered, especially near term.
- 4 or less (Abnormal): Indicates a high risk of fetal hypoxia or acidosis. Immediate further evaluation (e.g., Doppler studies, maternal assessment) or delivery is often indicated, particularly in term or near-term pregnancies.

Modified BPP: In some settings, a modified BPP is used, which includes only the NST and amniotic fluid volume assessment. A normal modified BPP (reactive NST and normal AFV) is highly reassuring, while abnormalities prompt a full BPP or further testing.

Physiological Basis

The BPP is grounded in the understanding that fetal hypoxia affects central nervous system functions in a predictable sequence. Acute hypoxia first impairs higher cortical functions (FHR reactivity, breathing movements), followed by gross body movements, and finally fetal tone. Amniotic fluid volume reflects chronic placental function and fetal renal perfusion, providing insight into long-term fetal well-being. The BPP's strength lies in its ability to combine acute and chronic markers to assess fetal status comprehensively.

Indications for Performing a BPP

The BPP is indicated in high-risk pregnancies where fetal compromise is a concern, including but not limited to:

Maternal conditions: Hypertension, diabetes, preeclampsia, systemic lupus erythematosus.

Fetal conditions: IUGR, decreased fetal movements, post-term pregnancy, multiple gestation.

Placental or umbilical cord issues: Oligohydramnios, polyhydramnios, abnormal Doppler studies.

Other: Previous stillbirth, maternal substance use, or trauma.

Procedure

1. Preparation: Explain the procedure to the patient, ensuring comfort and a relaxed environment.
2. Non-Stress Test: Perform the NST using an external fetal monitor to assess FHR reactivity.
3. Ultrasound Assessment: Conduct a real-time ultrasound to evaluate fetal breathing, movements, tone, and amniotic fluid volume over 30 minutes.
4. Scoring: Assign scores for each parameter and calculate the total BPP score.
5. Documentation: Record findings and communicate results to the clinical team for management planning.

Advantages of the BPP

Non-invasive and safe for both mother and fetus.

High sensitivity and negative predictive value (>99%) for fetal well-being when the score is normal (8–10).

Combines acute and chronic markers for a comprehensive assessment.

Guides clinical decision-making, reducing unnecessary interventions in low-risk cases.

Clinical Management Based on BPP

Score 8–10: Continue routine monitoring based on gestational age and maternal/fetal condition. Weekly or twice-weekly BPP may be indicated in high-risk cases.

Score 6: Repeat BPP within 24 hours or consider additional tests (e.g., umbilical artery Doppler). Delivery may be considered if near term or if oligohydramnios is present.

Score 4 or less: Urgent evaluation is required. Delivery is often indicated, especially at ≥36 weeks, after considering maternal and fetal factors. In preterm fetuses, corticosteroid administration and further testing may be warranted.

Oligohydramnios (AFV = 0): Regardless of other parameters, oligohydramnios is a strong indicator for delivery, especially in term pregnancies, due to the risk of cord compression and hypoxia.

Conclusion

The Fetal Biophysical Profile is a cornerstone of fetal surveillance in high-risk pregnancies, offering a reliable, non-invasive method to assess fetal well-being. By evaluating five key parameters, it provides critical information about fetal oxygenation and placental function, guiding timely clinical interventions. Its high negative predictive value makes it an essential tool for reassuring clinicians and patients while identifying fetuses requiring further evaluation or delivery.

13.9 Doppler Ultrasound

(*Doppler altrasound*)

Doppler ultrasound is a non-invasive imaging technique that measures blood flow velocity in fetal and maternal vessels to assess placental function, fetal well-being, and circulatory adaptations. By analyzing the Doppler shift of sound waves reflected by moving red blood cells, it provides critical information about vascular resistance and blood flow dynamics, particularly in high-risk pregnancies.

Physiological Basis

Doppler ultrasound is based on the Doppler effect, where the frequency of reflected ultrasound waves changes proportional to the velocity of moving blood cells. In obstetrics, it is used to evaluate blood flow in the umbilical artery, middle cerebral artery (MCA), ductus venosus, uterine arteries, and other vessels. Abnormal flow patterns may indicate placental insufficiency, fetal hypoxia, or fetal anemia.

Technique

Equipment: A real-time ultrasound machine with pulsed or continuous-wave Doppler capabilities.

Procedure:

Identify the target vessel using real-time ultrasound (e.g., umbilical artery in a free loop of the cord).

Apply the Doppler probe to measure blood flow velocity waveforms during fetal quiescence (to avoid motion artifacts).

Analyze waveforms for indices such as pulsatility index (PI), resistance index (RI), or systolic/diastolic (S/D) ratio.

Common Vessels Assessed:

Umbilical Artery: Reflects placental vascular resistance. Normal flow shows high diastolic flow; abnormal flow (e.g., absent or reversed end-diastolic flow) indicates placental insufficiency.

Middle Cerebral Artery (MCA): Assesses fetal brain sparing in response to hypoxia. Increased diastolic flow (low PI) suggests redistribution of blood to the brain.

Ductus Venosus: Evaluates fetal cardiac function. Reversed flow during atrial contraction indicates cardiac decompensation.

Uterine Artery: Assesses maternal placental perfusion. Persistent notching or high PI suggests inadequate trophoblast invasion.

Indications

Intrauterine growth restriction (IUGR).

Preeclampsia or maternal hypertension.

Suspected fetal hypoxia or anemia.

Twin-to-twin transfusion syndrome (TTTS).

Post-term pregnancy.

Maternal conditions affecting placental function (e.g., diabetes, lupus).

Interpretation

Umbilical Artery:

Normal: High diastolic flow, S/D ratio <3 (term), PI <1.1.

Abnormal: Increased S/D ratio (>3), absent end-diastolic flow (AEDF), or reversed end-diastolic flow (REDF). AEDF and REDF are associated with severe placental insufficiency and high perinatal mortality risk.

Middle Cerebral Artery:

Normal: High resistance (low diastolic flow, PI ~1.4–2.0).

Abnormal: Decreased PI (<1.4) or "brain-sparing effect" indicates fetal hypoxia with blood redistribution to the brain.

Ductus Venosus:

Normal: Forward flow throughout the cardiac cycle.

Abnormal: Reduced or reversed a-wave (atrial contraction) suggests fetal cardiac compromise.

Uterine Artery:

Normal: Low resistance, no diastolic notch after 24 weeks.

Abnormal: Persistent notching or high PI (>1.45) indicates increased risk of preeclampsia or IUGR.

Advantages

Non-invasive and safe.

Provides real-time assessment of fetal and placental hemodynamics.

High sensitivity for detecting fetal compromise in IUGR and preeclampsia.

Guides timing of delivery in high-risk cases.

Limitations

Operator-dependent; requires expertise for accurate vessel identification and waveform interpretation.

Normal Doppler findings do not rule out all fetal complications.

Limited predictive value in low-risk pregnancies.

Motion artifacts or maternal obesity may affect accuracy.

Clinical Applications

IUGR Management: Umbilical artery Doppler is a standard tool for monitoring IUGR. AEDF or REDF often prompts delivery, especially at term.

Preeclampsia Screening: Uterine artery Doppler in the second trimester identifies women at risk for preeclampsia.

Fetal Anemia: MCA peak systolic velocity (PSV) >1.5 MoM (multiples of the median) is diagnostic of fetal anemia (e.g., in Rh isoimmunization).

Timing of Delivery: Abnormal Doppler findings (e.g., REDF, reversed ductus venosus flow) guide decisions about preterm delivery versus continued monitoring.

13.10 Vibroacoustic Stimulation Test

(*Ikhtebar-e-ehterzi sautu*)

The Vibroacoustic Stimulation (VAS) Test is a non-invasive method used to stimulate fetal movement and heart rate reactivity during fetal monitoring, typically as an adjunct to the non-stress test (NST). It involves applying a brief acoustic and vibratory stimulus to the maternal abdomen to elicit a fetal response, reducing testing time and false-positive non-reactive NST results.

Physiological Basis

VAS stimulates the fetal central nervous system, eliciting a startle response, increased fetal movements, and heart rate accelerations. A reactive response indicates an intact neurologic and autonomic system, suggesting adequate fetal oxygenation. The test leverages the fetus's sensitivity to sound (100–120 dB) and vibration in the third trimester.

Technique

Equipment: A vibroacoustic stimulator (e.g., artificial larynx or specialized device) producing a sound of 80–120 dB and 20–100 Hz frequency.

Procedure:

Perform an NST to assess baseline fetal heart rate (FHR).

If the NST is non-reactive after 10–20 minutes, apply the VAS device to the maternal abdomen over the fetal head for 1–3 seconds.

Monitor FHR and fetal movements for 5–10 minutes post-stimulation.

Repeat up to 2–3 times if no response is observed, with 1-minute intervals.

Criteria for Normal Response:

At least two FHR accelerations (≥15 bpm above baseline for ≥15 seconds) within 10 minutes of stimulation.

Increased fetal movements.

Indications

Non-reactive NST to differentiate between fetal sleep cycles and hypoxia.

High-risk pregnancies requiring fetal surveillance (e.g., IUGR, diabetes, post-term pregnancy).

Reduced fetal movements reported by the mother.

Interpretation

Reactive (Normal): Two or more FHR accelerations post-stimulation indicate fetal well-being.

Non-Reactive (Abnormal): No accelerations or inadequate response after repeated stimulation suggests possible fetal compromise, warranting further evaluation (e.g., BPP, Doppler).

Advantages

Reduces false-positive non-reactive NSTs due to fetal sleep cycles.

Shortens NST duration, improving efficiency.

Safe and non-invasive with no significant maternal or fetal risks.

Limitations

Limited specificity; non-reactive VAS does not confirm fetal compromise and requires further testing.

Excessive stimulation may cause fetal tachycardia or distress (rare).

Not a standalone test; must be combined with NST or BPP.

Contraindicated in preterm premature rupture of membranes (PROM) or preterm labor due to potential uterine stimulation.

13.11 Contraction stress test

(*Ikhteabr-e- tqllus-e-jiahd*)

The Contraction Stress Test (CST), also known as the oxytocin challenge test, assesses fetal response to induced uterine contractions, which simulate the stress of labor. It evaluates the fetal heart rate response to transient reductions in placental blood flow during contractions, providing insight into fetal oxygenation and placental reserve.

Physiological Basis

Uterine contractions temporarily reduce placental blood flow, challenging fetal oxygenation. A healthy fetus with adequate placental function tolerates this stress, maintaining a stable FHR. Persistent late decelerations during contractions suggest reduced placental reserve or fetal hypoxia, indicating a fetus at risk during labor.

Technique

Equipment: External fetal monitor for FHR and tocodynamometer for uterine activity; oxytocin infusion (if needed).

Procedure:

Monitor baseline FHR and uterine activity for 10–20 minutes.

Induce contractions using nipple stimulation (preferred) or intravenous oxytocin (0.5–2 mU/min, titrated to achieve 3 contractions in 10 minutes, each lasting 40–60 seconds).

Continue monitoring FHR during and after contractions for 10–20 minutes.

Criteria for Adequate Test: At least three contractions in 10 minutes, each lasting ≥40 seconds.

Indications

Non-reactive NST or equivocal BPP results requiring further evaluation.

High-risk pregnancies (e.g., IUGR, diabetes, post-term pregnancy).

Suspected placental insufficiency.

History of previous stillbirth.

Interpretation

- Negative (Normal): No late or significant variable decelerations during contractions. Indicates fetal tolerance of labor-like stress.
- Positive (Abnormal): Late decelerations with ≥50% of contractions suggest fetal hypoxia or placental insufficiency.
- Equivocal: Inconsistent decelerations or inadequate contractions require repeat testing or alternative assessment (e.g., BPP, Doppler).
- Unsatisfactory: Inadequate contractions or poor FHR tracing quality.

Advantages

High negative predictive value (>99%) for fetal well-being when negative.

Directly assesses fetal response to labor-like stress.

Useful in high-risk pregnancies with equivocal NST or BPP results.

Limitations

Invasive and time-consuming (requires oxytocin infusion in some cases).

Contraindicated in conditions like preterm labor, PROM, placenta previa, or previous classical cesarean section due to risk of uterine rupture.

False-positive rate (20–40%) may lead to unnecessary interventions.

Requires skilled interpretation and monitoring.

Clinical Applications

Decision for Delivery: A positive CST often prompts delivery, especially at term, while a negative CST supports continued monitoring.

High-Risk Pregnancies: Used when other tests (e.g., NST, BPP) are inconclusive.

Rare Use: Largely replaced by BPP and Doppler in modern practice due to invasiveness and contraindications.

13.12 Amniotic Fluid Volume

(*Hijam-e-Rutubat-i-Aminusiyya*)

Amniotic Fluid Volume (AFV) assessment is a critical component of fetal surveillance, reflecting placental function, fetal renal perfusion, and overall fetal well-being. It is typically performed using ultrasound as part of the BPP or as a standalone test in high-risk pregnancies.

Physiological Basis

Amniotic fluid is primarily produced by fetal urine and lung secretions, with contributions from the placenta and fetal membranes. Adequate AFV indicates normal fetal renal function and placental perfusion. Oligohydramnios (low AFV) may result from placental insufficiency, fetal renal anomalies, or ruptured membranes, while polyhydramnios (excess AFV) may indicate fetal anomalies (e.g., gastrointestinal obstruction) or maternal diabetes.

Technique

Equipment: Real-time ultrasound with a high-frequency transducer.

Methods:

Single Deepest Pocket (SDP): Measure the deepest vertical pocket of amniotic fluid free of fetal parts or cord. Normal: ≥2 cm.

Amniotic Fluid Index (AFI): Divide the uterus into four quadrants and measure the deepest vertical pocket in each. Sum the measurements to calculate AFI. Normal: 5–25 cm.

Procedure:

Perform ultrasound in a supine patient.

Identify and measure fluid pockets perpendicular to the maternal abdomen.

Record SDP or AFI and note any cord or fetal parts in the pocket.

Indications

High-risk pregnancies (e.g., IUGR, preeclampsia, diabetes).

Decreased or excessive fetal movements.

Suspected fetal anomalies (e.g., renal agenesis, esophageal atresia).

Post-term pregnancy.

Suspected ruptured membranes.

Interpretation

Normal:

SDP: 2–8 cm.

AFI: 5–25 cm.

Oligohydramnios:

SDP: <2 cm.

AFI: <5 cm.

Associated with IUGR, placental insufficiency, fetal renal anomalies, or PROM.

Polyhydramnios

SDP: >8 cm.

AFI: >25 cm.

Associated with fetal anomalies (e.g., neural tube defects, gastrointestinal obstruction), maternal diabetes, or TTTS.

Advantages

Non-invasive and safe.

Provides insight into chronic fetal and placental status.

High negative predictive value when normal.

Easily integrated into BPP or routine ultrasound.

Limitations

Operator-dependent; measurements may vary with technique or maternal factors (e.g., obesity).

SDP and AFI may yield discordant results, complicating interpretation.

Oligohydramnios or polyhydramnios requires further investigation to determine etiology.

Transient changes (e.g., maternal dehydration) may affect results.

Clinical Applications

BPP Component: AFV is a key parameter in the BPP, with oligohydramnios prompting urgent evaluation or delivery.

Screening for Anomalies: Abnormal AFV triggers detailed fetal anomaly scans (e.g., for renal or gastrointestinal defects).

Management Decisions: Oligohydramnios often indicates delivery, especially in term pregnancies, due to risks of cord compression and hypoxia. Polyhydramnios may require amnioreduction or specific management based on etiology.

Conclusion

Doppler ultrasound, vibroacoustic stimulation, contraction stress testing, and amniotic fluid volume assessment are essential tools in obstetric fetal surveillance, each offering unique insights into fetal health. Doppler ultrasound excels in assessing vascular dynamics, VAS enhances NST efficiency, CST evaluates labor tolerance, and AFV reflects chronic fetal status. Together, they guide clinical decision-making in high-risk pregnancies, balancing the need for timely intervention with the goal of minimizing unnecessary procedures.

Long Answer Questions (LAQs)

Define fetal surveillance. Describe the indications, methods, and importance of antenatal assessment of fetal well-being.

Describe Biophysical Profile (BPP). Discuss its components, scoring system, interpretation, indications, and limitations.

Explain cardiotocography (CTG). Describe the principles, interpretation of fetal heart rate patterns, and clinical significance.

Describe Doppler ultrasound in obstetrics. Discuss its principle, indications, commonly studied vessels, and interpretation of abnormal findings.

Describe non-stress test (NST). Explain its procedure, interpretation, advantages, disadvantages, and clinical applications.

Short Answer Questions (SAQs)

Components of biophysical profile.

Indications for fetal surveillance.

Clinical importance of fetal movement count.

Causes of abnormal Doppler findings.

Methods of assessment of amniotic fluid volume.

Multiple Choice Questions (MCQs)

1. Most commonly used method of antenatal fetal surveillance is:

A. Amniocentesis B. Biochemical tests

C. Non-stress test D. Cordocentesis

Answer: C

2. Normal biophysical profile score is:

A. 4/10 B. 6/10

C. 8/10 D. 8–10/10

Answer: D

3. A reactive NST is defined by:

A. No accelerations B. One acceleration in 30 minutes

C. Two accelerations in 20 minutes D. Persistent decelerations

Answer: C

4. Which vessel is most commonly assessed in Doppler ultrasound?

A. Middle cerebral artery B. Ductus venosus

C. Umbilical artery D. Renal artery

Answer: C

5. Reduced fetal movements indicate:

A. Fetal maturity B. Polyhydramnios

C. Fetal hypoxia D. Normal pregnancy

Answer: C

6. Loss of end-diastolic flow in umbilical artery Doppler suggests:

A. Normal placental function B. Post-term pregnancy

C. Severe placental insufficiency D. Fetal macrosomia

Answer: C

7. Vibroacoustic stimulation test is used to:

A. Induce labor B. Stimulate fetal activity

C. Reduce uterine contractions D. Measure AFI

Answer: B

8. Amniotic fluid index (AFI) less than 5 cm indicates:

A. Polyhydramnios B. Normal liquor

C. Oligohydramnios D. Multiple pregnancy

Answer: C

9. Contraction stress test assesses:

A. Fetal movements B. Placental location

C. Uteroplacental reserve D. Amniotic fluid volume

Answer: C

10. Most sensitive test for detecting chronic fetal hypoxia is:

A. NST B. Fetal movement count

C. Doppler ultrasound D. Vibroacoustic test

Answer: C

14

Pharmacotherapeutics in Obstetrics

(Ilm al- Qabalat me musta'mal advia)

14.1 Mhall-i-estemalat aur mamnuaat (Indicated & Contraindicated Unani & Contemporary Medicines)

Learning Objective (At the end of the session, the students should be able to)

Enlist & classify the Indicated & Contraindicated drugs (Unani and allopathic both) in pregnancy and lactation.

14. Pharmacotherapeutics in Obstetrics

(*Ilm al- Qabalat me musta'mal advia*)

Introduction

Pharmacotherapeutics in obstetrics involves the use of medications to manage maternal and fetal conditions during pregnancy, labor, delivery and the postpartum period. Pregnancy introduces unique challenges due to physiological changes that affect drug pharmacokinetics and pharmacodynamics, as well as the need to balance maternal therapeutic benefits with potential fetal risks.

Principles of Pharmacotherapy in Pregnancy

1. Physiological Changes in Pregnancy

Pregnancy alters drug absorption, distribution, metabolism, and excretion, necessitating careful dose adjustments:

Absorption: Delayed gastric emptying and increased gastric pH may reduce oral drug absorption. Increased skin and mucosal blood flow enhances transdermal and vaginal absorption.

Distribution: Increased plasma volume (by 30–50%) and decreased albumin levels increase the volume of distribution for water-soluble drugs and the free fraction of protein-bound drugs.

Metabolism: Hepatic cytochrome P450 enzyme activity (e.g., CYP3A4, CYP2D6) increases, accelerating metabolism of some drugs. Conversely, reduced activity of other enzymes (e.g., CYP1A2) may prolong drug half-lives.

Excretion: Increased glomerular filtration rate (by 50%) enhances renal clearance of drugs like penicillins and digoxin.

2. Fetal Considerations

Placental Transfer: Most drugs cross the placenta via passive diffusion, influenced by molecular weight, lipophilicity and ionization. Low-molecular-weight (<500 Da), lipophilic and non-ionized drugs cross more readily.

Teratogenicity: The risk of congenital anomalies is highest during organogenesis (weeks 3–8 of gestation). Later exposure may affect fetal growth or organ function.

FDA Pregnancy Categories (Historical Context): Although replaced by the Pregnancy and Lactation Labeling Rule (PLLR) in 2015, categories A, B, C, D, and X were historically used to guide risk assessment. The PLLR provides narrative risk summaries instead.

Breastfeeding: Drugs may pass into breast milk, with potential effects on the neonate. The milk-to-plasma ratio and neonatal clearance rates guide safety assessments.

3. General Principles

Use medications only when benefits outweigh risks.

Select drugs with established safety profiles in pregnancy (e.g., Category A or B historically, or favorable PLLR data).

Use the lowest effective dose and shortest duration necessary.

Monitor maternal and fetal responses closely.

Consider non-pharmacologic alternatives when possible.

Placental Transfer of Drugs

Mechanisms

Passive diffusion (most common)

Facilitated diffusion

Active transport

Pinocytosis

Factors Affecting Placental Drug Transfer

Molecular weight (<500 Da crosses easily)

Lipid solubility (lipophilic drugs cross faster)

Ionization (non-ionized cross better)

Protein binding (free drug crosses)

Placental blood flow

Gestational age

Teratogenesis

Definition: Teratogenesis is the ability of a drug to cause structural or functional abnormalities in the fetus.

Critical Period: Day 17–56 (3–8 weeks) → organogenesis

Maximum risk of congenital anomalies

FDA drug risk classification

Category	Description
A	Controlled human studies show no risk
B	No risk in animals / no human evidence
C	Risk cannot be ruled out
D	Positive evidence of fetal risk
X	Contraindicated; risk outweighs benefit

Common Pharmacotherapeutics in Obstetrics

1. Antenatal Corticosteroids

Indications: Preterm labor (24–34 weeks), planned preterm delivery, or conditions risking preterm birth (e.g., preeclampsia).

Drugs

Betamethasone (12 mg IM, two doses 24 hours apart) or dexamethasone (6 mg IM, four doses 12 hours apart).

Mechanism: Stimulate fetal lung maturation by inducing surfactant production, reducing the risk of respiratory distress syndrome (RDS). Also decrease the incidence of intraventricular hemorrhage (IVH) and necrotizing enterocolitis (NEC).

Benefits: Reduce neonatal mortality by 31%, RDS by 44%, and IVH by 46% (Cochrane reviews).

Risks

Maternal: Transient hyperglycemia, increased infection risk (rare).

Fetal: No significant teratogenic risks. Repeated courses may reduce fetal growth or affect neurodevelopment (controversial).

Considerations: Optimal effect occurs 24 hours to 7 days post-administration. Use in preterm premature rupture of membranes (PPROM) requires balancing infection risk.

2. Tocolytics

Indications: Preterm labor (to delay delivery for 48 hours, allowing corticosteroid administration or transfer to a tertiary center).

Drugs

Nifedipine (Calcium Channel Blocker): 10–20 mg orally every 4–6 hours. Inhibits uterine contractions by reducing calcium influx.

Indomethacin (NSAID): 50–100 mg loading dose, then 25–50 mg every 6 hours (≤48 hours). Inhibits prostaglandin synthesis.

Terbutaline (Beta-Agonist): 0.25 mg SC every 20–30 minutes (up to 3 doses). Stimulates beta-2 receptors, relaxing uterine smooth muscle.

Magnesium Sulfate: 4–6 g IV bolus, then 1–2 g/hour. Exact mechanism unclear but may reduce calcium-dependent contractions.

Benefits: Delay delivery by 48–72 hours, improving neonatal outcomes with corticosteroids.

Risks

Nifedipine: Maternal hypotension, headache.

Indomethacin: Fetal oligohydramnios, premature closure of ductus arteriosus (avoid after 32 weeks).

Terbutaline: Maternal tachycardia, pulmonary edema, hyperglycemia.

Magnesium Sulfate: Maternal flushing, respiratory depression, fetal hypotonia (rare).

Considerations: Contraindicated in advanced labor, chorioamnionitis, or fetal distress. No evidence supports prolonged tocolysis beyond 48 hours.

3. Magnesium Sulfate for Neuroprotection

Indications: Preterm delivery (<32 weeks) to reduce the risk of cerebral palsy.

Regimen: 4–6 g IV bolus over 20–30 minutes, followed by 1–2 g/hour maintenance until delivery or for 24 hours.

Mechanism: Stabilizes neuronal membranes, reduces excitotoxicity, and improves cerebral blood flow regulation.

Benefits: Reduces cerebral palsy risk by 30% in preterm infants (Cochrane reviews).

Risks: Maternal flushing, nausea, respiratory depression (rare). Fetal hypotonia (minimal with standard dosing).

Considerations: Monitor for toxicity (e.g., loss of reflexes, respiratory rate). Calcium gluconate is the antidote for overdose.

4. Antihypertensives

Indications: Chronic hypertension, gestational hypertension, or preeclampsia.

Drugs

Methyldopa: 250–500 mg orally 2–4 times daily. Central alpha-2 agonist, reduces sympathetic outflow.

Labetalol: 100–400 mg orally 2–3 times daily or IV for severe hypertension. Combined alpha- and beta-blocker.

Nifedipine: 10–20 mg orally every 4–6 hours (extended-release preferred). Calcium channel blocker.

Hydralazine: 5–10 mg IV for acute severe hypertension. Vasodilator.

Benefits: Control maternal blood pressure, reduce risk of stroke, placental abruption, or eclampsia.

Risks

Methyldopa: Maternal sedation, depression (rare).

Labetalol: Fetal bradycardia (rare), avoids reflex tachycardia.

Nifedipine: Maternal hypotension, headache.

Hydralazine: Maternal tachycardia, headache; limited fetal data.

Considerations: Avoid ACE inhibitors and ARBs due to teratogenicity (renal dysgenesis, oligohydramnios). Target BP <160/110 mmHg in severe cases, avoiding over-correction to prevent placental hypoperfusion.

5. Anticonvulsants for Eclampsia/Preeclampsia

Indications: Prevention or treatment of seizures in preeclampsia or eclampsia.

Drug: Magnesium Sulfate (4 g IV bolus over 15–20 minutes, then 1–2 g/hour maintenance).

Mechanism: Reduces neuronal excitability by antagonizing NMDA receptors and stabilizing membranes.

Benefits: Reduces seizure recurrence by 50% and maternal mortality in eclampsia (MAGPIE trial).

Risks: Maternal respiratory depression, hypotonia; fetal hypotonia (rare).

Considerations: Monitor serum magnesium levels (therapeutic range: 4–7 mEq/L). Use levetiracetam or phenytoin as alternatives in rare cases of magnesium intolerance.

6. Antibiotics

Indications

Group B Streptococcus (GBS) prophylaxis: Intrapartum penicillin G (5 million units IV, then 2.5–3 million units every 4 hours) or ampicillin to prevent neonatal GBS sepsis.

PPROM: Erythromycin or amoxicillin-clavulanate to prolong latency and reduce neonatal morbidity.

Chorioamnionitis: Ampicillin + gentamicin IV to treat maternal and fetal infection.

Benefits: Reduce neonatal sepsis, meningitis, and maternal postpartum infections.

Risks: Allergic reactions, gastrointestinal upset, rare fetal effects (e.g., aminoglycoside ototoxicity with prolonged use).

Considerations: Adjust for penicillin allergy (e.g., clindamycin or vancomycin for GBS prophylaxis). Avoid tetracyclines (fetal bone/teeth effects) and fluoroquinolones (cartilage damage).

7. Antenatal Medications for Specific Conditions

Folic Acid: 400–800 mcg daily (4 mg in high-risk cases, e.g., prior neural tube defect). Prevents neural tube defects.

Iron Supplementation: Ferrous sulfate 325 mg daily or IV iron for anemia. Improves maternal hemoglobin, reduces preterm birth risk.

Aspirin: Low-dose (81–150 mg daily) from 12–16 weeks in high-risk women (e.g., preeclampsia history). Reduces preeclampsia risk by 17% (USPSTF guidelines).

Thyroid Medications: Levothyroxine for hypothyroidism; propylthiouracil or methimazole for hyperthyroidism (first trimester). Maintains maternal euthyroidism, supports fetal neurodevelopment.

Antidiabetic Agents: Insulin (preferred) or metformin for gestational diabetes. Glyburide is less commonly used due to fetal transfer.

8. Labor Induction and Augmentation

Indications: Post-term pregnancy, preeclampsia, PPROM, or fetal compromise.

Drugs

Oxytocin: 0.5–2 mU/min IV, titrated to achieve adequate contractions. Stimulates uterine contractions via oxytocin receptors.

Dinoprostone (PGE2): Intravaginal gel or insert for cervical ripening.

Misoprostol (PGE1): 25–50 mcg vaginally or orally every 4–6 hours. Promotes cervical ripening and uterine contractions.

Benefits: Facilitate vaginal delivery, reduce cesarean section rates in appropriate cases.

Risks: Uterine hyperstimulation, fetal distress, postpartum hemorrhage (oxytocin). Misoprostol is contraindicated in prior cesarean due to uterine rupture risk.

Considerations: Monitor FHR and uterine activity closely. Contraindicated in non-reassuring fetal status or placenta previa.

9. Postpartum Medications

Oxytocin: 10–40 units IV or 10 units IM post-delivery to prevent postpartum hemorrhage.

Methylergonovine: 0.2 mg IM every 2–4 hours for postpartum hemorrhage (contraindicated in hypertension).

Tranexamic Acid: 1 g IV for postpartum hemorrhage refractory to oxytocin. Inhibits fibrinolysis.

NSAIDs: Ibuprofen or ketorolac for postpartum pain. Safe in breastfeeding.

Antibiotic: For postpartum endometritis (e.g., clindamycin + gentamicin).

Indicated (Safe / Relatively safe) medicines (In short)

1. Supplements & prophylactic drugs

Folic Acid

- Dose: 0.4 mg/day (routine), 5 mg/day (high risk)
- Prevents neural tube defects
- Start preconceptionally
- Category A

Iron

- Ferrous sulfate / fumarate
- Prevents iron deficiency anemia
- Safe throughout pregnancy

Calcium

- 1000–1500 mg/day
- Reduces risk of preeclampsia
- Prevents maternal bone loss

Vitamin D

- Safe in recommended doses
- Avoid megadoses

2. Analgesics & Antipyretics

Paracetamol

- Drug of choice for pain & fever
- Safe in all trimesters
- Overdose → hepatotoxicity

3. Antibiotics (safe / preferred)

Penicillins

- Amoxicillin, Ampicillin
- Category B
- No teratogenicity

Cephalosporins

- Ceftriaxone, Cefixime
- Safe throughout pregnancy

Macrolides

- Erythromycin, Azithromycin
- Alternative in penicillin allergy

Clindamycin

- Anaerobic infections
- Safe

4. Antihypertensives (pregnancy-safe)

Methyldopa

- Drug of choice
- Longest safety record
- Central alpha-agonist

Labetalol

- Alpha + beta blocker
- First-line in modern practice

Nifedipine

- Calcium channel blocker
- Also used as tocolytic

5. Antidiabetic drugs

Insulin

- Gold standard
- Does not cross placenta
- Safe

Metformin

- Increasingly accepted
- Used in GDM and PCOS

6. Antiemetics

Doxylamine + Pyridoxine

- Drug of choice for hyperemesis gravidarum

Ondansetron

- Used after first trimester with caution

7. Anticoagulants

Unfractionated Heparin / LMWH

- Do not cross placenta
- Safe in pregnancy
- Preferred over warfarin

8. Antithyroid drugs

Propylthiouracil (PTU)

- Preferred in first trimester
- Lower teratogenic risk

9. Corticosteroids

Betamethasone / Dexamethasone

- Used for fetal lung maturity
- Safe when indicated

Contraindicated medicines in pregnancy

1. Absolute contraindications (Category X)

Isotretinoin	Severe craniofacial, cardiac defects
Thalidomide	Limb deformities (phocomelia)
Methotrexate	Abortifacient, Neural tube defects
Warfarin	Fetal warfarin syndrome

2. Antibiotics (Avoided)

Tetracyclines	Teeth discoloration, Bone growth inhibition
Fluoroquinolones	Cartilage damage
Aminoglycosides	Ototoxicity (dose-dependent)

3. NSAIDs

Aspirin (High dose) Premature ductus arteriosus closure

Ibuprofen (3rd trimester)-Oligohydramnios, Prolonged labor

4. Antihypertensives (Contraindicated)

ACE Inhibitors	Renal dysgenesis, Oligohydramnios
ARBs	Fetal renal failure

5. Antiepileptics (High risk)

Valproate	Neural tube defects
Phenytoin	Fetal hydantoin syndrome

6. Hormones

Androgens	Virilization of female fetus
DES	Vaginal adenocarcinoma

7. Psychotropic drugs

Lithium	Ebstein anomaly
Benzodiazepines	Neonatal withdrawal, hypotonia

8. Anti-thyroid drugs

Methimazole (1st trimester) Aplasia cutis

9. Trimester-wise drug effects

First Trimester	Congenital malformations
Second Trimester	Growth restriction
Third Trimester	Functional toxicity, Neonatal depression

Indicated Unani Medicines in Obstetrics

Unani medicine employs a holistic approach in obstetrics, focusing on preventive, promotive, and curative care. Treatments are tailored to the patient's temperament (Mizaj), humoral balance and physiological state. Below are key indicated medicines and their applications in obstetrics:

***Majoon-e-Hamal* (Uterine Tonic)**

Composition: Includes herbs like Zanjabeel (Zingiber officinale), Asaroon (Asarum europaeum), and Abhal (Juniperus communis).

Indications: Strengthens the uterus, promotes fetal growth, and prevents miscarriage by balancing humoral imbalances (e.g., excess cold or moist temperament). Used for general weakness in pregnancy and to support uterine health.

Dosage: Typically 5–10 g daily with milk or water, adjusted to patient's temperament.

Rationale: These herbs are warm in temperament, counteracting cold and moist imbalances common in pregnancy.

(https://www.amazon.in/Handbook-Medicines-Formulae-Processes-Analysis/dp/8178330423)

***Sharbat-e-Anar* (Pomegranate Syrup)**

Composition: Pomegranate (*Punica granatum*) juice, sugar, and sometimes rose water.

Indications: Used for nausea, vomiting, and anemia in pregnancy due to its cooling and astringent properties. It supports digestion and improves blood quality (sanguine humor).

Dosage: 10–20 ml diluted in water, twice daily.

Rationale: Pomegranate's cold and moist temperament helps balance hot and dry conditions like nausea.

(https://www.amazon.in/Handbook-Medicines-Formulae-Processes-Analysis/dp/8178330423)

Majoon-e-Dabeedul Ward

Composition: Contains Ward (Rosa damascena), *Sandal* (Santalum album), and Zafran (Crocus sativus).

Indications: Promotes uterine involution, reduces postpartum bleeding, and alleviates inflammation. It is also used for general debility post-delivery.

Dosage: 5–10 g with warm water or milk.

Rationale: Its cooling and astringent properties help restore uterine temperament and prevent excessive blood loss.

(https://www.scribd.com/doc/314063520/Unani-Medicine)

Qurs-e-Saleh

Composition: Includes Habb-e-Hamal (a compound of iron and herbal extracts).

Indications: Enhances lactation, strengthens the reproductive system, and corrects humoral imbalances post-delivery.

Dosage: 1–2 tablets daily.

Rationale: Supports the sanguine humor to improve milk production and maternal recovery.

(https://www.nhp.gov.in/unani_mty)

Habb-e-Mudir

Composition: Saffron (Crocus sativus), Aloe vera, and Myrrh (Commiphora myrrha).

Indications: Regulates menstruation, treats amenorrhea, and supports ovulation in cases of infertility. It is used cautiously in early pregnancy to avoid overstimulation.

Dosage: 1–2 pills daily with water.

Rationale: Its warm and dry properties stimulate blood flow and correct cold humoral imbalances.

(https://www.amazon.in/Handbook-Medicines-Formulae-Processes-Analysis/dp/8178330423)

***Sharbat-e-Faulad* (Iron Tonic)**

Composition: Iron-based compounds with *Gulab* (Rosa damascena) and *Qand* (sugar).

Indication: Treats anemia in pregnancy and postpartum, improving blood quality and vitality.

Dosage: 10–15 ml daily.

Rationale: Enhances the sanguine humor, addressing deficiencies common in obstetric patients.

(https://www.nhp.gov.in/unani_mty)

Khamira Abresham Hakim Arshad Wala

Composition: Silk cocoon, saffron, and amber.

Indications: Boosts immunity, supports cardiovascular health, and reduces stress during pregnancy and postpartum.

Dosage: 3–5 g with milk or water.

Rationale: Its warm temperament strengthens vital spirit (*Arwah*) and balances humors.

(https://www.nhp.gov.in/unani_mty)

Contraindicated Unani Medicines in Obstetrics

Unani medicine emphasizes caution in prescribing drugs during pregnancy and lactation due to potential adverse effects on the fetus or mother. Contraindications are based on the drug's temperament, potency (*Darjat-e-Advia*), and potential to disrupt humoral balance or organ function. Below are key contraindicated medicines and conditions:

Habb-e-Ayarij

Composition: Aloe vera, *Hing* (Ferula asafoetida), and *Sumbul* (Nardostachys jatamansi).

Contraindications: Avoided in pregnancy due to its strong purgative and hot temperament, which may induce uterine contractions or miscarriage. It is also contraindicated in early lactation as it may pass through breast milk, causing digestive upset in infants.

Rationale: Excessive heat and dryness can disrupt the moist and cold temperament needed for fetal development.

(https://pmc.ncbi.nlm.nih.gov/articles/PMC3038517/)

***Qurs-e-Musaqqit* (Abortifacient Pills)**

Composition: Safflower (Carthamus tinctorius), Rue (Ruta graveolens).

Contraindications: Strictly contraindicated in pregnancy as it is designed to induce abortion or premature labor. It is also avoided in lactation due to potential toxicity.

Rationale: Its potent hot and dry properties overstimulate the uterus, risking fetal loss.

(https://www.ncbi.nlm.nih.gov/pmc/articles/PMC3038517/)

Safoof-e-Turbud

Composition: Turbud (Operculina turpethum).

Contraindications: Contraindicated in pregnancy and early postpartum due to its strong purgative action, which may cause dehydration or uterine overstimulation.

Rationale: Purgatives disrupt the humoral balance and may lead to electrolyte imbalances harmful to the fetus or mother.

(https://pmc.ncbi.nlm.nih.gov/articles/PMC3038517/

Majoon-e-Ushba

Composition: Ushba (Smilax china), Bikh-e-Anjbar (Polygonum bistorta).

Contraindications: Avoided in pregnancy due to its diuretic and detoxifying effects, which may stress maternal kidneys or affect fetal fluid balance.

Rationale: Its cold and dry temperament can exacerbate dehydration in pregnant women.

(https://www.amazon.in/Handbook-Medicines-Formulae-Processes-Analysis/dp/8178330423)

Kushta* Preparations (e.g., *Kushta-e-Gaodanti)

Composition: Calcined gypsum or other minerals.

Contraindications: Avoided in pregnancy and lactation due to potential heavy metal content and unknown toxicological effects on the fetus or infant.

Rationale: Mineral-based drugs require strict pharmacovigilance due to risks of toxicity, especially in sensitive populations.

(https://en.wikipedia.org/wiki/Unani_medicine)

Habb-e-Mako

Composition: Mako (Solanum nigrum).

Contraindications: Contraindicated in pregnancy due to its potential hepatotoxicity and ability to disrupt humoral balance.

Rationale: Its cold and dry temperament may cause adverse effects in the fetus or maternal liver function.

(https://www.amazon.in/Handbook-Medicines-Formulae-Processes-Analysis/dp/8178330423)

Drugs in Extremes of Age or Altered Organ Function

Unani formularies caution against using potent drugs (third or fourth degree in potency) in pregnant women, lactating mothers, or those with compromised liver or kidney function. For example:

Ispand (Peganum harmala): Contraindicated due to its neurotoxic and abortifacient properties.

Azaraqi (Strychnos nux-vomica): Avoided due to its high toxicity and potential to cause convulsions or fetal harm.

(https://www.amazon.in/Handbook-Medicines-Formulae-Processes-Analysis/dp/8178330423)

Pharmacovigilance and Safety Considerations

Unani medicine emphasizes pharmacovigilance to ensure safety, particularly in obstetrics. Key points include:

Adverse Drug Reactions (ADRs): Monitoring for ADRs is critical, as some Unani drugs (e.g., mineral-based *Kushtas*) may contain heavy metals or toxins. Pregnant and lactating women are particularly vulnerable due to altered pharmacokinetics.

(https://pmc.ncbi.nlm.nih.gov/articles/PMC3038517/)

Correctives (*Muslehat*): Unani practitioners use correctives like honey or rose water to mitigate adverse effects of potent drugs. For example, *Zanjabeel* may be combined with cooling agents to reduce its heat in pregnancy.

(https://www.ncbi.nlm.nih.gov/pmc/articles/PMC3038517/)

Dietary Restrictions (*Parhez*): Specific diets are prescribed to complement treatments and avoid food-drug interactions. For instance, hot and spicy foods are avoided with warm-tempered drugs to prevent humoral imbalance.

(https://www.nhp.gov.in/unani_mty)

Clinical Studies: Limited clinical data exists on Unani drugs in obstetrics. Further research is needed to validate efficacy and safety, especially for herbal extracts with potential toxicity.

(https://www.ncbi.nlm.nih.gov/pmc/articles/PMC4253292/)

Conclusion

Unani medicine offers a rich pharmacopeia for obstetric care, with formulations like *Majoon-e-Hamal* and *Sharbat-e-Anar* supporting pregnancy and postpartum recovery, while emphasizing humoral and temperamental balance. However, potent drugs like *Habb-e-Ayarij* and *Qurs-e-Musaqqit* are contraindicated due to risks of miscarriage, toxicity, or humoral disruption. Practitioners must adhere to Unani formularies, employ correctives, and integrate pharmacovigilance to ensure safety, particularly in sensitive populations like pregnant and lactating women. Further clinical research is needed to standardize these treatments for modern obstetric practice.

(https://pmc.ncbi.nlm.nih.gov/articles/PMC3038517/)[](https://www.nhp.gov.in/unani_mty)

(https://en.wikipedia.org/wiki/Unani_medicine)

Disease	**Drug of Choice**
Fever	Paracetamol
UTI	Amoxicillin
Hypertension	Methyldopa
Diabetes	Insulin
Nausea	Doxylamine
Anticoagulation	Heparin
Anemia	Iron

Long Answer Questions (LAQs)

Classify the indicated and contraindicated drugs used during pregnancy. Discuss them under allopathic and Unani systems of medicine.

Describe drug therapy in pregnancy. Enlist safe and contraindicated allopathic drugs with suitable examples.

Explain the principles of drug use in pregnancy and lactation. Enumerate Unani drugs indicated and contraindicated during these periods.

Discuss the effects of drugs on the fetus and neonate. Classify drugs used during pregnancy and lactation with examples.

Write in detail about drugs contraindicated in pregnancy and lactation. Include both modern (allopathic) and Unani medicines.

Short Answer Questions (SAQs)

Enlist drugs safe for use in pregnancy.

Name four drugs absolutely contraindicated in pregnancy.

Write the drug of choice for fever and pain in pregnancy.

Mention Unani drugs contraindicated in pregnancy.

Enlist drugs contraindicated during lactation.

Multiple Choice Questions (MCQs)

1. Drug of choice for pain and fever during pregnancy is:

A. Aspirin B. Ibuprofen

C. Diclofenac D. Paracetamol

Answer: D

2. Which drug is absolutely contraindicated in pregnancy?

A. Heparin B. Insulin

C. Isotretinoin D. Methyldopa

Answer: C

3. Drug of choice for hypertension in pregnancy is:

A. ACE inhibitors B. Propranolol

C. Methyldopa D. Atenolol

Answer: C

4. Which anticoagulant is safe in pregnancy?

A. Warfarin B. Aspirin

C. Low molecular weight heparin D. Clopidogrel

Answer: C

5. Tetracyclines are contraindicated in pregnancy because they cause:

A. Renal failure B. Cardiac anomalies

C. Discoloration of teeth and bone defectsD. Neural tube defects

Answer: C

6. Which Unani drug is considered abortifacient and contraindicated in pregnancy?

A. Khamira Gaozaban B. Sharbat Faulad

C. Sibr (Aloe) D. Roghane Badam

Answer: C

7. Which drug causes fetal warfarin syndrome when used in pregnancy?

A. Heparin B. Aspirin

C. Warfarin D. Clopidogrel

Answer: C

8. Preferred antidiabetic drug during pregnancy is:

A. Glibenclamide B. Metformin

C. Insulin D. Pioglitazone

Answer: C

9. Which Unani drug is used as a galactagogue during lactation?

A. Sana Makki B. Turbud

C. Saunf (Foeniculum vulgare) D. Hiltit

Answer: C

10. Which drug should be avoided during lactation due to neonatal toxicity?

A. Paracetamol B. Penicillin

C. Chloramphenicol D. Cephalosporin

Answer:

www.ingramcontent.com/pod-product-compliance
Lightning Source LLC
LaVergne TN
LVHW060014210926
848481LV00013B/3705